Fl...**es of**
SURGERY

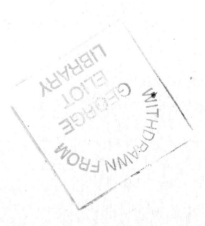

Commissioning Editor: **Timothy Horne**
Development Editor: **Barbara Simmons**
Copy Editor: **Jane Ward**
Project Manager: **Frances Affleck**
Designer: **Jayne Jones**

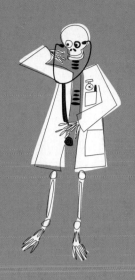

Flesh and Bones of
SURGERY

Aneel A Bhangu MBChB
Foundation Year 2 Doctor
West Midlands Deanery

M R B Keighley MS FRCS
Emeritus Professor
University of Birmingham;
Formerly Barling Professor and Head of Surgery
University of Birmingham;
Honorary Academic Faculty Professor of Surgery
Christian Medical College
Vellore, South India;
Chairman
Colorectal Research Foundation GB and Ireland

Illustrations by Jenni Miller

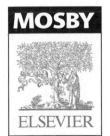

Edinburgh   London   New York   Oxford   Philadelphia   St Louis   Sydney   Toronto   2007

The right of Aneel Bhangu and Michael Keighley to be identified as authors of this work has been asserted by them in accordance with the Copyright, Designs and Patents Act 1988.

First published 2007

ISBN-13: 978-0-7234-3376-7
ISBN-10: 0-7234-3376-3

British Library Cataloguing in Publication Data
A catalogue record for this book is available from the British Library

Library of Congress Cataloging in Publication Data
A catalog record for this book is available from the Library of Congress

Notice:
Neither the Publisher nor the Authors assume any responsibility for any loss or injury and/or damage to persons or property arising out of or related to any use of the material contained in this book. It is the responsibility of the treating practitioner, relying on independent expertise and knowledge of the patient, to determine the best treatment and method of application for the patient.
The Publisher

Printed in China

The publisher's policy is to use **paper manufactured from sustainable forests**

Working together to grow libraries in developing countries

www.elsevier.com | www.bookaid.org | www.sabre.org

ELSEVIER   BOOK AID International   Sabre Foundation

 your source for books, journals and multimedia in the health sciences

www.elsevierhealth.com

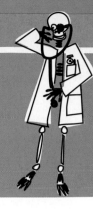

Contents

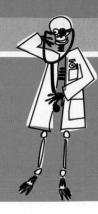

Preface

The modern medical student is training in an exciting and challenging time where large volumes of information must be taken in and understood rapidly, continuously and comprehensively. Surgery is covered in all the clinical years, with specialties (such as orthopaedics) often being covered in separate blocks. Surgery remains a core medical school topic, as it must be, even at a time when the medical school syllabus is expanding and becoming more varied.

The *Flesh and Bones* format is a unique approach to surgery, providing an initial overview of features common to all surgery, The big picture, followed by chapters containing, in a double page spread per topic, the focused, essential knowledge required. Section two shows how the chapters in Section three are grouped and gives the core 'high return facts' of each area. This progression from the general to the particular aims to maximize a student's learning. The decision to include orthopaedics and trauma in this text is important (it is often left out of such 'core' surgical textbooks) as, although it significantly lengthens the text, its inclusion makes this book a 'one-stop introduction' to a surgical syllabus.

It is important to remember that surgery is a rapidly evolving specialty and new surgical techniques are constantly developed. Many diseases are now being treated in new ways and diseases once considered incurable are now curable. This is particularly true of many forms of cancer surgery.

During training, all students are attached to surgical firms and this provides opportunities for theatre time, clinics, ward rounds and acute surgical takes. You should aim to split your time appropriately in order to attend all of these opportunities. Being 'on take', where new surgical patients are referred to hospital, is one of the most valuable ways to experience the workings of a surgical firm. When you have some confidence on a surgical firm (and certainly by your final year), you should aim to be the first to clerk in these patients and then present the case (with a differential diagnosis and suggested management plan) at the subsequent ward round. This volume will form the basis of developing the core knowledge needed for these skills, giving lists of clinical features, investigations and management that can then be expanded using more detailed texts and experience in the hospital.

This book is intended to provide the necessary, focused information regarding the core topics of the surgical syllabus in a unique and interesting way. It is naive to think that your primary aim at medical school is not to pass examinations (primarily the MCQ and OSCE) and this book provides a basis for this in a succinct way. However, the other, *just as important*, aim of a medical student is to gain the best knowledge in order to become a good clinician.

Aneel Bhangu and Michael Keighley

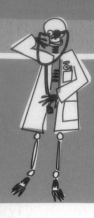

Acknowledgements

We are indebted to the following (alphabetical order) for their help in preparing the manuscript and for providing some fantastic images:

Mr Donald Adam, Consultant Vascular Surgeon

Mr Zaki Almallah, Consultant Urologist

Miss Sonia Bhangu, Basic Surgical Trainee

Mr Chris Bradish, Consultant Orthopaedic Surgeon

Dr Sally Bradley, Consultant Radiologist

Dr Swarup Chavda, Consultant Neuroradiologist

Dr Roy Cockel, Consultant Gastroenterological Physician

Dr Mark Davies, Consultant Radiologist

Miss Adele Francis, Consultant Breast Surgeon

Mr Graham Flint, Consultant Neurosurgeon

Dr Jason Goh, Consultant Gastroenterological Physician

Mr Robert Grimer, Consultant Orthopaedic Surgeon

Dr Peter Guest, Consultant Radiologist

Mr Mike Hallissey, Consultant General and Breast Surgeon

Dr Shauna Irgin, Consultant Anaesthetist

Dr Mark Ranjan Jesudason, Senior Lecturer in Surgery, Christian Medical College, Vellore, India

Mr Micheal Kuo, Consultant ENT Surgeon

Dr Jerry Marsden, Consultant Dermatologist

Mr Dion Morton, Consultant General and Colorectal Surgeon

Mr Keith Porter, Consultant Trauma and Orthopaedic Surgeon

Mr Anand Sachithanandan, Cardiothoracic Specialist Registrar

Mr Malcolm Simms, Consultant Vascular Surgeon

Dr Naomi Slator, F1 Doctor (for her tireless hours, patience and lower limb modelling skills)

Mr Paul Super, Consultant Upper GI Surgeon

Dr Douglas Thorburn, Consultant Physician

Miss Ruth Waters, Consultant Plastic Surgeon

Colorectal nurse specialists, University Hospital Birmingham

Birmingham Breast Screening Service

All those not mentioned who reviewed the manuscript and gave advice/comments

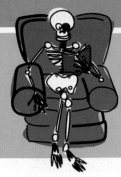

The big picture

Surgery is a core topic in medical training: forming a vital part of the knowledge needed to be a good clinician and appearing in many examinations. All students will require surgical knowledge regardless of any later specialization. The common aspects to any surgical situation- preoperative assessments, comorbidity, anaesthetics and analgesia, fluid management, recovery and complications-are covered in Section one. Section two gives the 'high return facts' of specific topics. These points can be used to identify areas where your knowledge is weak and to see what are the core facts that will be expanded in the corresponding chapters in Section three. The clinical images are all situations that will be seen on the wards and potentially in an OSCE station. The text is deliberately light on specific surgical technique unless this is a topic likely to form part of an examination.

No matter the specialty, there are certain surgical principles that both clinicians and students need to know. These principles involve an in-depth preoperative assessment of the patient (to identify potential problems and prepare the patient for theatre), postoperative care (including the ability to recognize, investigate and treat complications), and the basics of surgical procedures, such as wound management. The Big picture covers the general principles of:

- preoperative assessment
- fluid management
- postoperative care
- surgical complications
- basic surgical principles.

■ PREOPERATIVE ASSESSMENT

History and examination

A complete history (including drug history) is vital in all patients, checking for pregnancy, allergies, previous myocardial infarction (MI; especially within 6 months) and problems with previous anaesthesia. **Respiratory**, **cardiovascular** and **abdominal** examinations should be performed in all patients.

Investigations

The following investigations are basic.

Blood samples. Full blood count (FBC), urea and electrolytes (U&E) and serum glucose should be measured for most patients who are to undergo major surgery. If the patient is anaemic (haemoglobin, < 10 g/dl (< 100 g/l)), senior team members and the anaesthetist will decide about further investigations and preoperative transfusion.

Liver function tests. Standard liver function tests and serum amylase levels are required in jaundice, liver disease or malignancy.

Preparation for possible blood transfusion. **Group and save** (G&S) is used when blood loss is not expected. Blood group is determined and recorded but blood bags are only prepared if they are requested, which takes some time (bags selected, unfrozen and cross-matched before being sent out). This is used for mastectomy and cholecystectomy. **Cross-match** is used when blood loss is expected. The blood bags are cross-matched against the blood sample, and these bags of blood are unfrozen and saved for this patient. The amount of blood cross-matched depends on the procedure: for example, 6–8 units for abdominal aortic aneurysm repair; 2 units for neck of femur fracture. All colorectal cancer resections require cross-matching except for right hemicolectomy (where G&S suffices).

Chest radiograph. Any patients with an indication of respiratory disease should have chest X-ray examination.

Electrocardiography (ECG). This is required for all patients over 50 years, those with heart disease (e.g. previous MI or hypertension) and those with diabetes mellitus.

Consent. Informed consent should be obtained, preferably by the person performing the operation. The discussion with the patient should include the intended benefits of the operation, the likely success rate and the potential complications, with percentage probabilities. The document is merely a summary of the preoperative counselling process.

Assessment for fitness for major surgery

For elective surgery (e.g. elective repair of an abdominal aortic aneurysm), the fitness of the patient for the procedure should be assessed.

History and examination. These are carried out as described above.

Cardiac status. An ECG and an echocardiogram are taken if the patient has a history of cardiac problems, congestive heart failure or if a murmur is found. Fitness for surgery is sometimes assessed by 24-hour ECG monitoring and an exercise tolerance test. Patients can often report their own exercise ability, such as activities of daily living (tolerance of walking on flat and on incline, ability to walk to the shops, etc.).

Respiratory status. Measurement of arterial blood gases while breathing air is a useful indicator of resting oxygen and carbon dioxide partial pressures in the lungs. **Spirometry** (lung function testing) can be used for further investigation.

Renal status. U&E and serum creatinine indicate kidney function.

Coexisting medical conditions

Cardiovascular conditions

Myocardial infarction. If possible, there should be a delay of 6 months before surgery, although this depends on the urgency of the surgery and the risk:benefit ratio. The wait is to reduce the high risk of perioperative reinfarction, which most commonly occurs on the third postoperative day. This plan can be modified by preoperative stenting.

Hypertension. Medical control of hypertension should be optimized as there is a high risk of MI or stroke with surgery and uncontrolled hypertension; surgery may be cancelled if diastolic pressure is greater then 110 mmHg.

Valvular heart disease. An echocardiogram assesses current valvular disease. Warfarin is stopped 3 days before surgery and is replaced by intravenous heparin. Antibiotic prophylaxis is essential to reduce the risk of infective endocarditis in both high- and low-risk procedures. The management involves antibiotics at induction and possibly postoperatively (e.g. 3 mg oral amoxicillin 1 h before dental procedures under local anaesthetics in low-risk patients); the British National Formulary gives the latest recommended protocols.

Respiratory conditions

Upper and lower respiratory tract infection. Elective surgery should be deferred for 6 weeks as there is a serious risk of respiratory complications (e.g. secondary infection) under a general anaesthetic. It is imperative to explain to the patient the reason for the cancellation, that the surgery will be rescheduled as soon as possible after the time lapse, and to inform the GP.

Chronic obstructive pulmonary disease. Affected patients should be advised to stop smoking at least 8 weeks before

Table 1.1 A SLIDING SCALE FOR INSULIN DOSAGE UNTIL A PATIENT CAN EAT AND DRINK

Blood glucose (mmol/l)	Insulin dose (IU/h)[a]
< 4	0 (and a clinician should be called)
4.1–7.0	1
7.1–11.0	2
11.1–14.0	3
14.1–17.0	4
17.1–21.0	5
21.1	6 (and a clinician should be called)

[a]*Actrapid, a short-acting insulin.*

the operation, be admitted before the day of surgery and their condition optimized with nebulisers and physiotherapy.

Diabetes mellitus

It is important to optimize diabetic control before surgery and it may be necessary to admit patients 2–3 days preoperatively to gain tight control. The patient should be scheduled as first on the operating list. Diabetic control is monitored by measuring blood glucose and a **sliding scale** may be necessary to titrate an intravenous infusion of Actrapid against the patient's blood glucose level (Table 1.1). Actrapid is a short-acting insulin and 50 IU is made to 50 ml with normal saline (so 1 ml contains 1 IU). It should always be administered via a separate venflon to the intravenous infusion. For standard fluids, if the blood glucose is < 15 mmol/l, the patient should be given 5% dextrose, and if > 15 mmol/l, 0.9% saline is given instead.

Minor surgery

Type 1 diabetes. Omit the morning dose of insulin and commence the sliding scale for insulin dosage. The sliding scale should be continued until the patient is eating and drinking, when normal medication regimen is resumed.

Type 2 diabetes. Omit morning tablets if the patient is scheduled for the morning operation list and monitor blood glucose. If the patient is scheduled for an afternoon list, they can have an early breakfast and normal medication in the morning. The patient should be encouraged to eat and drink as soon as possible postoperatively.

Major surgery

Type 1 diabetes. The patient is admitted before the day of operation and started on the sliding scale for insulin dosage on the day before their operation.

Type 2 diabetes. The normal medication is omitted the night before the operation and the sliding scale for insulin dosage is commenced on the day as described above.

Obesity

The body mass index (BMI) defines the level of obesity (> 25 is overweight, > 28 is obese and > 30 is morbid obesity). Being obese puts the patient at higher risk of developing:

- **general risks**: diabetes, ischaemic heart disease, hypertension and heart failure
- **obstructive sleep apnoea**: increasing the risk of developing pulmonary hypertension
- **increased perioperative morbidity and mortality**: perioperative MI, arrhythmias, heart failure, deep vein thrombosis (DVT) and pulmonary embolism
- **respiratory problems**: difficult airway, aspiration and the development of atelectasis and postoperative pneumonia
- **wound problems**: infections and dehiscence.

The patient's BMI should be calculated and all overweight and obese patients should be encouraged to lose weight before surgery.

Alcohol

Patients with alcohol dependence syndrome who are admitted to hospital may go into an acute withdrawal state, developing acute confusion, tremors, hallucination and fits (delirium tremens). This is a medical emergency and treatment is with immediate diazepam (intravenous if the patient is having fits; otherwise orally or rectally).

Existing medication

Patients should be asked to detail all medications they are taking, including prescription and non-prescription drugs and homeopathic remedies.

Anticoagulants (warfarin). Patients taking warfarin should be admitted before the day of surgery and converted to an intravenous heparin infusion. The reason for taking warfarin guides how important it is to maintain anticoagulation once the patient is admitted; for example, it is more important to maintain adequate anticoagulation in patients with valvular disease or thrombosis and potentially less important in patients with atrial fibrillation. Patients taking warfarin may be contraindicated for an epidural, although there are circumstances where it can be permitted. Usually warfarin is stopped 3 days before an operation and heparin is commenced based on the results of coagulation tests (if necessary by a haematologist). The heparin infusion should be stopped 4 h before surgery, and clotting rechecked.

Oral contraceptive pill. Oral contraceptives should be stopped 4 weeks before major elective surgery or surgery to the legs to decrease the risk of DVT.

Insulin. Insulin dosage is managed as described above for diabetes mellitus.

Digoxin. Levels of digoxin should be measured (especially in high-risk patients) as it has a narrow therapeutic window. It can also accumulate in patients with renal dysfunction and cause it to worsen. It is, therefore, important to measure U&E daily in these patients.

Steroids. Any patient taking steroids within the previous 3 months and who is undergoing major surgery is given steroids perioperatively to prevent disruption of the hypothalamic–pituitary adrenal axis and the stress response initiated by the surgery. These intravenous steroids are continued for 48 h or until the patient has resumed their diet.

Diuretics and angiotensin-converting enzyme (ACE) inhibitors. These are continued but U&E values are measured and monitored for electrolyte disturbances.

Aspirin and clopidogel. These drugs interfere with platelet function and should be stopped at least 5 days before an operation; otherwise there is a risk of bleeding during or early after the procedure.

Prophylaxis for deep vein thrombosis

All surgical patients are at risk of developing a DVT but the risk is increased in the obese and in smokers; where there is prolonged immobility or malignancy; in large operations (including pelvic and orthopaedic surgery); in patients taking hormone replacement therapy or the oral contraceptive pill; and patients who are dehydrated or septic.

Risk factors can be modified in advance. The oral contraceptive pill is stopped 6 weeks before surgery. Loss of excess weight and stopping smoking before surgery is advised and adequate hydration should be ensured.

At the time of surgery, risks can be reduced by:

- compression stockings: all patients should wear compression, TED stockings
- low-molecular-weight heparin (LMWH; e.g. enoxaparin): given subcutaneously 12 h before the operation and continued until the patient is mobile
- active calf compression: inflatable stockings used during surgery to prevent venous stasis.

Nutrition

Enteral feeding is the usual and preferred method of feeding as it uses the patient's own gastrointestinal tract. This should be normal oral intake via the mouth if possible or by nasogastric tube, gastrostomy (a tube inserted via the anterior abdominal wall directly into the stomach; percutaneous endoscopic gastrostomy) or jejunostomy (tube into the jejunum).

Total parenteral nutrition (TPN) is used less commonly and only when the gastrointestinal tract is dysfunctional (e.g. ileus, short bowel syndrome and high-volume enterocutaneoous fistula), when the bowel needs to be rested postoperatively, or to supplement the malnourished patient's oral intake. It is administered via a central vein, such as the subclavian vein. It carries a significant risk of infection and sepsis and can cause liver damage if used for an extended period. There is also the risks of insertion of a central venous line, such as pneumothorax, haemothorax, air embolism, nerve injury and arterial puncture; therefore, it should only be used when absolutely necessary.

Bowel preparation

Bowel preparation is the process of removing faecal matter from the gastrointestinal tract before left-sided operations and colonoscopy. The main indications are:

- elective left-sided colorectal surgery (rectal, sigmoid, left and colon surgery) to prevent faecal matter contaminating the abdomen; there is no evidence that it reduces sepsis or anastomotic breakdown
- to allow loop ileostomy to be used safely to protect a rectal anastomosis
- colonoscopy: to allow visualization of the bowel wall, which is otherwise obscured by faeces.

Methods used are:

- **chemical preparation**: commonly Picolax, which contains sodium picosulphate and causes diarrhoea, is taken 24 and 12 h preoperatively; no solids should be taken in the 24 h before the procedure but oral fluid intake should be high and intravenous fluids should be given preoperatively to correct dehydration
- **mechanical preparation**: using serial enemas for anal surgery (e.g. fistula surgery)

- **antibiotic prophylaxis**: required for all colorectal surgery, usually single doses of cefuroxime and metronidazole at induction.

Antibiotic prophylaxis is also used in all other gastrointestinal surgery and whenever implants are being used (e.g. hip replacements, mesh repairs, Dacron arterial prostheses). Prophylaxis is with a cephalosporin with or without metronidazole, depending on whether anaerobes are likely to be encountered, or with flucloxacillin if skin organisms might infect an inplant.

FLUID MANAGEMENT

An understanding of the fluid compartments (Fig. 1.1) guides which fluid to give in which circumstance. About 60% of body weight is water; therefore, a 70 kg man has about 42 litres of water.

Fluids are given to patients who are 'nil by mouth' or when their oral diet needs to be supplemented. Preoperative patients are 'nil by mouth' for at least 6 h before an operation but often this may extend to 12–18 h of starvation, particularly in patients undergoing surgery in an emergency. Postoperatively, patients may have no oral intake for some time but modern minimally invasive surgery aims to commence fluids and diet in the first postoperative day, even after gastrointestinal surgery. Those who are too ill or weak to eat or those with persistent vomiting also need fluid supplementation. Fluid requirements are calculated to replace the fluids lost (Table 1.2). The total fluid lost per day is between 2500 and 3000 ml (without abnormal losses), which must be routinely replaced, either orally or intravenously. As a guide, *healthy adults require 3 litres per day (2.5 litres in the elderly or frail).*

Caution should be taken in the elderly and in patients with a history of heart failure as they are more likely to be precipitated into pulmonary oedema. Long-standing fluid deficits should be replaced slowly.

Fig. 1.1 Fluid compartments.

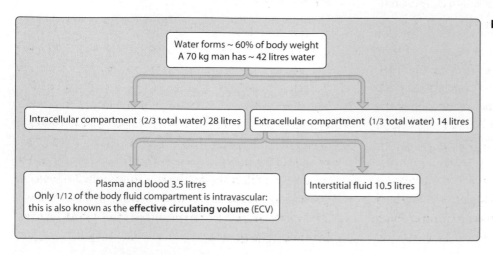

Table 1.2 LOSS OF FLUIDS

Loss	Example	Approximate volume (ml/day)
Measurable losses	Urine output	~1500
Insensible losses	Sweating, breathing, faeces; increased with fever	~1000–1500
Abnormal losses	Surgical drains, stomas, nasogastric tube aspirate, vomit, fistulae	Variable (can be measured and replaced by normal saline with potassium)

Electrolyte requirements

The two electrolytes most commonly replaced are sodium and potassium. The normal daily requirements are:

- sodium 0.7–1 mmol/kg
- potassium 0.7–1 mmol/kg

Remember where the fluid will be distributed before prescribing.

Normal serum potassium ranges vary at every laboratory, although a normal range is considered to be 3.5–5.5 mmol/l. Malnourished patients and patients taking diuretics are often hypokalaemic preoperatively. When treating hypokalaemia, potassium replacement can be given orally in patients who are tolerating oral intake and intravenously in patients who cannot tolerate oral intake or whose potassium is particularly low. Patients with profound hypokalaemia (e.g.< 2.5 mmol/l) may require replacement via a central line in an intensive-treatment unit (ITU). Premixed bags of fluid and potassium are found on the wards.

Classification of fluids

Fluids are broadly classified as crystalloid, colloid or blood products. The debate about whether to use crystalloids or colloids in acute trauma resuscitation and intensive care continues.

Crystalloids

Saline 0.9%. This contains 154 mmol/l sodium and 154 mmol/l chloride. It expands the extracellular compartment (interstitial 75%, plasma 25%), and so only 25% of the volume given will expand the plasma; hence four times as much crystalloid must be given as colloid to gain the same effect in acute blood loss.

Dextrose 5%. This contains 50 g/l glucose. The dextrose is readily metabolized by the liver leaving only water, which expands total body water (extracellular and intracellular fluid), thus only 1/12 remains in the extracellular volume.

The main purpose of administering dextrose is to replenish a water deficit.

Dextrose saline (0.18% saline/4% dextrose). This is sometimes given in place of 0.9% saline and 5% dextrose routines. It contains 30 mmol/l sodium chloride and 40 g/l glucose.

Hartmann's solution. This is an attempt to be more physiological in content and it contains 131 mmol/l sodium, 111 mmol/l chloride, 5 mmol/l potassium, 2 mmol/l calcium and 29 mmol/l lactate. However, once given, it behaves like 0.9% saline and expands the extracellular compartment. Excess administration may cause lactic acidosis.

Dextrose 50%. This is only used in the management of hypoglycaemia (50 ml given intravenously).

Colloids

A colloid is a substance that is unable to pass through a semipermeable membrane, and thus remains in the extracellular volume; colloids are useful when replacing a deficit in the extracellular volume, such as in haemorrhage or hypotension but are not used as a means of general fluid replacement. Their ability to expand the extracellular volume (often in excess of the volume administered) is based on their greater osmolality than plasma. They can be subdivided into three types.

Gelatin derivatives. The average molecular mass of these products (e.g. Gelofusin, Haemaccel) is 35000 daltons and they have half-lives of approximately 4.5 h. They are made from animal gelatine, and anaphylactic reactions have followed rapid infusion. Solutions contain the same amount of sodium (154 mmol/l).

Starch. The starch products have longer half-lives and the expansion lasts for 18–24 h (e.g. Hetastarch, Pentastarch).

Human albumin solution (HAS). This is available as 4.5% or 20% solutions. There is some controversy as there are suggestions of increased mortality in patients who are in intensive care; consequently it is only used at a consultant's express request.

Blood products

Packed red cells. These are used for acute blood loss, acute and chronic anaemia and during surgery. The universal donor blood is O-negative and is given to replace serious blood loss before cross-matched blood arrives. It contains the pellet from centrifuged whole blood and is routinely depleted of leucocytes; it is also fairly deplete of any platelets or clotting factors. A group-specific match takes about 15 min and a full cross-match takes 30–40 min. It is better to give group-specific blood than O-negative *if time allows.* When used to correct anaemia, 1 unit of blood (500 ml) increases haemoglobin content by 1 g/dl (10 g/l).

Fresh frozen plasma (FFP).   This is rich in clotting factors and so is given to improve clotting. It requires full thawing before it can be administered. It is given for oozing during an operation and in postoperative wounds, disseminated intravascular coagulation (DIC), single factor deficiencies and reversal of warfarin action.

Platelets.   These have a short shelf life of 5 days and so are not often given. Platelets are used for thrombocytopenia, DIC and specific platelet defects.

Cryoprecipitate.   Rapid thawing of fresh frozen plasma provides cryoprecipitate, which is rich in factor 8 and fibrinogen. It is used where fibrinogen is low, for DIC and in haemophilia.

Blood factors.   Various factors may be given for a specific deficiency.

Complications of blood transfusions

There are a number of potential complications in blood transfusions:

- human error (common)
- infection and prion transmission
- haemolytic transfusion reaction (acute < 24 h, delayed ~2 weeks)
- severe allergic reaction/alloimmunization
- immunosuppression
- volume and iron overload
- marrow suppression
- graft-versus-host disease.

Fluid regimens

The most commonly used fluid regimens when a patient is nil by mouth are:

- 1 litre of 0.9% saline + 2 litres of 5% dextrose, or
- 3 litres of 0.18% saline/4% dextrose.

The key message is to use:

- crystalloids for general fluid replacement and in the dehydrated patient
- colloids for hypovolaemia (from haemorrhage) or hypotension.

Measurement of fluid balance

An accurate fluid balance chart (all input and outputs) should be kept for each patient to be combined with clinical assessments:

- clinical judgement: evidence of dehydration clinically (dry mucus membranes, sunken eyes, decreased skin turgor); a general examination should be performed, looking for

evidence of increased heart rate, decrease in blood pressure, wide pulse pressure (systolic to diastolic blood pressure)

- urine output: minimum 0.5–1.0 ml/h per kg body weight (thus a minimum of 30 ml/h)
- bowel losses: variable
- drains, stomas, vomit, fistula: variable
- fluid charts: fluid input minus fluid output (stoma output, urine output, fistula losses, nasogastric aspirates and incidences of diarrhoea and vomiting)
- fluid overload: oedema (ankles and lungs), increased jugular blood pressure (signs of heart failure).

If urine output is low or falls in the postoperative patient, the first thing to do is to examine the patient:

- assess **ABC**
- exclude **hypovolaemic shock**: check blood pressure, heart rate, actively bleeding wounds/drains
- assess for **acute urinary retention**: feel for a palpable bladder and positive fluid balance (on fluid charts); a catheter may also be blocked, and so perform a bladder washout.

If there are no signs of urinary retention or hypovolaemia, the cause may be dehydration and a lack of fluids; intravenous infusion may be increased, and the patient reassessed, possibly with central venous pressure (CVP) monitoring. If the CVP is normal or if there has been a response to a fluid challenge, then acute renal failure should be suspected.

■ POSTOPERATIVE CARE

The level of postoperative monitoring needs to be appropriate to the patient's condition. The majority of postoperative patients are suitable for ward-based care. The minimum monitoring required immediately postoperatively is ECG, pulse oximetry, blood pressure, temperature and respiratory rate. Glasgow Coma Score (GCS) assessment is needed in some circumstances. All patients should receive postoperative oxygen for at least 4 h.

The patient will be reviewed by the nursing staff and a clinician postoperatively and again on regular ward rounds, where the key factors to review are:

- blood pressure, pulse, temperature: is the patient shocked?
- drains and wounds: is there more bleeding or drainage than expected?
- pain status: is more pain relief needed?

Levels of care

Most patients receive adequate care on the surgical wards, where the nursing ratios are 4:1 in the UK. Those who have had major surgery (e.g. repair of an abdominal aortic aneurysm) or are anticipated to develop surgical complications may require more intensive monitoring and treatment in a high-dependency unit (HDU) or ITU.

An HDU has a 2:1 nurse to patient ratio and an ITU a 1:1 ratio, but both allow continuous monitoring of blood pressure, heart rate and pulse oximetry and fluid balance. The former are used for patients with single-system failure and so are ideal to manage most postoperative patients, whereas ITU are used to treat patients with more than one system failure; they tend to be reserved for patients who require ventilation postoperatively or who have developed major complications such as cardio-respiratory complications (adult respiratory distress syndrome (ARDS) or requiring inotrope support) or septic shock.

Nowadays, most special care units in the UK are critical care units, which combine high-dependency and intensive-care facilities and so allow the level of care to be stepped up or down easily as needed.

Pain management

Pain management is a vital aspect of care in patients postoperatively, after trauma, in chronic disease and for palliation.

There are three grades of analgesic available (Fig. 1.2). The type of surgery and the severity of pain determine whether the patient is started at the top or bottom of the ladder. The patient moves up and down the ladder according to their pain, although non-opiates should be used in conjunction with opiates.

Non-opiates. Normally patients are started with paracetamol given regularly rather than as required in order to achieve maximum effect. It can be given orally, enterally or rectally to a maximum of 8 g/24 h. Non-steroidal anti-inflammatory drugs (NSAIDs) are often very effective and are excellent in patients with orthopaedic pain; they can be given orally, intramuscularly or as suppositories. They should not be given to those with asthma, renal dysfunction or a history of peptic ulceration.

Weak opiates. **Paracetamol** combined with codeine preparations (**codeine phosphate** (Co-codamol), **dihydrocodeine** (Co-dydramol)) are often used once paracetamol alone proves ineffective but they do cause constipation.

Strong opiates. The main form of immediate postoperative pain relief is strong opiates. **Morphine** can be given orally, enterally, intramuscularly, subcutaneously and intravenously, and also via a continuous infusion or as patient-controlled analgesia. Side effects of morphine are respiratory depression (care is needed in trauma victims and the elderly), hypotension, nausea and constipation.

Epidural analgesia. This is an excellent method that can be used to provide analgesia intraoperatively instead of a general anaesthetic (e.g. in a femoral bypass) but is most often used with a general anaesthetic to provide both intra- and postoperative analgesia. **Bupivacaine** (a local anaesthetic) is most often used, and it is commonly mixed with **diamorphine** to enhance the analgesia; this mixture is infused via a catheter into the epidural space. It is contraindicated if there is a clotting disorder or if the patient is taking warfarin or heparin and has an international normalized ratio (INR) > 1.5. This is because there is risk of causing an epidural haematoma and thus the risk of paraplegia. Epidurals can also cause hypotension and urinary retention. There is also a small risk of infection (epidural abscess).

Epidural analgesia in patients taking warfarin. Although warfarin is theoretically an absolute contraindication for an epidural, there is a risk:benefit ratio and patients undergoing major abdominal or thoracic surgery benefit significantly from a working epidural, which allows early mobilization and cough without pain, thus reducing the risk of a postoperative pneumonia. The heparin infusion should be stopped 4 h before surgery and then the clotting rechecked. If the INR and activated partial thromboplastin time (APTT) are < 1.5, an epidural can be inserted.

Patient-controlled analgesia. This technique allows the patient to feel that they are in control of their pain relief and is commonly used postoperatively. The patient presses a button that delivers a bolus of morphine intravenously, normally 1 mg every 5 min, with a maximum of 12 mg/h. In this way, the patient cannot accidentally overdose. The patient must have the physical ability to press the button (e.g. it may not be suitable for those with severe rheumatoid arthritis and those with dementia, who may lack the mental capacity to understand how to use it properly).

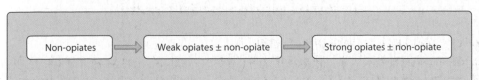

Fig. 1.2 Pain management ladders. NSAIDs, non-steroidal anti-inflammatory drugs.

■ COMPLICATIONS

Surgical complications

Rapid identification of surgical complications is vital to prevent a patient deteriorating and even dying. High suspicion is indicated by the time after surgery at which the complication becomes apparent and also by the operation performed. Any description of complications should always be structured by the time at which complications occur, mostly either early or late (Table 1.3).

There are also operation-specific complications, for example:

- **bowel**: faecal peritonitis from anastomotic breakdown or bowel ischaemia, ileus, fistulae, ureteric damage
- **gastric**: vitamin B_{12}-deficient anaemia, dumping syndrome, malabsorption, iron-deficiency anaemia
- **orthopaedic**: compartment syndrome, fat embolism, deep infection, aseptic loosening
- **thyroidectomy**: laryngeal oedema (tracheal compression), recurrent laryngeal nerve damage, thyroid crisis (storm), hypothyroidism
- **abdominal aortic aneurysm graft**: haemorrhage, MI (as the cross-clamped aorta is released, suddenly increasing cardiac load), thrombus, embolus (gut ischaemia, acute ischemic limb, stroke), graft rejection/infection, acute renal failure, aortoduodenal fistula (presents with haematemesis and has high mortality), reperfusion injury
- **cholecystecomy**: retained stones (ongoing jaundice), bile leakage
- **prostatectomy**: haemorrhage, transurethral resection of the prostrate (TUR) syndrome, retrograde ejaculation (80%), impotence
- **mastecomy**: arm lymphoedema, long thoracic nerve damage (supplying serratus anterior and causing a winged scapula), brachial nerve damage (very rare).

Infectious complications

Cellulitis

Cellulitis is a non-suppurative infection of tissues, usually with β-haemolytic streptococci, staphylococci or *Clostridium perfringens*; it is associated with lymphangitis and septicaemia. There may be tissue destruction and necrosis (usually from anaerobic organisms).

Gangrene

Gangrene occurs in tissues that have compromised blood supply or from gas-forming necrotizing infections. Ischaemic gangrene is commonly seen in the distal limbs, gut (appendix and gall bladder), and sometimes in the testis. Causes include:

- thrombosis of an atherosclerotic artery
- embolus from atrial fibrillation
- Buerger's disease
- trauma: crush injuries, pressure sores
- physical: burns, scalds, frostbites.

Examples of soft tissue infections and necrotizing infection are boils/carbuncles, gas gangrene, gangrene of the scrotum (Fournier's gangrene). There are three types of gangrene: dry, wet and gas.

- **Dry gangrene**. Tissue death is caused by a gradual reduction in the blood supply (typically atherosclerosis); the

Table 1.3 COMPLICATIONS OF SURGERY

Time of occurrence	Complication
Intraoperative	Intraoperative haemorrhage: leading to hypovolaemic shock Fluid balance: dehydration and decreased organ perfusion Faecal contamination (becomes apparent in days 1–4) Incidental, e.g. myocardial infarction
Early (< 24 h)	Haemorrhage Respiratory: atelectasis, adult respiratory distress syndrome Fluid balance: with poor urine outputs and dehydration
Middle (days 1–4)	Urinary retention (can also occur in the first 24 h) Respiratory: pneumonia Thromboembolic: deep vein thrombosis, pulmonary embolism Gastrointestinal: paralytic ileus Operative sepsis (endogenous): faecal contamination during bowel surgery Non-operative sepsis (exogenous): respiratory infection via ventilation, urinary tract infection via a catheter
Before discharge (days 4–14)	Wound complications: anastomotic breakdown[a], faecal fistula[a], wound dehiscence resulting in incisional hernia later
Late (weeks to months)	Incisional hernia Obstruction from adhesions

[a]Complicated by severe sepsis and multiorgan failure, peritonitis, acidosis, ARDS, marrow depression, abscesses, bleeding.

affected part becomes dry, wrinkled and blackened from the disintegration of haemoglobin.

- **Wet gangrene**. Death and putrefactive decay of tissue is caused by bacterial infection, giving rise to moist and infected areas.
- **Gas gangrene**. This typically results from infection of deep wounds or the abdominal cavity (e.g. bowel) with *Clostridium performans* or other gas-forming organisms (usually anaerobes). The pathogenic process involves tissue enzymes (proteases, collagenase, hyaluronidase) and α-toxin. It is a complication of trauma, vascular disease (amputations) and intestinal disease or intestinal operations. Risk factors for gas gangrene are diabetes mellitus, immunosuppression, malignancy and acute kidney disease. The clinical features are an infected wound and spreading cellulitis. The prognosis is poor unless it is treated aggressively with penicillin and repeated debridement.
- **Fournier's gangrene**. This is a spreading cellulitis of the peritoneum and scrotum, which may involve the thighs and abdominal wall. It can result in necrotizing fasciitis, which can be fatal if it spreads systemically. The causative organisms are *Clostridia* and *Bacteroides* spp., streptococci, coliforms, peptostreptococci; treatment is with broad-spectrum intravenous antibiotics and aggressive debridement (see Ch. 31).
- **Melaney's gangrene**. This is like Fournier's gangrene but involving the abdominal wall.

Management of gangrene is as follows.

Peripheral ischaemia. Limb salvage is the primary aim:
- the area is kept absolutely dry
- the zone of demarcation is monitored and pressure sores are prevented
- the blood supply needs to be restored for arterial disease (otherwise amputation)
- a life-saving amputation is required for major crush injury where symptomatic gangrene is rapidly spreading.

Gut ischaemia. This is often difficult to diagnose until systemic sepsis intervenes. Treatment is rapid resuscitation and bowel resection (Ch. 9).

Soft tissue infections. Boils, carbuncles and abscesses require surgical drainage and antibiotic therapy.

Soft tissue anaerobic synergistic infections and gas gangrene. These require an emergency resection (debridement and repeat debridement) of all infected and dead tissue, high-dose intravenous metronidazole, amikacin and penicillin plus hyperbaric oxygen if possible.

Other comorbidities. Other system dysfunction must be managed usually on an ITU: heart failure, arrhythmias, respiratory support, renal function, nutritional and diabetic control. Most patients will need correction of acidosis, inotropes and ventilation. Mortality rates are high for advanced disease.

Hospital-acquired sepsis

Hospitals are reservoirs of multiresistant bacteria owing to the prolonged and extensive use of antibiotics, particularly in ITU with immunocompromised patients: diabetes mellitus, malignancy, transplant recipients, human immunodeficiency virus (HIV) infection, steroid therapy or immunosuppressive therapy. These patients may have open wounds and areas of tissue necrosis.

Multiresistant Staphylococcus aureus *(MRSA)*. This organism is carried by patients and staff in the nose and oropharynx and on the skin and perineum. MRSA will infect implants and non-healing wounds as in sepsis and may be fatal.

Pseudomonas aeruginosa. *Ps. aeruginosa* often infects urine in immunocompromised hosts. It is also found in burns units. It is a common bacteria infecting the bronchial tree and open wounds of patients in the ITU. Most organisms are multiresistant and difficult to eradicate.

Pseudomembranous colitis. Clostridium difficile is now a common cause of acute diarrhoeal illness in hospitalized patients particularly if they are immunocompromised. The organism is carried by patients and is reintroduced on admission to hospital. It is difficult to eradicate even using specific therapy (oral (where possible) vancomycin and/or metronidazole). Pseudomembranous colitis may cause toxic dilatation and fulminating colitis with a risk of perforation, leading to emergency colonectomy, as in ulcerative colitis (Ch. 17).

Boils and carbuncles. See Ch. 70.

Closed space infections. See Ch. 48.

Abscesses

An abscess is a collection of pus and may be uni- or multi-locular. Abscesses may occur in specific sites (e.g. subphrenic spaces, empyema thoracis) or may be non-localized (e.g. inter-loop, pelvic, lower limb abscesses).

The features are swinging pyrexia, tachycardia, localized signs, swelling, redness, loss of function, pain and pressure symptoms. Treatment is by surgical drainage after localization (CT or ultrasound) or by radiographically guided percutaneous drainage under broad-spectrum antibiotic cover.

Tetanus

Tetanus is an infection by *Clostridium tetani* (a spore-forming organism); the bacterium produces an endotoxin, tetanospasmin, that inhibits cholinesterase at the motor end plates. Excess tetanospasmin travels along the nerves to cause hyperexcitability of the anterior horn cells and spasm. Tetanus can be prevented by tetanus toxoid.

Presentation is with dysphagia, jaw stiffness, muscle pain, respiratory problems, muscle spasms, risus sardonicus and opisthotonus. Treatment is with antitoxin (of uncertain value), muscle paralysis and positive ventilation. The prognosis depends on the time from first symptoms to muscle spasms (< 48 h has poor prognosis).

Chronic infection

In patients with infection, the following should always be considered in the differential diagnosis:

- **tuberculosis**: may be pulmonary or may infect almost any tissue, especially paraspinal areas, joints, soft tissue, perioral region and lymph nodes, leading to lymphadenopathy, ascites and bowel obstruction; diagnosis is by testing for acid-fast bacilli or by histopathology of caseating granulomas
- **leprosy**: infection by *Mycobacterium leprae* is becoming rare; it leads to lepromatous or tuberculoid forms of leprosy, resulting in deformities, peripheral nerve paralysis, Charcot's joints and neuropathic ulcers
- **syphilis**: infection by *Treponema pallidum* leads initially to a primary chancre and then to the secondary features of a rash and papules (highly infectious); latent disease causes vasculitis, tissue necrosis, fibrosis, neurological disease, cardiovascular disease and gumma
- **lymphogranuloma venereum**: infection by *Chlamydia trachomatis* leading to painless genital papules and enlarged lymph glands
- **actinomycosis**: persistant subcutaneous infection associated with deep sinuses especially in the right iliac fossa and caused by *Actinomyces israelii*.

Acquired immunodeficiency syndrome

The acquired immunodeficiency syndrome (AIDS) is the clinical manifestation of infection by HIV, a retrovirus that is transmitted sexually and intrauterinely during childbirth and by infected needles or blood products. The surgical presentation of AIDS can be as

- **anal disease**: anal warts, perianal sepsis with poor perineal healing, anorectal ulceration, anal neoplasms (sqamous cell carcinoma, lymphoma, Kaposi sarcoma), faecal incontinence
- **acute abdomen**: infective colitis (also caused by cytomegalovirus and other infective diarrhoeal illnesses), secondary infection by *Mycobacterium avium intracellulare*, non-Hodgkin's lymphoma
- **cholangitis**: similar to sclerosing cholangitis
- **non-Hodgkin's lymphoma**.

Prevention of infection during surgery requires:

- avoidance of needlestick injuries
- using double gloves with at-risk patients
- eye protection
- waterproof protection
- disposable instruments and drapes.

The protocol for staff that may have been infected is therapy with zidovudine, lamivudine and indinavir for 1 month plus prophylaxis for hepatitis within 1 h.

Treatment of HIV infection is with multidrug combinations known as highly active antiretroviral therapy (HAART). Both treatment and prognosis is guided by the CD4 cell count (falls as disease progresses) and the plasma viral load.

Circulatory complications: shock

Shock is a syndrome in which the perfusion of tissues is inadequate for their metabolic requirements. It is divided into types (Table 1.4):

- hypovolaemic shock
- cardiogenic shock
- septic shock
- others: including anaphylactic shock and neurogenic shock.

The diagnosis is made by rapidly assessing the patient with a combination of:

- **history**: trauma, recent surgery, chest pain (MI), insect bite, peanuts
- **observations**: charted values for blood pressure, heart rate, temperature, urine output

Table 1.4 DIFFERENTIATING THE TYPES OF SHOCK

Type	Blood pressure	Pulse	Temperature	Jugular venous pressure
Hypovolaemic	↓	↑	↓	–
Cardiogenic	↓	↓/↑ may be irregular)	↓	↑
Septic	↓	↑ (↓ late)	↑ (in severe cases, WBC and temperature ↓)	–

Table 1.5 CLASSIFICATION OF HYPOVOLAEMIC SHOCK

Class	Blood loss	Signs	Urine output (ml/h)	Patient response
1	15% (750 ml)	Mild tachycardia	> 30	Alert
2	15–30% (750–1500 ml)	Moderate tachycardia, falling blood pressure, falling capillary return	20–30	Anxious, aggressive, thirsty
3	30–40% (1500–2000 ml)	Hypotension, tachycardia, low urine output	5–15	Drowsy, aggressive
4	> 40% (> 2000 ml)	As above with profound hypotension	0–10	Drowsy, unconscious

- **examination**: active bleeding, heart rate, respiratory rate, blood pressure, oximetry, conscious level (a good indicator of adequate brain perfusion), jugular venous pressure, skin perfusion and peripheral temperatures, drains, scars, urine output (minimum 0.5 ml/h per kg body weight)
- **monitor**: blood pressure, heart rate, temperature, urine output
- **investigations**: FBC, U&E, cross-match, arterial blood gases, ECG, chest radiograph, blood cultures, ultrasound to identify abdominal bleeding

Hypovolaemic shock

Hypovolaemic shock can be identified (Table 1.5) with

- a positive **history** (postoperative, trauma)
- a **rising pulse** with a decreasing **blood pressure**
- falling or absent **urine output** (shown on observation charts).

Multiple organ dysfunction syndrome (MODS) may follow, with ARDS, renal failure and multiple system organ failure (MSOF) being frequent occurrences.

Hypovolaemic shock is caused by haemorrhage (postoperative or traumatic; 1.5 litres of blood can be lost with a hip fracture), abdominal aortic aneurysm rupture, dehydration (postoperative patient), major burns, pancreatitis (large third-space losses).

Management of hypovolaemic shock comprises:

- ABC with fluid resuscitation; simultaneously trying to find and correct the cause
- oxygen: 15 l/min oxygen via a facemask
- setting up intravenous access: two large-bore cannulae in two large veins (a **saphenous cutdown** or **intraosseous line** may be needed)
- fluid resuscitation: crystalloids or colloids are started (neither has been proved superior); if losses are severe (e.g. trauma) a 200 ml fluid bolus and O-negative blood are given before cross-matched blood arrives
- monitoring observations: heart rate, blood pressure, urine output, blood oxygen saturation, temperature.

Once treatment has been initiated, drains and wounds should be checked for bleeding. The patient should be monitored closely for a response, aiming for a *minimum* urine output of 0.5–1 ml/h per kg body weight (minimum 30 ml/h).

Surgery may be required to arrest internal bleeding, and dehydration should be corrected with fluid balance.

Cardiogenic shock

Cardiogenic shock occurs when the heart cannot pump enough blood to satisfy the body's immediate needs. Causes include:

- MI, ischaemia, arrhythmias: identify on ECG
- obstructive disorders, cardiac tamponade: identify on clinical examination, looking for a Beck's triad, hypotension, raised jugular venous pressure and muffled heart sounds; pulsus paradoxus and an increase in jugular venous pressure on inspiration (Kussmaul's sign) may also be present
- pulmonary embolus: can cause a variety of ECG abnormalities of which sinus tachycardia (most common), right axis deviation and right bundle branch block are seen far more commonly than the classic 'S1 Q3 T3' (rarely seen).

Management of cardiogenic shock comprises:

- ABC
- oxygen: 15 l/min oxygen via a facemask
- arrhythmias and electrolyte imbalance should be corrected
- finding and correcting the cause.

If the patient has had an MI, thrombolysis should be considered. Serial ECGs need to be done and troponin should be measured at 12 h. An echocardiograph is useful to assess the contractility of the heart and to assess for any valvular damage.

Septic shock

Septic shock is the most common cause of mortality in the ITU; it is characterized by:

- hypotension despite adequate fluid resuscitation
- evidence of inadequate perfusion
- the presence of sepsis.

There is a continuum of clinical manifestations from the systemic inflammatory response syndrome (SIRS) to sepsis to severe sepsis to septic shock to multiple organ dysfunction syndrome (MODS). SIRS is the systemic outcome of sepsis and is probably caused by a toxin. It may be associated with bacterial translocation from the gut. It is commonly associated with ARDS and MSOF. It is characterized by two of the following:

- hypo- or hyperthermia (< 38°C or > 36°C)
- tachycardia (> 90 beats/min)
- white blood cell count > 12×10^9 or < 4×10^9 cells/l.

The patient with sepsis is often **pyrexial** (although may occasionally be hypothermic). The peripheries are warm and vasodilated; hypotension is present, and tachycardia may occur. Sweats, chills and rigors may be present.

Most sepsis is caused by bacterial infection. Infections can be initiated operatively (e.g. faecal leakage and peritonitis) or result from non-operative factors (e.g. respiratory infections, urinary tract infections, patients with burns and pancreatitis).

Management of sepsis comprises:

- ABC with aggressive fluid management
- use of inotropes (adrenaline (epinephrine) or noradrenaline (norepinephrine)) may be used to maintain arterial pressure
- a **septic screen**: samples from blood, sputum, urine and wounds are cultured
- the chest is examined and a chest X-ray ordered
- intravenous antibiotics are required to treat the infective source (guided by microbiology)
- admission of the patient to the critical care unit for optimal care and fluid management, with central and arterial line insertion and regular monitoring of blood gases.

Surgical intervention is likely to be necessary to drain an infective source or to ensure that there is no intestinal ischaemia or continued contamination of the peritoneal cavity.

Anaphylactic shock
Anaphylactic shock is a **type 1 hypersensitivity reaction**, resulting from an antigen–antibody reaction on the surface of mast cells, leading to their degranulation and histamine release. Anaphylaxis requires prior exposure to the antigenic agent. It may be caused by insect bites, food reactions and drug reactions.

Anaphylaxis results in a variety of symptoms, which may be manifested in various degrees of severity: skin redness, urticaria, angioedema, bronchospasm and cardiovascular collapse.

Management of anaphylactic shock comprises:

- ABC
- adrenaline (epinephrine): this is the mainstay of treatment (intramuscular, 0.5–1.0 ml of 1:1000 solution; intravenous, 1 ml of 1:10 000 solution) and is repeated every 10 min as required
- oxygen: 15 l/min of high-flow oxygen via facemask
- aggressive fluid resuscitation.

Secondary treatment includes **antihistamine drugs** (e.g. chlorpheniramine 10–20 mg given intravenous slowly), **H$_2$ receptor antagonists** (e.g. rantidine 50 mg intravenous slowly) and **hydrocortisone** (100–200 mg intravenous). The patient may require admission to a critical care unit.

Respiratory complications

Atelectasis
Atelectasis is the absence of gas from part or all of the lung. It is caused by insufficient aeration of the alveoli, with consequent malabsorption of the gas. It occurs most commonly in the dependent areas of the lung and is common after a general anaesthetic. It is more common in patients with preexisting lung disease and sputum retention and in patients who have had abdominal or thoracic surgery and are unable to cough or deep breathe because of pain. Deep breathing exercises are encouraged postoperatively to reduce the incidence. Treatment is with oxygen therapy and physiotherapy.

Pneumonia
A postoperative pulmonary infection will cause numerous symptoms including general malaise, pyrexia and tachycardia. The patient may develop a cough, with sputum or haemoptysis, and may also have chest pain and be hypoxic. It may also follow aspiration (inhalation of acidic stomach contents), causing a lobar pneumonia; this is why patients are starved before surgery.

The source is likely to be a hospital-acquired bacterial pneumonia, and a clinical finding of consolidation is confirmed with chest radiograph.

Pneumonia is more common in the elderly, the infirm, patients in a poor nutritional state, following major abdominal and thoracic surgery and in patients with poor pain control who are reluctant to cough. Mortality from postoperative pneumonia is 10% and it also delays recovery from surgery; poor tissue oxygenation may contribute to delayed wound healing.

Initial management is to give the patient high-flow oxygen, to take sputum and blood cultures and an FBC to measure the white cell count, and then to start antibiotics (adjusted to culture results). All patients should be given regular physiotherapy and have their blood gas saturations monitored.

Acute respiratory distress syndrome
ARDS is the most severe form of acute lung injury. It is associated with sepsis, multiple trauma, major surgery, pancreatitis, massive transfusion, burns and smoke or chemical

inhalation. The onset is usually within 2–3 days of the original insult or injury. ARDS has:

- an acute onset
- bilateral diffuse infiltrates on chest radiograph
- pulmonary artery wedge pressure < 18 mmHg
- arterial hypoxaemia that is resistant to oxygen therapy: partial arterial oxygen pressure (PaO_2) < 27 kPa or a ratio of PaO_2 to fraction of inspired oxygen (FiO_2) < 200.

Management is supportive in a critical care setting, with the aim to optimize oxygen delivery. The patient will commonly need a period of endotracheal intubation and ventilation.

Renal complications

Acute urinary retention

Urine output should be carefully recorded following surgery: hourly in the case of major surgery. If the urine output is less than 0.5 ml/h per kg body weight, the cause may be:

- **insufficient fluid replacement,** the most likely cause
- **acute urinary retention**: there is a palpable bladder (and the patient may have the urge but inability to pass urine); a catheter should be passed and if one is already in place, a bladder washout should ensure it is not blocked (if a urethral catheter cannot be passed (e.g. because of benign prostatic hyperplasia), a suprapubic catheter may be needed)
- **renal shutdown**: if the bladder cannot be palpated and a catheter is in place, failure to pass urine may indicate renal failure (see below)
- **hypovolaemic shock**: identified by examining the hydration status of the patient and finding a decreasing blood pressure and increasing pulse rate, with a widened pulse pressure (systolic to diastolic blood pressure); drains and wounds are checked for active bleeding (see above).

Acute renal failure

Acute renal failure usually develops over a few days and may develop with or without preexisting renal impairment. The causes can be divided into:

- **prerenal**: hypoperfusion, e.g. shock, hypovolaemia, cardiogenic shock
- **renal**: glomerular causes, e.g. glomerulonephritis and tubulointerstitial causes (acute tubular necrosis accounts for 75% of acute renal failure in the hospital setting)
- **postrenal**: obstruction in the urinary collection system.

There are numerous risk factors, for example the elderly, diabetes mellitus, preexisting renal impairment, dehydration, overlong use of NSAIDs or ACE inhibitors and prolonged periods of intra or postoperative hypotension.

The patient may present with oliguria, with increasing urea and creatinine. The patient may also have a worsening metabolic acidosis owing to the accumulation of metabolic waste products.

Management initially is by giving a fluid challenge and assessing the response whilst trying to elicit the cause. Once the cause is known, specific treatment can be initiated. Hyperkalaemia is a potential emergency and must be treated rapidly. If there is no improvement, referral to the renal unit is needed for further management, which may include urgent dialysis.

Thromboembolic complications

Deep vein thrombosis

DVT often presents with sudden-onset calf tenderness, with a swollen limb and tight skin, although it may be asymptomatic. A Duplex scan should be performed to identify the thrombosis. Initial management is with low-molecular-weight heparin (LMWH), which is subsequently converted to warfarin therapy. Warfarin is continued for 3 months after the first DVT but is needed lifelong after the second. Further details and risk factors are given on p. 3 and in Ch. 27.

Pulmonary embolism

The symptoms of pulmonary embolism are sudden-onset pleuritic chest pain with cyanosis, tachypnoea, haemoptysis, tachycardia, elevated jugular venous pressure and cardiovascular collapse, although symptoms vary with severity. A pulmonary embolism may result from an embolus that has broken off from a thrombus in a deep vein. Pulmonary embolism can be excluded by a negative assay for D-dimer; it can be diagnosed with either ventilation–perfusion scan (showing a mismatch) or spiral computed tomographic (CT) scan, although both these investigations may be inconclusive. The definitive test for pulmonary embolism is CT pulmonary angiography; in addition:

- measurement of arterial blood gases will identify respiratory failure
- ECG commonly shows a sinus tachycardia, right bundle branch block or right axis deviation; it rarely shows the characteristic S1 Q3 T3 pattern
- chest radiograph will show a wedge-shaped infarct in only 10%.

Management is with anticoagulation and intravenous low-molecular-weight heparin (1.5 mg/kg enoxaparin), followed by conversion to warfarin. Massive pulmonary embolism requires thrombolysis with tissue plasminogen activator or surgical embolectomy.

Wound complications

Dehiscence and infection can affect wounds and these are dealt with later in this section.

■ BASIC SURGICAL PRINCIPLES

Wound management

Wound management is an essential principle of surgery, since surgeons both create and treat wounds. There are three main types of wound:

- **incisional wounds**: caused by a sharp object, such as a knife (either traumatic or surgical)
- **lacerations**: injuries caused by blunt objects or tearing of the skin in which the skin is stretched and the dermis and underlying blood vessels tear; **degloving** occurs when skin is removed from the fascia, usually by a rotational force
- **burns**: these can be thermal, electrical or chemical; superficial burns are treated conservatively but deep burns require specialist surgical intervention.

Making incisions

When making a wound, the incision line should be made along lines of tension of the normal skin (**Langer's lines**). In the face, incisions should be made along lines of skin folds. In the hands, incisions crossing the palmar creases should be avoided since the skin may contract and limit function. If possible, incisions should be made in natural skin folds for cosmetic purposes. When accessing the abdomen, the abdominal fascias and muscles should be bluntly dissected (as in appendicectomy) so that when the wound is closed, a strong grid is formed, preventing breakdown and incisional hernias. Midline incisions are generally preferred to paramedian incisions for laparotomy. Transverse incisions (Pfannensteil) are used for pelvic surgery, some abdominal procedures and to expose the kidneys.

Wound healing

Superficial wounds often heal spontaneously, but deep wounds (those which cross the dermis and pass into the subdermis) require surgical closure. There are two physiological ways a wound can heal:

- **primary intention**: the two edges of skin are brought together and healing occurs rapidly between the two sides
- **secondary intention**: if the two wound edges cannot be brought together or are deliberately left open (because of sepsis or swelling), the wound is kept clean and granulation tissue forms in the gap (e.g. wound dehiscence); eventually this fills the space and the wound heals slowly by secondary intention.

Healthy wound healing is promoted by:

- good blood supply
- no foreign material or infection
- no excess tension of the wound/skin
- accurate apposition (aligning of the skin).

Materials for closing wounds

Sutures.   These are classified as either absorbable or non-absorbable.

- absorbable sutures (e.g. Polyglactin) are biological and are broken down by enzymatic action leaving no foreign material; they do not need to be removed but they provide support for the wound for a limited period
- non-absorbable sutures are non-biological materials (e.g. silk, nylon, prolene) and provide permanent wound support but there is potential for a foreign body reaction and infection; superficial sutures are removed after 10 days if on the limbs or 5 days if on the face.

Steri-Strips.   These are used to close small skin wounds (e.g. non-complicated superficial arm wound) and non-gaping scalp injuries.

Tissue glue.   This is often used for superficial scalp wounds.

Metal clips.   These resemble metal staples and are often used for large abdominal or thoracic surgery; if there are no complications, they are removed after 10 days.

Special wounds

Abdominal wounds.   These usually close well, particularly oblique incisions, as the abdominal wall forms a grid, thus preventing incisional hernias.

Head injuries.   Any wound to the scalp that penetrates the aponeurosis subsequently gapes open and needs to be closed with sutures (Fig. 1.3). Any wound above the aponeuroris can be closed using tissue glue or Steri-Strips.

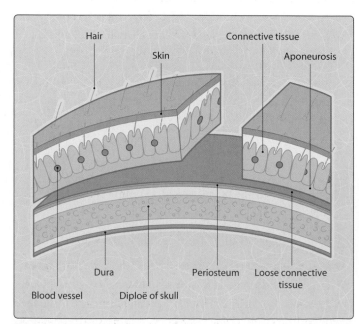

Fig 1.3 Scalp injuries.

Wound complications

Healing can be delayed by:

- infection or foreign body
- steroids: inhibit collagen synthesis and cytokine function
- tissue hypoxia: poor blood supply or respiratory failure
- systemic disease: jaundice, diabetes, cancer and malnutrition
- previous radiation to the damaged area
- sepsis
- poor surgical technique.

Wound infection

Wound infection is a middle-period complication. The origin can be exogenous (usually *Staphylococcus aureus* or *Staphylococcus epidermis*) or endogenous: usually gut organisms after bowel surgery (e.g. *Escherichia coli*, *Klebsiella*, *Proteus*, *Pseudomonas*, *Bacteroides* or *Clostridia* spp., anaerobic streptococci), urinary pathogens after open urology (e.g. *E. coli*, enterococci) or vaginal pathogens after gynaecological operations (anaerobic or aerobic streptococci and yeasts). The infected wound should be opened and washed out with either surgical toilet or surgical debridement. Dressings should be changed regularly, and antibiotics given according to wound swabs taken for culture and sensitivity (intravenous if infection is severe). Wound dehiscence is a serious sequelae.

Wound dehiscence

Wound dehiscence is a middle-period complication that occurs in 2–10% of abdominal wounds, which completely break down. For example, if a laparotomy wound dehisces and exposes loops of bowel. It occurs from wound infection or when sutures tear through weak tissues (steroids, malnourishment, the elderly, malignancy). Treatment is to return the patient to theatre and resuture abdominal wounds or to allow healing by secondary intention. Open laparotomy might be indicated if there is severe sepsis or a fistula.

Incisional hernia

An incisional hernia is a late-period complication that occurs when an abdominal wound closure becomes infected or breaks down. Underlying contents (such as gut) protrude through the wound defect. It is more common in the obese, the elderly, the malnourished, when the wound becomes infected or after poor surgical technique.

Anastomoses

An anastomosis is formed between two ends of a tube (Fig. 1.4), commonly between the divided ends of bowel or blood vessels. The factors that inhibit healing of an anastomosis are the same as for any wound: sepsis, ischaemia, local physical tension,

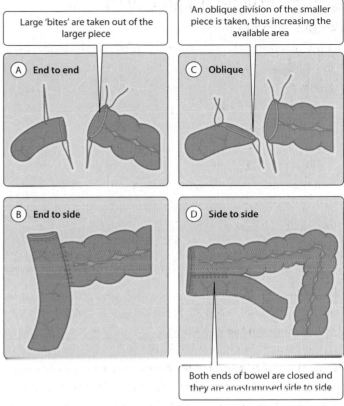

Fig. 1.4 Anastomoses

steroids, hypotension, blood clot, foreign material, severe contamination, poor technique.

Drains

Drains are placed into surgical wounds at the end of the operation. They allow excess blood and pus to drain out of the body, thus preventing their accumulation and subsequent abscess formation.

The most commonly used drain is the **closed suction drain** (e.g. an urinary catheter, a chest drain, or a T-tube connected to a bile drain). For a closed non-suction drain, the bottle is kept below the patient, and fluid drains into it by gravity.

Drains are usually removed once < 25 ml is draining per day. Patients may be allowed home with drains attached, and the community nurse will remove them at home. T-tubes are removed after 10 days if the T-tube cholangiogram shows a patent duct.

The possibility of a blocked drain can be assessed by:

- swing test: hold the drain where fluid is present; by moving the drain from side to side ('swinging' it), the fluid level should move within the tube if the drain is not blocked
- if the patient coughs, the increase in pressure will cause the fluid level in the drain to shift; this is best for abdominal drains.

Table 1.6 POTENTIAL OSCE STATIONS IN SURGERY

	Station	Chapter in Section 3
Abdominal	Organomegaly, mass, ascites/ distension, jaundice	6
	Stomas: ileostomy versus colostomy	16
Groin lump	Hernia (inguinal or femoral), other groin lump	33
Neck	Thyroid goitre	40
	Other neck lump (lymph nodes, salivary glands)	42
Vascular	Varicose veins/chronic venous insufficiency	22
	Peripheral vascular disease	24
	Ulcers	28
	Swollen leg (cellulitis, DVT, lymphodema)	27
	Diabetic foot: Charcot's joints, neurpathy, ulcers	28
Breast	Single lump, multiple lumps, nipple change/discharge	39
Orthopaedic	Hip	59
	Knee	61
	Shoulder/ankle/elbow/spine	63
	Nerve palsy	57
	Carpal tunnel syndrome	57
Postoperative patient: inspection, investigations and complications of surgery	Gallstones: open and laparoscopic cholecystectomy	
	Colorectal cancer resection	
	Obstruction (inspection of a stoma, interpretation of radiographs)	
Urology	Testicular lump (+/- hernia), urinary stone (nephrostomy with IVU)	32
Lumps and bumps	Subcutaneous cyst, lipoma, etc.	70, 71

THE OSCE STATION

The surgical examination station may take the classical form of examining a system, presenting the findings, and then answering the examiner's questions. In some stations, the student is asked to observe a patient, comment on what they see and answer the examiner's structured questions. These patients may have obvious features such as wounds, drains, stomas, scars or ulcers.

However, in the modern OSCE, the student is more likely to encounter a simulated patient (who may be able to simulate mild to severe abdominal pain) or a mannequin (such as a breast or scrotal model), where the examiner can insert abnormalities, such as lumps. Also data stations, such as interpreting radiographs, may be present; here an examiner is not needed. The modern OSCE is constantly assessing communication skills in addition to clinical skills.

Some surgical OSCE stations are structured so that the history is already given to the student and marks are allocated for the following:

- general demeanour between student and patient, communication, gentle examination; building a *rapport* with the patient
- inspection
- examination and special tests

- diagnosis and differential diagnosis
- knowing potential benefits and likely outcomes of treatment
- knowing possible risks and complications of treatment.

Answers on management should be structured with the general principles of **conservative, medical and surgical management options** for most conditions, and **curative or palliative management** for cancer.

An OSCE station should follow best practice for examining a patient. The student should always address the patient before attempting to examine in any way. Any examination must follow the steps of *introduction*, obtaining *consent* and then *exposing* the relevant area. The patient should be asked about any pain or tenderness first. A student would then indicate the area to be examined, such as 'I would like to expose the patient from nipples to knees'. An examiner may ask for just the abdomen to be exposed.

Table 1.6 lists the chapters in Section 3 that cover potential OSCE stations in surgery.

GETTING STARTED

It is important to know by heart the 'surgical sieve' before getting started. When confronted by a 'lump' and you have no idea of what it is, you can say so (it is well to be honest) but you could then go on to say that there are a number of things it could be. The list below gives such possibilities with examples (Ch. 20 also uses this approach for anal fistulae).

- congenital: a good example is dermoid (dermoid cyst of the ovary)
- acquired:
  — traumatic: old injury such as an atrioventricular fistula
  — metabolic: parathyroid lump if the swelling is in the neck
  — degenerative: nodule on the finger (Heberden's nodes)
  — autoimmune: midline swelling in the neck (thyroiditis)
  — ischaemic: avascular necrosis, osteoarthritis
  — inflammatory: trigger finger secondary to rheumatoid arthritis
  — infective, acute: non-specific (e.g. orbital cellulitis) or specific (e.g. mumps, enlarged lymph nodes)
  — infective, chronic: non-specific (e.g. osteomyelitis) or specific (e.g. tuberculous cold abscess)
  — benign neoplasm: e.g. osteoma
  — primary malignant neoplasm: e.g. cancer of the breast
  — secondary malignant neoplasm: depends on the primary; using breast cancer as the example, there may be local invasion (e.g. chest wall tethering), mesothelial (pleural) or lymph node involvement (near in the pectoral node, intermediate in the apical node and distant in the left supraclavicular node), or distant sites (commonly lungs, liver, bone, brain, adrenal glands, skin).

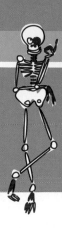

High return facts

2

General abdominal surgery

1 The acute abdomen is an extremely common surgical presentation that is characterized by pain: it has a wide differential diagnosis. Presentation varies from mild abdominal pain through to peritonitis and shock. Pain is best considered by dividing the abdomen into regions, although radiating pain must be considered. If a diagnosis cannot be reached immediately, observation is warranted and further investigations may be performed. If the patient does not improve or worsens, surgery to identify a cause may be necessary.

2 Appendicitis is the most common surgical emergency. Abdominal pain typically starts as a dull, central pain as the visceral peritoneum is irritated; as inflammation continues, the parietal peritoneum is irritated, causing a sharp, localized pain in the right iliac fossa, maximal over McBurney's point. However, diagnosis can prove difficult, as only 50% of patients present with typical features. If the appendix perforates, the patient may develop peritonitis. Appendicectomy is the definitive treatment and is performed either in an open procedure or laparoscopically.

3 Gallstones are very common, although 80% of stones remain asymptomatic. Most (80%) are mixed stones where cholesterol is the main component, with bile pigments and calcium salts. Ultrasound is the best test in the acute phase. The complications of gallstones are best considered by the level at which the stones may impact: either in the gallbladder/cystic duct or in the common bile duct. Biliary colic, acute cholecystitis and obstructive jaundice are common presentations.

4 The treatment of gallstone disease depends on possible complications. Most acute events can be managed conservatively, where 90% of stones pass spontaneously. If the stone does not pass (indicated by the patient's condition and no improvement in liver function tests), endoscopic retrograde cholangiopancreatography can be used in the first instance to retrieve the stone, although cholecystectomy (surgical removal of the gall-bladder) is definitive treatment. Open cholecystectomy may be required; 90% of cholecystectomies are performed laparoscopically.

5 A hernia is an abnormal protrusion of a viscus through its containing cavity wall. The four most common types of abdominal hernia in adults are inguinal, femoral, umbilical and incisional. Inguinal hernias are classified as either direct or indirect and are either reducible or irreducible. The treatment of choice is surgery, even in the elderly if fit, as there is risk that the hernia will strangulate if left alone, which is a surgical emergency.

6 Examination of the abdomen is common and important, as it is a frequent OSCE station and it is a very common examination performed by clinicians in all specialties. It is important to know the differential diagnosis of pain and masses and how to test for shifting dullness.

Surgery of the upper gastrointestinal tract

7 Dyspepsia is a broad term that encompasses a range of symptoms, including epigastric pain, heartburn and bloating. A patient of any age with alarm symptoms is investigated endoscopically within 2 weeks; such symptoms are chronic gastrointestinal bleeding, weight loss, dysphagia, persistent vomiting, iron-deficiency anaemia or an epigastric mass. Unexplained and persistent dyspepsia without alarm symptoms in a patient over 55 years warrants endoscopy within 2 weeks to exclude cancer. Both gastro-oesophageal reflux disease and peptic ulcer disease are common diagnoses; their management is mostly medical. Haemorrhage, perforation and pyloric stenosis are the three relatively common complications of peptic ulcers.

8 Common causes of upper gastrointestinal bleeding include Mallory–Weiss tears, bleeding peptic ulcers, oesophageal varices and oesophagitis/acute gastritis. The patient may present with a range of symptoms, from unexplained anaemia ranging to acute haematemesis causing haemodynamical instability. A digital rectal examination must be performed, which often reveals malaena. Patients are resuscitated and stabilized before endoscopy, which is the investigation of choice and is also therapeutic to arrest the bleeding.

9 Disorders affecting the oesophagus include cancer, achalasia, strictures and perforation. Dysphagia means difficulty in swallowing and requires urgent investigation with endoscopy. Progressive dysphagia and weight loss in the elderly is assumed to be oesophageal cancer until proved otherwise. Although most tumours are squamous cell carcinomas, the incidence of adeno-carcinoma is rapidly rising because of the occurrence of Barrett's oesophagus.

10 Stomach cancer is the second most common cancer worldwide. Although the frequency of stomach cancer in the UK is falling, there is currently a sharp rise in the incidence of adenocarcinoma of the gastro-oesophageal junction. Presentation is often late, when cancer is advanced and prognosis poor.

11 Portal hypertension and ascites are commonly caused by chronic conditions of the liver. Secondary tumours of the liver are more common than primary tumours in the UK, although primary tumours are the most common worldwide. The main operation for the spleen is splenectomy, which is either performed electively for lymphoma or blood disorders or as an emergency, when the spleen ruptures following blunt trauma to the abdomen. Patients should be counselled about complications of infection and can be started on long-term prophylactic antibiotics.

12 Acute pancreatitis is most often caused by gall-stones or alcohol, and it may range from mild to life threatening. Treatment is conservative, and surgery is only required when complications occur. Chronic pancreatitis results from repeated acute attacks and is commonly caused by alcohol use; the majority of patients are managed conservatively for long periods. Pancreatic tumours most often present late and have an extremely poor prognosis.

Lower gastrointestinal tract: colorectal surgery

13 Colorectal cancer is the second most common cause of death from malignancy in developed countries, and its incidence is increasing. Suspicious features include weight loss, altered bowel habit and blood passed per rectum; patients with these symptoms should be seen within 2 weeks in cancer clinics for investigations. Among patients with colorectal cancer, 30% present as an emergency, with obstruction, perforation or haemorrhage. Curative surgical resection is attempted in 80% of patients.

14 Bowel obstruction is broadly classified as affecting either the small or the large bowel and being either mechanical or functional. The key investigation is the plain film abdominal radiograph, which differentiates between small and large bowel obstruction. Initial treatment is conservative and surgery is indicated if an obstructing tumour is present, there is strangulation (e.g. of a hernia causing obstruction) or if there is no clinical improvement.

15 Diverticular disease is very common, although symptoms only occur in 20% of patients. There are a wide variety of presentations and symptoms; investigations can be performed to exclude colorectal cancer when a change in bowel habit is present. Conservative treatment is satisfactory for most patients; surgery may be required when complications occur. If infection and peritonitis is present, a two-stage resection of the affected sigmoid colon with a Hartmann's procedure (end-colostomy and oversewn rectal stump) may be required; the sections are rejoined 3–6 months later.

16 Stomas are surgically created openings in the body between the skin and a hollow viscus. A colostomy is used to divert faeces from the large bowel, and an ileostomy is used for the small bowel. These stomas are either permanent or temporary. Other types of stoma include an ileal conduit (following bladder cancer resection), a gastrostomy and a jejunostomy (both allow enteral feeding directly into the gut).

17 Ulcerative colitis is a chronic inflammatory bowel disease that causes inflammation of the mucosa and submucosa of the large bowel only, starting in the rectum and progressing distally. Presentation is commonly with gradual-onset diarrhoea, abdominal pain and weight loss. Toxic dilatation is a complication that requires urgent surgery, although the main long-term complication is malignant change.

18 Crohn's disease is a chronic inflammatory disease that can affect any part of the gastrointestinal tract from mouth to anus. It affects the full thickness of the bowel wall and is most common at the ileocaecal junction. Colonic disease is similar to ulcerative colitis, although Crohn's disease may also present with recurrent perianal disease. It is usually treated medically and with diet. Surgery is required for complications of stenosis, perforation, abscess or fistula.

19 Rectal bleeding is a common presentation, and the differential diagnosis is determined by the patient's age. Colorectal cancer must be excluded in those over 45 years. Haemorrhoids are also a common cause; these are treated either conservatively or surgically, depending on symptoms and patient preference.

20 The conditions that occur around the anus are very common but are very distressing for the patient. In patients who present with recurrent perianal disease, Crohn's disease, HIV infection and diabetes mellitus should be excluded.

Vascular surgery

21 Varicose veins are tortuous dilatations of veins, commonly affecting the veins of the lower limbs. The most commonly affected vein is the great saphenous vein. The majority of varicose veins are idiopathic, although occasionally there is an underlying cause. Management is conservative, medical or surgical.

22 The aim of examining for varicose veins is to identify which vein is affected and the level at which incompetence is occurring. The patient may have simple varicose veins (which appear as tortuous, dilated veins) or may have signs of chronic venous insufficiency, characterized by long-standing changes to the limb, including ulcers and lipodermatosclerosis.

23 Peripheral vascular disease occurs when there is narrowing of the arteries. There are two main clinical states. Intermittent claudication is a cramp-like pain that occurs in a group of muscles upon exercise and is relieved by rest. Critical limb ischaemia is rest pain, ulceration or gangrene that has been occurring for 2 weeks or more. Intermittent claudication is managed by optimization of medical management; critical limb ischaemia is managed by best medical management, angioplasty, bypass surgery and amputation.

24 The examination of the peripheral vascular system requires palpation of the pulses in order to identify the level of any blockage and to determine the severity of disease. The absence of pulses should enable the clinician to predict the level of the blockage as seen on an angiogram.

25 An ulcer is a full-thickness loss of an epithelial surface. The most common leg ulcers are venous (70% of all leg ulcers), arterial, neuropathic and mixed ulcers. The foot in diabetic patients is a vulnerable area because of the presence of peripheral neuropathy, peripheral vascular disease and infection. A Charcot's joint may develop secondary to neuropathy.

26 Aneurysms are permanent localized dilatations in an arterial wall. An abdominal aortic aneurysm typically produces an expansile, pulsatile abdominal mass. Surgical repair can either be performed electively or as an emergency. If the aneurysm ruptures, the patient presents with severe abdominal or back pain, peritonitis and is in hypovolaemic shock; this is a surgical emergency that requires immediate laparatomy and has an associated mortality of 75–85%.

27 Carotid artery disease is a common cause of stroke, stenosis often occurring at the carotid bifurcation. The indications for surgery are when the stenosis is greater than 70% or when symptoms are present.

28 An acute ischaemic limb occurs when an embolus or thrombus causes sudden blockage of an artery, with rapid necrosis of distal tissues. It is characterized by pain, pallor, pulselessness, perishingly cold, paralysis, paraesthesia (remembered as the 6Ps). Management is urgent reperfusion of the limb, although amputation may be required in late cases. Deep vein thrombosis and cellulitis can also cause a hot, swollen, painful limb.

Urology

29 Benign prostatic hyperplasia of the prostate tissue is extremely common, affecting 50% of men over 50 years of age. Approximately 50% of those affected deteriorate, 30% remain stable and 20% improve. Medical management is sometimes possible; trans-urethral resection of the prostate is the gold standard and is very commonly performed. Acute urinary retention is the sudden inability to pass urine and is a urological emergency where a urinary catheter should be passed without delay.

30 Prostate cancer is the second most common cancer in men. Up to 80% of men over 80 die *with* prostate cancer, but not necessarily *of* it. It may present following screening for prostate-specific antigen (PSA), with urinary symptoms or with lower back pain, indicating metastatic spread. PSA is an imperfect marker of prostate cancer. Management is either curative or non-curative, when 'active surveillance' (no active treatment) is an acceptable option for many patients.

31 Although rare, testicular cancer is the most common cancer in men aged 20–40 years. The incidence is increasing, but the overall 5 year survival is excellent (> 95%). Treatment is with radical orchidectomy and adjuvant treatments are used according to pathology and stage. Penile cancer is rare and almost always affects uncircumcised men.

32 A testicular lump is treated as a tumour until proved otherwise. If any suspicion of malignancy exists, lumps should be scanned with ultrasound at rapid-access clinics. Hydroceles, varicoceles and epididymal cysts all cause lumps; these can be surgically removed if problematic. Testicular torsion and epididymitis both cause scrotal pain. Torsion is a surgical emergency and requires immediate surgery based on a positive clinical diagnosis alone.

33 There are many causes of a lump in the groin. Examination of inguinal hernias and scrotal lumps often go together and should be well practiced. Examination of inguinal hernias is to determine whether the hernia is direct or indirect, whether it is reducible or irreducible, and whether it extends into the scrotum. There is a scheme of questions to answer when examining scrotal lumps, including whether it is possible to feel above the lump and whether the lump is separate from the testis.

34 Haematuria is the presence of blood in the urine; it can be either macroscopic (visible to the naked eye) or microscopic (blood is only detectable on dipstick). Macroscopic haematuria is a common presentation of bladder tumours, and treatment is determined by whether the tumour is superficial (75%) or if there is muscle invasive. Renal cancer is often found incidentally while investigating other problems, and treatment is primarily surgical.

35 Urinary stone disease ('kidney stones') is a common disorder, although stones may remain asymptomatic. Stones typically produce 'loin to groin' pain, and microscopic haematuria is present in more than 90% of those with urinary stone disease. Plain radiograph will detect 90% of stones, and an intravenous urogram or computed tomography can establish the exact location of the stone and whether the stone is obstructing the kidney. Most stones < 5 mm in diameter pass with conservative management; if the stone does not pass or is > 5 mm, then active measures to remove it may be required. (Obstruction of a kidney is a urological emergency that may need to be relieved with a percutensous nephrostomy.)

36 Urinary tract infection (UTI) is very common. *Escherichia coli* is the causative organism in 80% of cases, and UTIs are much more common in women (because of their shorter urethra). A course of trimethoprin for 3 days is adequate for simple cystitis. When UTIs occur in children and men, they are almost always abnormal and can be caused by anatomical abnormalities, hence further investigated is warranted.

37 Urinary incontinence is the involuntary loss of urine and is a common and often embarrassing problem. The main types are stress incontinence (abdominal pressure overcomes urethral closing pressure), urgency incontinence (caused by detrusor muscle overactivity) and overflow incontinence (caused by high residual volume bladder). A neuropathic bladder occurs when there is damage to the nervous supply of the bladder. Stress and urgency incontinence may occur together.

Breast surgery

38 Breast cancer is the commonest cancer affecting women. All women aged 50 to 70 years in the UK are currently screened with mammography. A suspicious lump is assessed with triple assessment: clinical examination, imaging (mammography or ultrasound) and biopsy (fine needle or core biopsy). Treatment depends on the pathology and stage, and the prognosis is determined by the Nottingham Prognostic Index.

39 The majority of women who present with a breast problem have a benign breast disease. They can present with a lump, breast enlargement, pain, nipple changes or discharge. Any suspicious lump should be investigated with triple assessment to exclude malignancy.

Neck and endocrine surgery

40 Patients with thyroid disease typically present with symptoms of hyperthyroidism, hypothyroidism or a thyroid enlargement. Treatment is with medications or surgery. A single thyroid lump should be investigated further to exclude malignancy; 10-20% are malignant. The complications of thyroid surgery is a common examination question.

41 The lymph glands of the neck are common sites of metastases and they are also enlarged in infection, sarcoidosis and leukaemia/lymphoma. Dysfunction of the endocrine glands can have major systemic effects and they are also the sites for tumours. Knowledge of disorders of the parathyroid, pituitary and adrenal glands is important, particularly Cushing's disease and syndrome.

42 Neck lumps can broadly be classified as being midline or non-midline, or in the anterior or posterior triangles of the neck. The lump's characteristics guide the diagnosis. When considering salivary gland tumours, 80% of all tumours are in the parotid glands, 80% are benign and 80% are pleomorphic adenomas.

43 Neck palpation is carried out while standing behind the patient. The examination is to determine whether a neck lump originates from the thyroid gland or other structures, and then to establish the other characteristics to guide the diagnosis. Examination is also to determine whether a thyroid goitre is causing tracheal deviation, and whether there is any retrosternal extension, which may compress the superior vena cava.

Trauma

44 Management of trauma follows a set pattern to ensure a team's priorities so that nothing is missed. The primary survey is performed first in all patients before addressing any obvious fractures, and follows an ABC pattern: airway with cervical spine control, breathing and circulation. This is repeated as many times as is necessary until the patient has been stabilized. Only then is the secondary survey started, where the patient is examined meticulously from head to toe, including a log-roll to inspect the back, and all orifices are examined.

45 A fracture is a soft tissue injury with a disruption in the continuity of a bone; the soft tissue injury is just as important as the break in the bone. Fractures should be described in terms of whether they are open or closed, what bones and what sides of bones are involved, and whether the proximal, middle or distal portion is involved. The shape and deformity accurately describe the fracture.

46 The initial management of any patient with a fracture is with a complete primary survey (ABC with cervical spine control), as there may be a potentially life-threatening problem, especially if the patient has a distracting injury. The overall management of a specific fracture is to reduce, immobilize and rehabilitate the fracture. Open reduction and internal fixation (ORIF) may be required for some fractures.

47 Trauma to the shoulder is common, most often as a result of falls either directly onto the shoulder or onto an outstretched hand. Fractured clavicles are very common, and treatment is conservative with a broad arm sling. The shoulder joint sacrifices stability in favour of a wide range of movement; consequently the shoulder is the most commonly dislocated joint, with anterior shoulder dislocations being much more common than posterior dislocations. Humeral shaft fractures are common in patients with osteoporosis, and even when displaced are treated by a collar and cuff with gravity providing the traction to reduce the fracture.

48 There are many types of fracture of the forearm and hand and these can be complicated. They can be considered as five groups: around the elbow, in the mid shaft, of the distal radius, of the carpals, and of the hand. If a single fracture of the forearm is found, it is important to look for another and also for a dislocation; radiographs of the distal and proximal joint must be taken. A Colles' fracture is a fracture of the distal radius and is very common. An associated tendon injury should be sought when examining a patient with a forearm or hand fracture; if present, surgical exploration and repair is required.

49 Fractures of the lower limb are common, and since they are often caused by high-energy impacts, initial ABC with cervical spine control principles take priority over the limb injury. Hip dislocation typically occurs after a road traffic accident, where most are posterior. Life-threatening injuries are assessed first and other fractures should be sought. Tibial shaft fractures are common and may be open; even with undisplaced fractures, a compartment syndrome must be considered.

50 Neck of the femur fractures are very common, typically affecting females over 80 years as a result of osteoporosis; they are most often a result of a fall. Both morbidity and mortality are very high, with only 60% surviving to 1 year. Treatment depends on the specific type of fracture and on the quality of the blood supply to the femoral head. Non-displaced intracapsular fractures can be fixed in situ with cannulated screws. Displaced intracapsular fractures disrupt the blood supply to the femoral head, meaning that avascular necrosis and non-union are common, and so treatment with hemi-arthroplasty is needed. Extracapsular fractures are much less likely to disrupt the blood supply, so non-union is a lesser problem and fixation with a dynamic hip screw is used.

51 The skull, spinal column and pelvis help to maintain posture, allow articulation of the limbs and protect the spinal cord. All spinal trauma must be managed with ABC principles; it should be assumed that all unconscious patients have a spinal injury and that all vertebral fractures are unstable until proved otherwise. Pelvic fractures can cause considerable blood loss, which may be life threatening. The pelvis is considered as a solid ring, hence if there is one obvious fracture visible on the radiograph, then there will be a second smaller fracture or sacroiliac joint disruption.

52 Paediatric fractures are common and differ from adult fractures in terms of type, healing and involvement of growth plates. Greenstick fractures are common, where one side of the cortex breaks but the other stays intact. The most common site of fracture is at the distal radius; other sites include supracondylar fractures of the elbow, femoral shaft fractures and pulled elbows.

53 Orthopaedic complications are best considered by the time at which they occur: early and late. Compartment syndrome occurs when increasing pressure within a fascial compartment disrupts blood flow into that compartment. It is characterized by pain that is unresponsive to opiates and worsens on passive flexion. The first step is to split the plaster cast down to the skin since it may be too tight. Urgent fasciotomy may also be necessary for all types of compartment syndrome. It is indicated if elimination of local pressure factors does not achieve immediate resolution. The complications of fracture healing include malunion, delayed union and non-union. Fat embolism is a potentially life-threatening complication that typically follows long bone fractures.

Orthopaedics

54 Back pain is extremely common and 90% is mechanical, where there is no specific underlying pathology. Surgery for back pain is almost never appropriate, and only 0.5% of patients require surgery. In fact, 90% of back pain resolves in 6 weeks with or without any treatment. There are 'red flag' signs of back pain that should raise a suspicion of malignancy or infection: weight loss, active/previous history of cancer, night/rest pain, fever, recent bacterial infection, back pain that persists for more than 3 months, aged under 20 or over 50 years.

55 Shoulder pain is the second most common cause of orthopaedic pain presentation to a GP. Anatomically, stability at the shoulder is sacrificed to allow a wide range of movement. Painful arc syndrome is a common complaint. Frozen shoulder is also common; it is self-limiting although may take some time. Arthroplasty is effective for advanced arthritis of the shoulder.

56 Disorders of the elbow, wrist and hand often present when they interfere with the patient's function. A good understanding of the anatomy of the region is important to understand and diagnose these conditions. Rheumatoid arthritis is extremely common in the hand and elbow. Osteoarthritis is common in the hand but not the elbow. Treatment is aimed to maximizing functionality, not to correcting the anatomy.

57 Peripheral nerve palsies are particularly common in the upper limb. Carpal tunnel syndrome is compression of the median nerve at the wrist. The ulnar nerve can be damaged by trauma or compression, and distal lesions cause a characteristic 'claw hand', which is much less prominent with proximal lesions (ulnar paradox). Radial nerve compression causes wrist drop, and upper brachial plexus damage is called Erb's palsy.

58 Osteoarthritis is the most common chronic joint disease and is a major cause of morbidity and disability. The most commonly affected sites are the hips, knees, hands and spine. The four characteristic changes seen on radiography are loss of joint space, osteophytes, sclerosis and subchondral bone cysts (remember by LOSS). Early management is conservative. Surgery is reserved for late and advanced disease. Total hip replacement is the gold standard for hip osteoarthritis and is one of the most effective modern orthopaedic procedures.

59 Examination of the hip is a common orthopaedic examination. The general examination scheme for orthopaedics is look, feel, move, special tests, although for the hip the special tests are merged into the examination stages. Special tests include the Trendelenburg test and Thomas' test.

60 Knee pain is a common complaint and has a wide range of causes. Osteoarthritis of the knee is common, and knee replacement is a reliable and common treatment for advanced disease. There are four ligaments and two menisci of the knee. Damage to these in isolation or combination can result in pain and instability. Knee pain in children may have a serious underlying cause and warrants further investigation.

61 Examination of the knee follows a look, feel, move, special tests scheme, but, as for the hip, the special tests can be merged into the examination; these tests include identifying effusions and performing ligamentous stress tests. Typical examination cases include arthritis, effusions, ligamental tears and meniscal tears.

62 There are many disorders of the ankle and foot. Hallux valgus, osteoarthritis and rheumatoid arthritis are also common in this area. Achilles tendon ruptures are assessed using the 'calf-squeeze' test.

63 A general orthopaedic examination scheme follows a look, feel, move, special tests format. The hip and knee are most common in OSCE stations, but examinations of the shoulder, elbow, ankle and foot, and the spine (cervical and lumbar) should be known. Examination of the hands typically involves a patient with rheumatoid hands or with a peripheral nerve palsy.

64 The limping child is a common and important presentation to both general practice and accident and emergency departments. The age of the child is key to directing the differential diagnosis. Trauma is the most common cause, although if there is no history of trauma, transient synovitis is the next most frequent with the remainder being rare specific hip conditions. Paediatric hip disorders include developmental dysplasia of the hip, Perthes' disease, slipped upper femoral epiphysis and septic arthritis.

65 Osteoporosis is the most common metabolic bone disorder, affecting 25% of women over 50 years. Patients with osteoporosis typically present with low-energy fractures. Paget's disease and ankylosing spondylitis are less common, although their presentation and clinical features should be known.

66 Infections of joints (septic arthritis) and bones (osteomyelitis) are decreasing in incidence as living standards increase, although they are still to be considered in differential diagnoses of painful limbs. The consequences of missed or poorly treated infections are devastating, especially for children. A hot, swollen joint is typical of septic arthritis although there are other less-subtle presentations, such as infants not moving a particular limb. Urgent treatment is necessary for these infections, with antibiotics and surgical drainage.

67 Bone tumours are benign or malignant, primary or secondary. Primary bone tumours are very rare. Osteosarcoma is the most common malignant primary tumour; it has a peak of occurrence at approximately 16 years of age and most commonly affects the distal femur. Metastatic (secondary) tumours are much more common. The five most common tumours that metastasize to bone are breast, lung, prostate, kidney and thyroid cancers.

Plastic surgery

68 Burns are coagulative destruction of skin and are very commonly seen in A&E departments. The initial priority is to resuscitate the patient, secure an airway and gain prompt intravenous access. Management of the burns starts alongside this; specific management continues later. Close attention must be given to fluid management. Major skin and tissue losses need to be covered or replaced, with either skin grafts or tissue flaps.

69 The incidence of skin cancer is increasing; the main types are basal cell carcinoma, squamous cell carcinoma and melanoma. Melanoma affects young people, and the *history* of a new or changing mole is just as important as the *examination* in forming a diagnosis.

70 There are many lumps and bumps that may be found on the body. Sebaceous cysts, lipomas, lymph nodes and ganglia are common. A thorough history and examination (using an inspection, palpation, percussion and auscultation scheme) are used to exclude suspicious features and form a diagnosis.

71 Less than 1% of all lumps are malignant, although patients often present to their GPs worried about lumps they find. The suspicious features that should prompt further investigation by a specialist are rapid growth, > 5 cm in size and pain, deep seated or occurring at the site of a previous surgical excision. Soft tissue sarcomas are tumours affecting soft tissues and may be highly malignant, warranting referral to a specialist centre before biopsy. Treatment is with wide local excision and chemoradiotherapy.

Neurosurgery

72 Head injury is a common presentation to the A&E department. All unconscious patients are admitted to hospital, but difficulty arises in deciding which conscious patient requires further and urgent management. Rapid assessment is made with the Glasgow Coma Score. Primary brain damage occurs at the time of injury and is permanent, secondary injury occurs later and is preventable.

73 If a skull fracture is present, the risk of extradural haemorrhage is much increased, and this should be identified early to prevent secondary brain damage. Spontaneous intracranial haemorrhages may present very suddenly and dramatically. In subarachnoid haemorrhage, *primary* brain damage occurs; the key is to prevent rebleeding and *secondary* brain damage. Computed tomography identifies most; if negative, lumbar puncture after 12 hours is warranted.

74 Acute spinal cord compression is a surgical emergency and must be recognized early. Causes include trauma, prolapsed intravertebral discs, tumour and infection. Features include spinal pain and leg pain, sensory disturbance (buttock anaethesia) and sphincter disturbance. The perianal dermatomes must be tested for sensation and a digital rectal examination performed to assess anal tone. Treatment in most is with urgent surgical decompression.

75 The most common type of brain tumour is metastatic; gliomas are the most common primary brain tumours. Brain tumours present with three classic groups of signs: raised intracranial pressure, focal signs and epilepsy. The history and examinations identify what and where the lesion is. Treatment is with a combination of medicine, surgery and chemoradiotherapy. Hydrocephalus is defined as an increase in cerebrospinal fluid volume and presents with signs of raised intracranial pressure. Treatment includes ventricular shunts to divert excess cerebrospinal fluid to other locations, such as the right atrium or peritoneum.

Cardiothoracic surgery

76 Cardiothoracic surgery involves surgery of the thoracic cage and its contents. Surgical approaches to the thorax include a median sternotomy or a thoracotomy. Coronary artery bypass graft is used in the treatment of ischaemic heart disease when medical treatment fails. Congenital heart diseases affect 8 in 1000 births, and most patients now survive until adulthood with modern surgical techniques.

77 Thoracic surgery largely involves surgery of the lung. Lung tumours present late: only 10% of lung tumours are surgically respectable and the fitness of the patient must be considered. The indications for tracheostomy must be known as they are common surgical questions.

Transplantation

78 Transplantation may be from cadaver donors, if so the recipient will need immunosuppressive therapy and tissue/blood matching, or from related live donors, where the match may be closer and rejection less likely. Transplantation of the heart is used for end-stage pump failure and of the lung for chronic lung disease; a heart–lung transplantation may be indicated for cardiorespiratory failure. Kidney is the most common organ transplanted. It is used alone for renal failure and can be transplanted with the pancreas for some patients with diabetes. Liver transplantation is used for end-stage liver disease or acute liver failure. Other organ transplants include cornea, small bowel and skin. The main complications are infection and rejection.

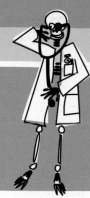

Fleshed out

3

This section contains chapters as double page spreads, each covering a single surgical topic but grouped together by system. Fitting single surgical topics (which are, by definition, huge subjects) into the useful double page spread format means that decisions had to be made about what to leave out, and thus the remaining text focuses on essential features. The chapters may concentrate on a specific topic such as colorectal cancer, on specific surgical presentations such as abdominal pain, or on specific surgical examination skills, such as palpating for peripheral pulses. The decision to include orthopaedics and trauma is important (it is often left out of such 'core' surgical textbooks) as it makes the book a 'one-stop introduction' to a surgical syllabus.

1. The acute abdomen

Questions
- What are the causes of an acute abdomen?
- What are the different types of pain?
- How would you manage an acute abdomen?

The 'acute abdomen' is the most common presenting surgical symptom. It can be defined as undiagnosed abdominal pain that has been present for less than 1 week, although the definition varies. Pain is the main symptom and it may vary from mild to severe. Surgical, medical and gynaecological causes must be considered when assessing such patients; if diagnosis proves difficult, careful observation and further investigation is warranted. The specific treatment depends upon the cause, so the differential diagnosis is critical.

Pathology
Pain originates from irritation of the peritoneum:

- visceral peritoneum (lining organs): innervation is autonomic and pain is deep, dull and poorly defined
- parietal peritoneum (underneath the abdominal wall): innervation is somatic and pain is sharp and well localized, with rebound tenderness (pain felt when release of the hand from the abdomen) and guarding (a board-like rigidity).

Clinical features
The cardinal symptom is pain (Fig. 3.1.1). Onset can be:

- explosive: suggests perforation of a viscus (e.g. appendix or colon) or sudden ischaemia (e.g. mesenteric)
- rapid: acute inflammation (appendicitis, cholecystitis)
- gradual or progressive: peritonitis (below).

The character of pain is also distinctive.

Colic. Contraction of a smooth muscle tube against an obstruction causes a cyclical on–off pain. The painful intervals are severe, and the patient may roll around without relief, but there are pain-free intervals. **Biliary colic** is not a true on–off colic, as it is gradual onset and then constant. A true colic is more likely to be **ureteric** (secondary to stones) or **intestinal colic**.

Peritonitis. Inflammation of the peritoneum is either general or localized and is characterized by continuous severe pain that is worse upon movement. Tenderness, guarding and rebound tenderness may be present. It can be caused by inflammation from chemicals (acid from a perforated ulcer or bile from the biliary system) or infection (appendicitis, pancreatitis, perforation, e.g. appendix or colon).

Associated symptoms. Diagnosis is assisted by the occurrence of associated symptoms: nausea and vomiting, retching,

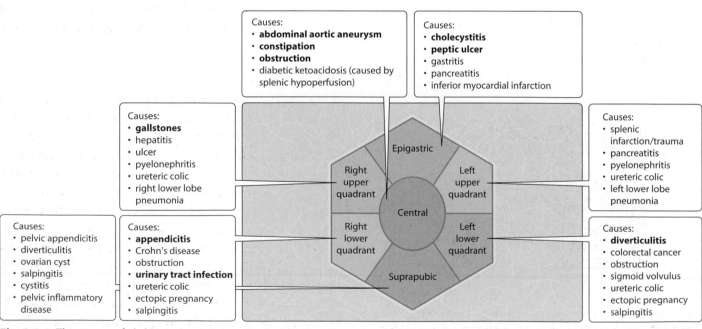

Fig. 3.1.1 The causes of abdominal pain by region (bold indicating common causes). Trauma can cause pain anywhere so the organs underneath the site of pain must be considered (e.g. left upper quadrant pain in a patient from a road traffic accident may be caused by a splenic rupture).

constipation or diarrhoea, haematemesis, melaena. Bleeding may be an emergency (Ch. 7). Menstrual status and gynaecological symptoms should be noted as should bowel sounds (obstruction) and pulse (tachycardia).

Pain out of proportion to signs. This is an indication of possible **mesenteric infarction**, produced by occlusion of the **superior mesenteric artery** or **vein**. It can be either *acute* or *chronic*. Acute occlusion may be caused by an arterial embolus (commonly from atrial fibrillation), venous thrombosis, vasculitis, volvulus or shock. The affected bowel infarcts and necrosis is rapid; mortality is high and total infarction is often fatal. Be suspicious of pain that is out of proportion to signs, particularly in an elderly patient, acidosis (found on arterial blood gas measurements) and tachycardia persisting in a rehydrated patient. The white cell count (WCC) is often raised.

A computed tomographic (CT) scan will identify air in the peritoneal cavity, retroperitoneum or a wall of the bowel. Urgent laparotomy is needed to remove the affected segment if possible. Revascularization (e.g. graft) may be possible in rare cases.

Differential diagnosis

Figure 3.1.1 gives the more common causes. Extra-abdominal causes are inferior myocardial infarction, lower lobe pneumonia, diabetic ketoacidosis, sickle crisis, porphorias, haemolysis, warfarin therapy and herpetic neuralgia.

Clinical examination

A complete abdominal examination should pay particular attention to:

- tenderness (pain upon palpation; look at the patient's face), rebound tenderness and guarding, all of which indicate peritonitis

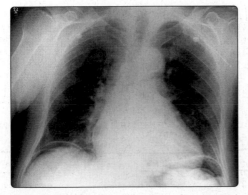

Fig. 3.1.2 Erect chest radiograph showing free air underneath the diaphragm (*pneumoperitoneum*). Remember that a gastric bubble underneath the right diaphragm is normal.

- strangulated hernias need to be sought actively: small, tense, painful masses
- rectal and vaginal examination
- the scrotum, as a torsion often causes referred pain to the abdomen.

Investigations

Bloods. Full blood count (FBC; e.g. anaemia of malignancy), WCC (e.g. leukocytosis in infection), urea and electrolytes (U&E), amylase (> 1000 U/l with pancreatitis), liver function tests (non-specific but may indicate an obstructive picture with cholecystitis), arterial blood gases (for sick patients; metabolic acidosis with no other signs may indicate mesenteric infarction).

Urinalysis. Haematuria (renal stones), infection, ketones (diabetic ketoacidosis can present as abdominal pain), pregnancy test (human β-chorionic gonadotrophins).

Electrocardiograph. This will identify a myocardial infarction (inferior MI can cause epigastric pain).

Abdominal radiograph. This may show faecal loading (constipation), dilated loops of bowel (obstruction), air in the biliary tree (gallstone complications), renal stones or calcification of an abdominal aortic aneurysm.

Erect chest radiograph. Free air underneath the diaphragm indicates perforation of an abdominal viscus (Fig. 3.1.2).

Ultrasound. Inflamed appendix, gallstones, free blood, abscesses, trauma (liver/spleen) and the size and state of an abdominal aortic aneurysm.

Endoscopy (oesophago-gastro-duodenoscopy (OGD)). Although endoscopy is not advisable when assessing for the presence of a perforated ulcer, it is useful for diagnosis and treatment of bleeding peptic ulcers.

Management

Initial management depends on the patient's state; resuscitation with ABC principles (Ch. 43) may be the first priority. Further management is directed by the working diagnosis (formed from history, examination and investigations). If a diagnosis still has not been formed, there should not be a rush to surgery; the patient is monitored and examined for 4–6 h (depending on their state) and CT scan performed for further information. If all investigations are negative, and depending on the patient's state, a diagnosis of exclusion can be reached, termed *non-specific abdominal pain*. If diagnosis is still in doubt and the patient has not improved or is worsening, diagnostic laparoscopy (Ch. 2) can be performed to try to identify a cause; laparoscopy may be therapeutic, for example identifying and removing an inflamed appendix.

2. Acute appendicitis

Questions
■ How can acute appendicitis present?
■ What is the initial management of these patients?
■ How are patients with typical and atypical features managed?

The appendix is an extension of the caecum with an average length of 6–10 cm (range, 2–20 cm). Its position is variable, but it is normally retrocaecal. (Fig. 3.2.1). Beware of a **pelvic appendix** (where the appendix points backwards) as there may be few abdominal signs and urinary symptoms. Inflammation of the appendix is the commonest surgical emergency.

Acute appendicitis can occur at any age but is seen more commonly in:

■ adolescents and young adults: acquire more infections and are thus more susceptible (rare before age 2 years)
■ elderly: more prone to constipation and faecoliths
■ inflammatory bowel disease: lymphoid hyperplasia.

Pathology

Although the cause of appendicitis is not definitely known, obstruction is found in 80% and the following are common.

Obstruction by faecolith. A faecolith is a solid mass within the appendix formed from precipitated calcium salts and fibre around a central matrix of dry faeces. The appendix mucosa continues to secrete mucus and fluid, and swelling with infection and inflammation rapidly set in.

Lymphoid hyperplasia. This causes obstruction, secondary to inflammatory bowel disease (ulcerative colitis, Crohn's disease) or infections (mononucleosis, measles, gastro-intestinal and respiratory infections).

Clinical features

The typical presentation is only seen in approximately half of presenting patients and diagnostic difficulties arise for the atypical presentations (Fig. 3.2.2).

Abdominal pain. Pain starts as a dull central pain as the autonomic visceral peritoneum (the inner peritoneum surrounding the organs) is irritated, causing referred pain to the T_{10} dermatome (around the umbilicus). As inflammation continues, the somatic parietal peritoneum (the outer layer of peritoneum) becomes irritated, causing a well-localized, sharp intense pain over the appendix, maximal at McBurney's point (right iliac fossa (RIF)).

Nausea and vomiting with anorexia. If inflammation continues, fever may develop.

Perforation. Thrombosis of the appendicular artery may occur, resulting in ischaemia, gangrene and perforation. Subsequent peritonitis causes increased pain, nausea and vomiting, guarding and systemic upset.

Appendix mass. Following perforation, a mass forms on day 3 that is localized by omentum and loops of bowel; by day 5, a central abscess forms. The patient is tachycardic with a fluctuating pyrexia.

Atypical presentation. Appendicitis may cause diarrhoea if the appendix lies near to the rectum or symptoms of urinary tract infection (dysuria) if close to the bladder. Other presentations vary upon the exact position of the appendix.

Differential diagnosis

The differential diagnosis is long and a thorough history is vital (Fig. 3.2.3).

Clinical examination

Pressing over McBurney's point causes maximal pain (Fig. 3.2.4). Pressing in the left iliac fossa causes pain in the RIF (Rovsing's sign) and a rectal examination will identify a pelvic appendicitis.

Investigations

Diagnosis is clinical (history and examination), so only preoperative tests are required: bloods (FBC, U&E, blood

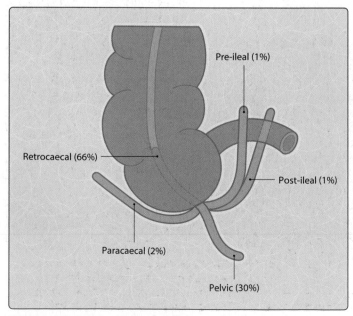

Fig. 3.2.1 Positions of the appendix.

Pre-ileal (1%)

Retrocaecal (66%)

Post-ileal (1%)

Paracaecal (2%)

Pelvic (30%)

grouping) and urinalysis (to exclude urinary tract infection or an ectopic pregnancy).

If appendicitis is *clinically* diagnosed, the patient goes to surgery. If there is still diagnostic confusion, observation is continued for 4–6 h, during which more tests are performed:

- ultrasound: a healthy appendix is not visible but *an inflamed appendix may also not be visible*; transvaginal ultrasound in women helps to identify a gynaecological cause
- CT: if diagnosis is still in question
- laparoscopy: if the patient does not improve and acute appendicitis cannot be excluded; laparoscopy is diagnostic, and therapeutic as an inflamed appendix is removed.

Laparoscopy is particularly suitable for children and females (undiagnosed pregnancy). The appendix should be removed even if it appears normal (to avoid diagnostic confusion if future episodes of pain arise), and the diagnosis reevaluated.

Management

Initial management. The patient may require urgent resuscitation using ABC principles.

Surgical management. Surgical removal (**appendicectomy**) is the definitive treatment. It is open or laparoscopic; the latter causes less pain and allows a shorter inpatient stay. Antibiotic prophylaxis (cefuroxime and metronidazole) is given pre- and postoperatively to all patients. An appendix mass is currently treated with surgery and antibiotics.

Open appendicectomy. McBurney's incision is made over McBurney's point (Fig. 3.2.4). The fascia and muscles below are divided (a **gridiron incision**: 'muscle-splitting'). The appendix and its vascular base are ligated and removed. Routine insertion of a drain is not required. As no muscles have been cut, a strong grid forms on closure, preventing incisional hernias. A cosmetic Lanz incision is a muscle-cutting incision in the RIF around the bikini line, for better appearance.

Laparoscopic appendicectomy. Three laparoscopic ports are used. The abdominal cavity is distended with carbon dioxide (forming a **pneumoperitoneum**) to give better views to the surgeon. The appendix is ligated, divided away and withdrawn. The cavity is thoroughly irrigated, the cannuale removed and the pneumoperitoneum reduced. The small abdominal wounds (port sites) are sutured.

Prognosis

Mortality is zero with an unperforated appendix; with a perforated appendix it is 1% (5% in the elderly).

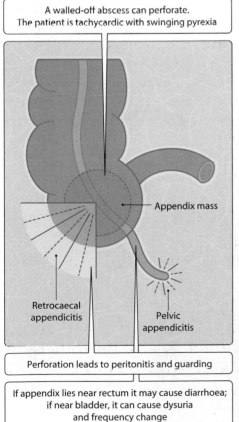

A walled-off abscess can perforate. The patient is tachycardic with swinging pyrexia

Appendix mass

Retrocaecal appendicitis

Pelvic appendicitis

Perforation leads to peritonitis and guarding

If appendix lies near rectum it may cause diarrhoea; if near bladder, it can cause dysuria and frequency change

Fig. 3.2.2 Other presentations of appendicitis.

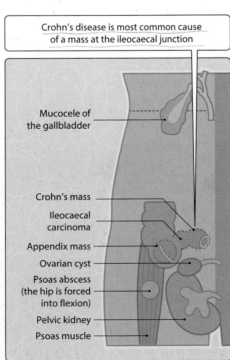

Crohn's disease is most common cause of a mass at the ileocaecal junction

Mucocele of the gallbladder

Crohn's mass

Ileocaecal carcinoma

Appendix mass

Ovarian cyst

Psoas abscess (the hip is forced into flexion)

Pelvic kidney

Psoas muscle

Fig. 3.2.3 Causes of a mass in the right iliac fossa (RIF).

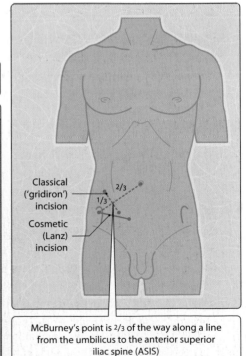

Classical ('gridiron') incision

Cosmetic (Lanz) incision

McBurney's point is 2/3 of the way along a line from the umbilicus to the anterior superior iliac spine (ASIS)

Fig. 3.2.4 McBurney's point. This is the point of maximal tenderness. If open surgery is being performed, a gridiron incision is made (at right angles to McBurney's point).

3. Gallstones

Questions
- What are the complications of gallstones in the cystic duct?
- What are the complications of gallstones in the common bile duct?
- What tests would you perform to confirm gallstones?

Gallstones are very common, with prevalence at postmortem of 15–25%. However, 80% of stones remain asymptomatic.

Aetiology

A number of factors are associated with the occurrence of gallstones (the 'Fs': fat, fertile females over forty):

- gender (female to male 2:1) and age (> 40 years) are the most important determinants
- obesity: increases hepatic synthesis/secretion of cholesterol
- pregnancy: increased oestrogen causes choleostasis
- diabetes mellitus
- ileal disease or resection: leading to bile salt loss
- total parenteral nutrition: owing to gallbladder stasis.

There are three types of stone:

- mixed (80%): cholesterol is the main component, with bile pigments and calcium salts
- pigmented (10%): contain calcium bilirubinate, are associated with haemolytic disorders (haemolytic anaemia, malaria) and are rare in Western countries
- pure cholesterol (10%).

Investigations

Blood tests. Liver function tests may be normal or show an obstructive picture (bilirubin, alkaline phosphatase, alanine aminotransferase or aspartate aminotransferase may be raised). Serum amylase excludes associated acute pancreatitis. Blood cultures identify septicaemia in the seriously ill.

Ultrasound. The best test in the acute phase as it demonstrates gallstones (as an 'acoustic shadow') in over 90% of patients. (Only 10% of stones are radioopaque and so plain radiograph is unsuitable.) Ultrasound also will show wall thickening, pericholecystic collections, dilatation of common bile duct (CBD) and intrahepatic biliary tree.

Endoscopic retrograde cholangiopancreatography (ERCP). This allows visualization of the CBD and pancreatic duct via the ampulla of Vater; additionally any stones can be retrieved (Fig. 3.3.1; see Ch. 4).

Magnetic resonance cholangiopancreatography (MRCP). Contrast dye is secreted in bile, allowing a three-dimensional view of the entire biliary tree and stones.

Percutaneous transhepatic cholangiography. This approach is only used when the above are unsuitable or have failed to visualize the stones; contrast dye is injected percutaneously into the liver and biliary tree, allowing direct visualization of stones on radiograph.

Complications of gallstones

Complications depend on the level at which the stones impact: in the **cystic duct** or (Fig. 3.3.2) in the **CBD**. Management options for each are dealt with in Ch. 4. Most stones (90%) remain in the gallbladder or cystic duct.

Stones in the gallbladder/cystic duct

1. *Biliary colic.* This is caused by a transient impaction in Hartman's pouch or the cystic duct. The patient often does not present to hospital. It is characterized by:
   - pain: episodic right upper quadrant or epigastric pain; it is not a 'colicky' pain but is progressive and then constant for around 1 to 4 h until the stone passes and pain is relieved; the pain radiates to the right shoulder (diaphragmatic irritation) and is provoked by fatty foods
   - nausea and vomiting
   - acute cholecystitis occurs if infection develops.

2. *Acute cholecystitis.* This is caused by an impacted stone in Hartmann's pouch with bacterial infection. There may be a previous history of biliary colic. Common infective

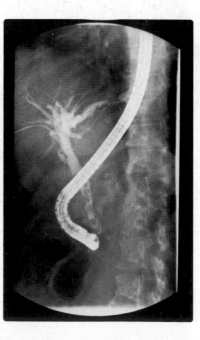

Fig. 3.3.1 Multiple gallstones in the common bile duct visualized with ERCP. Dye shows the biliary tree and a dilated proximal common bile duct.

organisms are Gram-negative gut flora (*Escherichia coli*), which reach the gallbladder via the blood or bile. Symptoms may occur as separate, repeated attacks:

- pain with fever: epigastric and/or right upper quadrant pain radiating to the right shoulder tip
- Murphy's sign: two fingers are placed in the right upper quadrant, pressing on the gallbladder; there is pain when the patient inhales that ceases when the patient breathes out (positive if no pain on left side)
- nausea and vomiting, with tachycardia and pyrexia.

Chronic cholecystitis leads to a fibrosed and enlarged gallbladder wall and atrophic mucosa. **Acalculous cholecystitis** is rare and occurs without stones; it can be caused by burns, sepsis and diabetes.

3. *Mucocele and empyema.* A mucocele occurs when a stone impacts in Hartmann's pouch; continued mucus secretion behind the stones causing distension and tenderness. An infected mucocele **abscess** (empyema), although rare, may cause perforation of the gallbladder. **Mirrizi's syndrome** is an uncommon complication of a stone impacted in the cystic duct. This causes swelling of the gallbladder and cystic duct, which then compress the CBD and lead to obstructive jaundice.

Stones in the common bile duct

Of patients with gallbladder stones, 10% also have stones in the CBD, which have almost always migrated from the gallbladder (rarely formed in the duct itself). Many small stones pass into the duodenum, causing mild colic or mild jaundice; the larger stones may cause blockage.

4. *Obstructive jaundice.* Impaction of a stone in the CBD leads to obstructive jaundice. A stone in the CBD causes biliary colic or acute cholecystitis plus obstructive jaundice, since the bile drainage of the gallbladder and liver are blocked. It may recur in repeated attacks. Management is similar to acute cholecystitis. Obstructive jaundice involves conjugated bile acids (water soluble), leading to **dark urine** (dissolve in the urine) and **pale stools**.

5. *Ascending cholangitis.* When obstructive jaundice occurs, the stagnant bile above the stone may become infected, producing cholangitis and signs of **Charcot's triad**: rigors (fever and chills), obstructive jaundice and pain (upper right quadrant, radiates to right shoulder). This infection may spread to the intrahepatic ducts (hence 'ascending' cholangitis), and may cause a liver abscess or septicaemia. It is life threatening so the biliary system needs urgent decompression with ERCP or surgery.

6. *Gallstone pancreatitis.* If a stone impacts at or beyond the point of drainage of the pancreatic duct into the CBD, symptoms of obstructive jaundice plus acute pancreatitis are seen as bile refluxes into the pancreatic ducts.

Other

7. *Gallstone ileus.* This is small bowel obstruction caused by a stone which has perforated directly through the gallbladder wall into the duodenum via a **cholecystoenteric fistula**. Gas is visible in the biliary tree on plain abdominal radiography. Some stones may obstruct the ileocaecal valve, causing small bowel obstruction. This is a rare complication occurring mainly in the elderly.

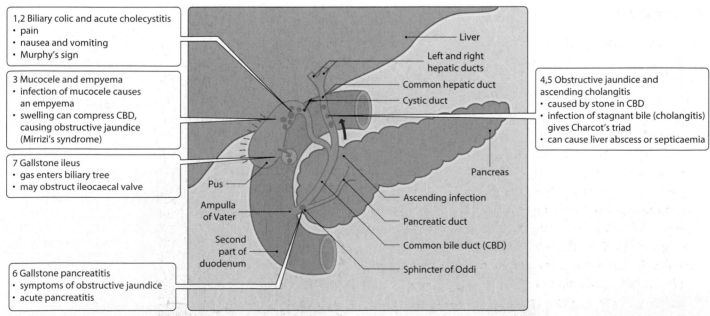

Fig. 3.3.2 The biliary tree and complications of biliary disease.

4. Management of gallstone disease

Questions
- What is a cholecystectomy and when is it performed?
- How would you treat common bile duct stones?
- What are the complications of cholecystectomy?

Cholecystectomy (surgical removal of the gallbladder) is the 'gold standard' of treatment for gallstone disease. Remember asymptomatic stones require no treatment. Figure 3.4.1 shows the algorithm for acute management:

- common acute gallstone disease (biliary colic, acute cholecystitis, obstructive jaundice) is managed conservatively initially to allow the stone to pass spontaneously
- mucoceles, empyemas or ascending cholangitis require immediate drainage of the biliary tree with endoscopic retrograde cholangiopancreatography (ERCP) or cholecystectomy (Table 3.4.1).

With conservative regimens, 90% of patients improve:

- fluid management and nil by mouth
- antibiotics: intravenous cefotaxime plus metronidazole (against Gram-negative organisms)
- analgesia: patients may require opiates.

If symptoms do not improve, further treatment is indicated, although the wide differential diagnosis for abdominal pain must be considered.

Endoscopic management
Indications for ERCP (Fig. 3.4.2) are:

- clinical, biochemical or sonological evidence of biliary obstruction; an emergency procedure if ascending cholangitis is suspected
- the need to remove ductal stones found during laparoscopic cholecystectomy
- urgent biliary tree drainage required for ascending cholangitis.

A tube is passed through the oesophagus into the duodenum to locate the **ampulla of Vater** in the second part of the duodenum:

- sphincterotomy: diathermy is used to cut open the **sphincter of Odi** to access to the biliary tree
- imaging: contrast dye is injected into the bile ducts and a plain radiograph illustrates any stones
- stones are retrieved using a dormia basket or balloons
- complications: perforation, haemorrhage, acute pancreatitis.

Stenting of tumours and balloon dilatation of biliary strictures are also possible.

Surgical management
Cholecystectomy is commonly performed laparoscopically (90% of cholecystecomies) but sometimes by open operation. The former allows a shorter stay in hospital, smaller portal scars and is safe (mortality of 0.1% versus 0.5% for open surgery). The procedure depends on the location of the stone.

Stones in the cystic duct. These are removed by laparoscopic cholecystectomy. The cystic artery and cystic duct are exposed and clipped, and the gallbladder removed. This is suitable as most stones remain in the gallbladder or cystic duct. It is performed:

- early: if no improvement with conservative management or ERCP; some surgeons also now perform it immediately in all patients when they present in the acute phase

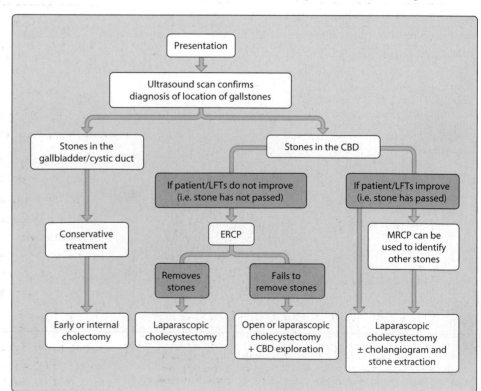

Fig. 3.4.1 Principles of treatment for acute biliary colic, acute cholecystitis and obstructive jaundice.

Table 3.4.1 SPECIFIC MANAGEMENT IN GALLSTONE DISEASE

	Management
Mucocele	Removed by urgent/early laparoscopic cholecystectomy
Empyema	Resucitate with fluids and antibiotics; requires urgent **cholecystectomy** or percutaneous drainage (**cholecystostomy**, under ultrasound guidance)
Ascending cholangitis	Urgent decompression of the biliary system using ERCP with antibiotics and fluid resuscitation; if unsuccessful then open surgery to remove stone in common bile duct
Gallstone pancreatitis	ERCP is required to remove the offending stone (open cholecystectomy if this fails)

ERCP, endoscopic retrograde cholangiopancreatography.

- late: performed electively after 3 months, allowing time for inflammation and infection to settle.

Stones in the common bile duct (CBD). Stones in the CBD are removed by one of two methods: a two-stage procedure (Fig. 3.4.2) or a one-stage open or laparoscopic cholecystectomy

A length of the CBD is opened and explored for stones. It is then sewn closed over the T-tube

The gallbladder is removed, and the cystic duct tied off to form a stump

Gall bladder (removed)

Skin

T-tube

To stoma bag

Stoma bag

Bile

Hepatic duct

Common bile duct

Pancreas

The T-tube allows the biliary tree to drain, preventing leaks . Dye can be injected into the T-tube, showing any remaining stones (cholangiogram) If the cholangiogram is clear on day 10, the T-tube is clamped off and removed

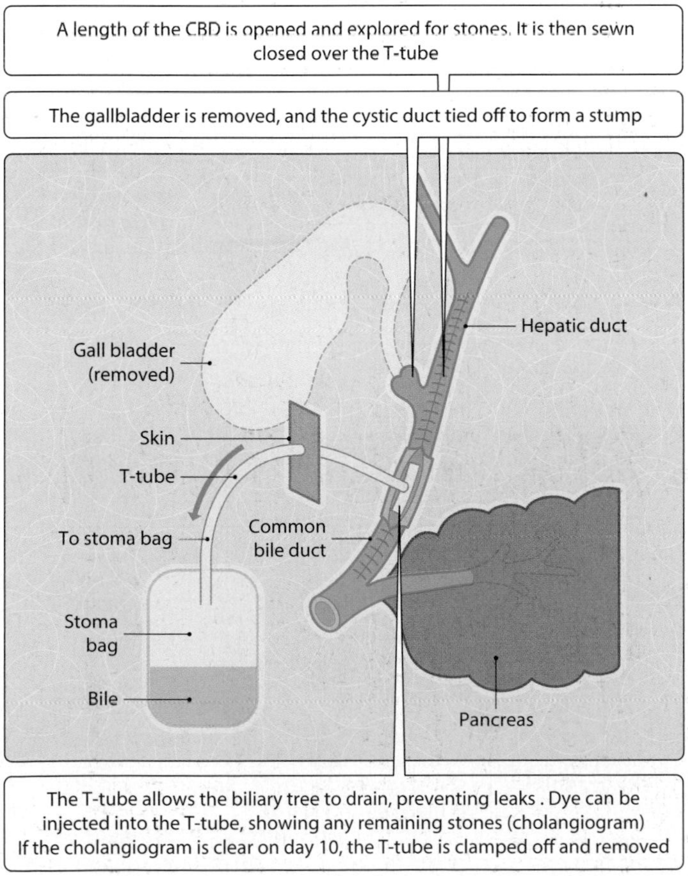

Fig. 3.4.2 Removal of gallbladder and insertion of a T-tube by ERCP.

with CBD exploration. Increased use of laparoscopy and ERCP means that stones in the CBD can often be retrieved without an open operation.

The two-stage procedure

During laparoscopic cholecystectomy, the surgeon may suspect stones in the CBD especially if the patient has a history of obstructive jaundice. Exploration of the CBD can be done laparoscopically where surgical expertise and equipment exist. At the end of the procedure, an intraoperative cholangiogram shows any stones in the CBD. If stones are found, the procedure is finished as normal and then in the next 2–3 days ERCP is performed to retrieve these stones. If ERCP fails, open exploration of the CBD may be performed.

One-stage open cholecystectomy

The open approach is indicated if ERCP failed to allow retrieval of stones. Approximately 5% of laparoscopic operations are converted to open operations owing to technical difficulties (e.g. adhesions). The abdomen is opened with a **Kocher's incision**. The gallbladder is excised and the CBD is opened and explored for stones. Any stones are removed, and then the duct is closed around a T-tube, which is connected to a **bile drain** (allowing the biliary tree to drain, preventing bile leakage).

Following the operation, a cholangiogram is performed via the T-tube (contrast dye is injected down the tube) to identify any missed stones, especially if jaundice persists after the operation. Missed stones can be retrieved by passing a Dormia basket down the T-tube; the cholangiogram is then repeated. If no stones are found, a final cholangiogram is performed at day 10 before the T-tube is clamped off and removed.

Complications of cholecystectomy

Recurrent symptoms similar to the original ones are termed **postcholecystectomy syndrome**.

Bile duct injury. This is the major complication of laparoscopic or open surgery, occurring in 0.5%. Immediate bile leakage may lead to infection, peritonitis and septicaemia, but if missed a stricture may form (below).

Retained stones. Obstructive jaundice is caused by stones retained in the CBD; they can be identified and retrieved via a ERCP or a T-tube cholangiogram. An on-table cholangiogram helps to prevent this.

Bile duct stricture. A bile duct injury not recognized at the time of injury may result in stricture, ascending cholangitis, hepatic abscess or secondary biliary cirrhosis.

Other complications. These include haemorrhage, infection, port-site hernia, bowel or vascular injury caused by pneumoperitoneum.

5. Hernias

Questions
- How can inguinal hernias be classified?
- What are the complications of hernia?
- How should groin hernias be managed?

A hernia is an abnormal protrusion usually of a viscus through its containing cavity wall (Fig. 3.5.1). Abdominal hernias are formed from peritoneum and may contain loops of bowel. The four most common types of hernia in adults are **inguinal**, **femoral**, **umbilical** and **incisional**.

Pathology

In infants, hernias are almost always caused by a patent process vaginalis in boys (9:1), leading to indirect inguinal hernias. In children, hernias occur because of developmental weaknesses in the abdominal wall. In adults, chronically raised abdominal pressure can cause hernias (obesity, straining, a single event such as lifting something heavy). Hernias are classified as **reducible** — can be pushed back into the containing sac (most commonly the abdomen), such as a reducible indirect inguinal hernia, or **irreducible** — cannot be pushed back into the abdominal cavity, thus predisposing to obstruction.

As hernias enlarge and adhesions form, complete reduction is less likely.

Types of hernia

Inguinal hernias

Inguinal hernias (direct and indirect) occur above and medial to the pubic tubercle (Fig. 3.5.2) and are more common in men. An **indirect inguinal hernia** arises through the deep ring, passes down the inguinal canal and protrudes through the superficial ring. It can be controlled by finger pressure over the deep ring (Gh. 33). These hernias result from congenital defects, regardless of age. A **direct inguinal hernia** arises straight through a defect in the posterior wall and then protrudes into the inguinal canal. These cannot be controlled by pressure over the deep ring. They result from weaknesses in the abdominal wall and are, therefore, more common in older patients. A **scrotal hernia** is an indirect inguinal hernia that continues down through the spermatic cord into the scrotum. A **pantaloon hernia** occurs when indirect and direct hernia occur together and are seen to 'straddle' the inferior epigastric vessels.

Femoral hernias

Femoral hernias occur through the femoral canal and are acquired. They are below and lateral to the pubic tubercle and are less common than inguinal hernias but occur more often in women than men. Hernias in the femoral canal are most at risk

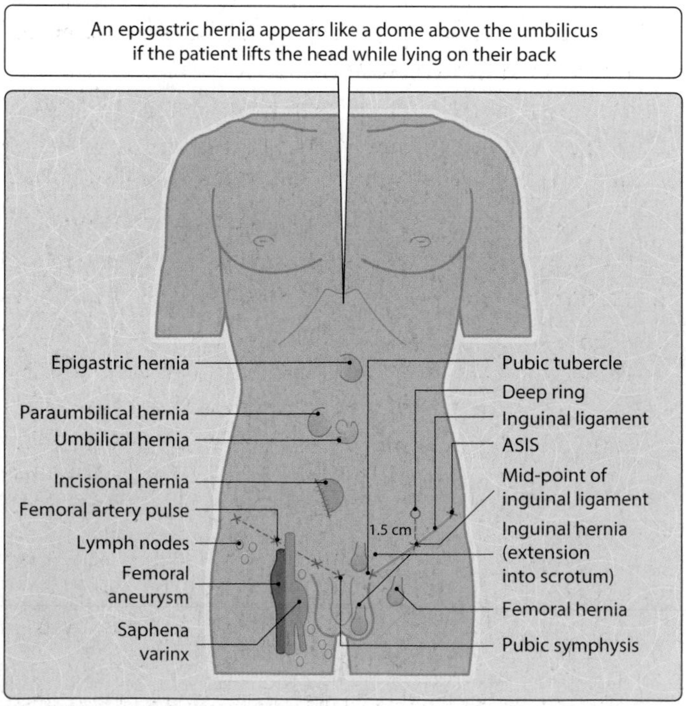

An epigastric hernia appears like a dome above the umbilicus if the patient lifts the head while lying on their back

Epigastric hernia
Paraumbilical hernia
Umbilical hernia
Incisional hernia
Femoral artery pulse
Lymph nodes
Femoral aneurysm
Saphena varinx

Pubic tubercle
Deep ring
Inguinal ligament
ASIS
Mid-point of inguinal ligament
1.5 cm
Inguinal hernia (extension into scrotum)
Femoral hernia
Pubic symphysis

Fig. 3.5.1 Landmarks of hernia bumps and groin pulses (see Fig. 3.24.2 for more detail).

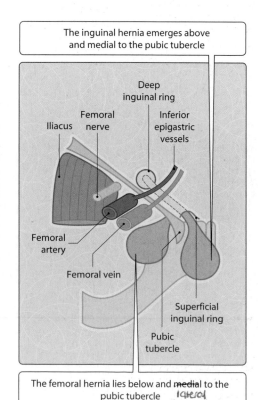

The inguinal hernia emerges above and medial to the pubic tubercle

Fig. 3.5.2 The relationship of indirect inguinal and femoral hernias to the pubic tubercle.

Deep inguinal ring
Femoral nerve
Iliacus
Inferior epigastric vessels
Femoral artery
Femoral vein
Superficial inguinal ring
Pubic tubercle

The femoral hernia lies below and medial to the pubic tubercle lateral

of strangulation (more so than inguinal hernias) as the femoral ring is tight.

Other types of hernia

Incisional hernia. This occurs when closure of an abdominal wound breaks down after the skin has healed. It is more common in the obese and when the wound becomes infected or it can follow poor surgical technique.

Umbilical hernia. This hernia is present at birth and arises from a congenital weakness of the umbilicus. It is more common in Afro-Caribbeans. Umbilical hernias are asymptomatic and may resolve spontaneously. Otherwise, they should be surgically corrected at 4 years.

Paraumbilical hernia. This hernia is most often acquired in adults and passes above or below the umbilicus, through the linea alba. It should be corrected surgically.

Spigelian hernia. This protrudes between the internal and external oblique, through defects in the lateral edge of the rectus sheath. It occurs above and medial to the normal inguinal ligament position but is difficult to palpate as it is covered by muscle layers.

Richter's hernia. This strangulated hernia involves part of the circumference of the bowel wall. Since the entire circumference is not involved, it does not affect the passage of bowel contents through the bowel lumen. Hence, despite strangulation, there is an absence of intestinal obstruction.

Epigastric hernia. The abdominal contents pass through the weakened fibres of the linea alba, above the umbilicus.

Obturator hernia. Abdominal contents pass through the pelvic obturator foramen, causing pain in the thigh or groin.

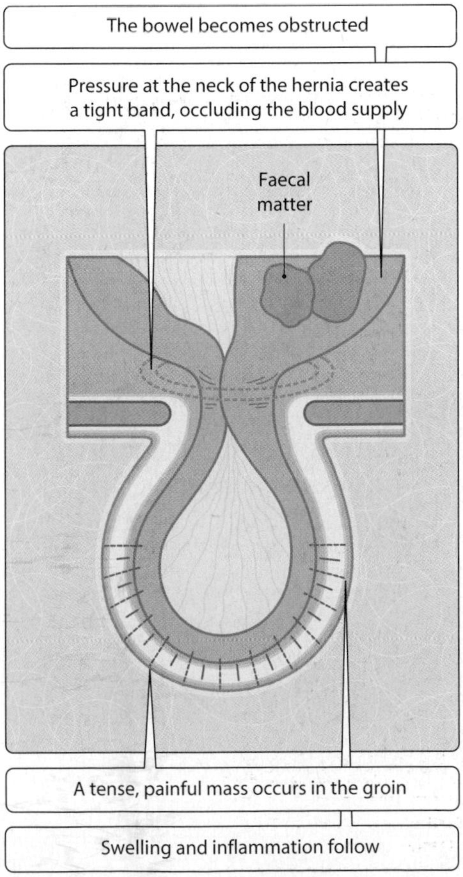

Complications of hernias

Irreducible hernias (which cannot be pushed back into the abdomen) predispose to obstruction of their contents because of their tight neck (also known as *incarcerated*: irreducible but not obstructed). The bowel contents of the hernia can become obstructed, predisposing to complete bowel obstruction and strangulation; therefore, prompt reduction is required. **Strangulation** occurs when the obstructed contents of a hernia become infected and swollen (Fig. 3.5.3). This causes pressure at the neck that occludes venous drainage, subsequently preventing arterial blood supply to the hernia wall. Infarction (with subsequent necrosis, peritonitis and sepsis) occurs if the hernia is not urgently relieved surgically.

Management

The treatment of choice is surgery as there is risk that a hernia will strangulate if left. Surgery is suitable even for the elderly if fit. Hernias in infants (under 1 year) mostly resolve spontaneously but should be fixed surgically if they persist after 1 year (**herniotomy**).

Conservative management. This comprises protection and reduction of stressing factors:
- truss: worn around the waist to hold the hernia in place, suitable for those unfit for surgery
- weight loss, stopping smoking (decreases coughing) and avoiding heavy lifting: required before and after surgery.

Surgical management. Surgery can be performed under local or general anaesthetic. **Mesh repairs** for inguinal hernia can be carried out laparoscopically or by an open operation under local or general anaesthesia as a day case, allowing faster recovery. The hernial sac is identified and reduced. A large piece of insoluble mesh is stapled to cover all areas affected by hernias in the groin region, reinforcing the abdominal wall (**Lichtenstein repair**). Recurrence occurs in < 1% and these are managed in the same way but usually laparoscopically. Patients may return to work 1 or 2 weeks after a mesh repair. **Laparoscopic hernia repair** is used increasingly, especially for recurrent inguinal hernias, affording all the benefits of laparoscopic surgery (e.g. small scar, shorter stay, less pain, faster return to work).

The bowel becomes obstructed

Pressure at the neck of the hernia creates a tight band, occluding the blood supply

Faecal matter

A tense, painful mass occurs in the groin

Swelling and inflammation follow

Fig. 3.5.3 Strangulation cuts off the blood supply to the hernia, producing intestinal obstruction with a painful mass in the groin.

6. Examination of the abdomen

Questions
- What are the hand signs of chronic liver disease?
- What are the methods for assessing ascites?
- What are the differences between a kidney and the spleen?

Certain cases might be expected to be in an OSCE: chronic liver disease, hepatomegaly, splenomegaly, hepatosplenomegaly, ascites, stomas, scars (fresh or old), drains, and past dialysis.

Introduction

Any examination *must* follow the initial steps of introduction, obtaining consent and then exposing the relevant area. The patient should be asked about any pain. A student would then indicate the area to be examined, such as 'I would like to expose the patient from nipples to knees'. The examiner may ask for just the abdomen to be exposed.

Inspection

General inspection. This starts from the end of the bed: anaemia, jaundice, cyanosis, pain, distressed, shortness of breath, raised jugular venous pressure. Obvious abdominal signs are scars, drains, stomas, distension, wasting, drips, feeding (enteral with nasogastric tubes or gastrostomy, or parenteral via central line). Obvious hernias are revealed if the patient coughs.

Hands. The hands can indicate a number of conditions
- clubbing: chronic liver diseases (cirrhosis); also indicative of gastrointestinal lymphoma and inflammatory bowel disease
- leukonychia: white nails (hypoalbuminaemia)
- koilonychia: spooned nails (iron-deficient anaemia)
- spider naevi: a dilated arteriole surrounded by capillaries that blanches and reappears when pressed; it is thought to be caused by oestrogen excess (the liver normally metabolizes oestrogen, and so liver damage reduces oestrogen removal) and occurs in the distribution of the superior vena cava (arms, face and chest above umbilicus); a normal adult may have up to five
- palmar erythema: reddening of the palms (of uncertain cause: it is seen in liver disease, rheumatoid arthritis, pregnancy, regional ileitis, some skin diseases)
- Dupuytren's contracture
- liver flap: arms straight with hands extended back (caused by hepatic encephalopathy).

Eyes. Signs of jaundice (yellow sclera), anaemia (pale conjunctivae), xanthalasmia, corneal arcus (hyperlipidaemia) may be seen.

Mouth. Ulcers (Crohn's disease, coeliac's disease, herpes), angular stomatitis (iron deficiency, alcoholism) or glossitis (bright, beefy tongue of iron- or B_{12}-deficient anaemia) may be noted.

Neck. Lymph nodes should be examined for lymphadenopathy whilst observing the head/neck region. An enlarged lymph node in the left supraclavicular fossa (**Virchow's node**) indicates possible stomach cancer (if found, this is **Troisier's sign**).

Chest. Spider naevi, gynaecomastia (any associated testicular atrophy?) and scratch marks may be observed in patients with chronic liver disease.

Abdomen. A closer inspection and description should indicate:
- scars and stomas (Figs 3.6.1 and 3.6.2)
- Grey–Turner's and Cullen's signs (Ch. 12)
- **caput medusa**: dilated veins around the umbilicus.

Palpation and percussion

The clinician kneels down at the level of the abdomen and asks if there is any pain while palpating (starting away from the pain, otherwise in the left iliac fossa). The patient's face should be watched for signs of discomfort during palpation.

1. Light palpation: screens for pain, guarding and rebound tenderness.

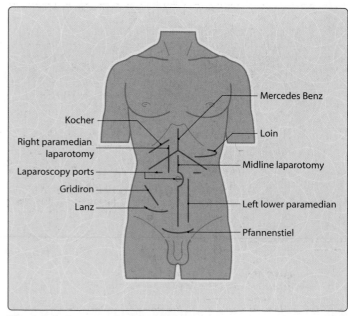

Kocher
Right paramedian laparotomy
Laparoscopy ports
Gridiron
Lanz
Mercedes Benz
Loin
Midline laparotomy
Left lower paramedian
Pfannenstiel

Fig. 3.6.1 Common incisions in surgery.

2. Deep palpation: screens for masses.

3. Liver palpation: starts in right iliac fossa, with patient breathing deeply; a normal liver is normally not palpable.

4. Spleen palpation: starts again in the right iliac fossa; a normal spleen is not palpable.

5. Liver percussion: moves down from the right nipple; a normal liver produces 3–4 finger-breadths of dullness.

6. Spleen percussion: as for the liver, starting at the left nipple.

7. Balloting the kidneys: large kidneys may indicate poly-cystic kidney disease, hydronephrosis, abscess or tumour.

8. Palpating for fluid in the abdomen (**ascites**): either test for shifting dullness (which is more commonly used) or a fluid thrill. **Shifting dullness** in the abdominal cavity should be tested even if there is no apparent distension; if the fingers are placed pointing upwards on the midline of the abdomen and percussed towards yourself, a dullness will indicates a fluid level. The hand is kept in place and the patient is asked to roll onto the side away from you; the fluid will move away from your hand. Percussion is now resonant and there is no fluid underneath your fingers. *The dullness has shifted.* **Fluid thrill** (tapping for ascites) is suitable when the abdomen is so distended that the fluid will not move and shifting dullness cannot be elicited. The patient is asked to place the edge of their own hand pointing downwards across their umbilicus. The clinician places a hand on either side of the abdomen, tapping with one while keeping the other still. The abdominal fluid transmits the tap underneath the patient's hand to the clinician's other hand. (The patient's hand stops the tap being transmitted through fat or skin.)

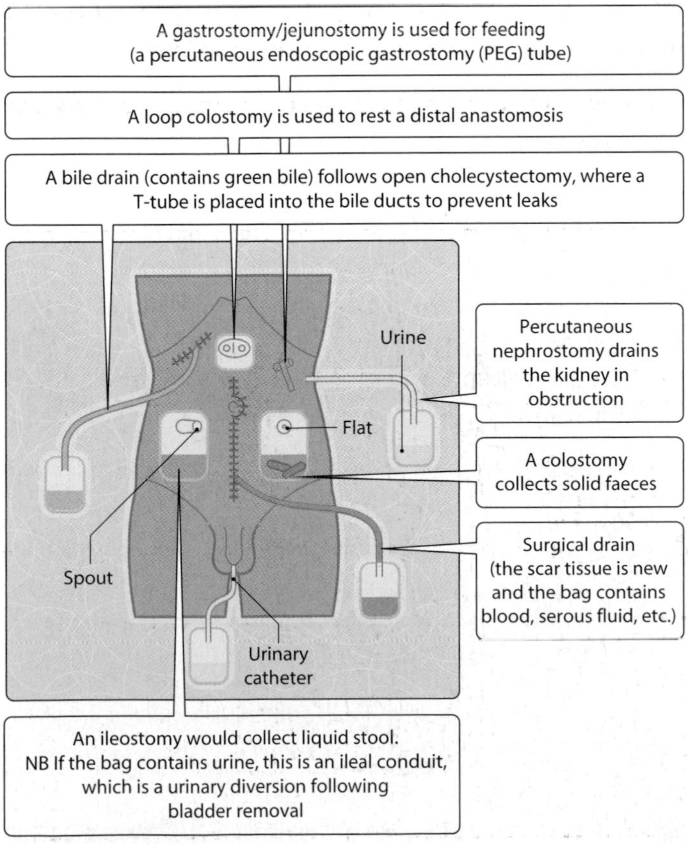

Auscultation
The normal presence of bowel sounds should be assessed at two places; absence suggests a functional obstruction, and high-pitched (tinkling) sounds suggest mechanical obstruction.

Concluding the examination

A clinician can palpate centrally for an abdominal aortic aneurysm and screen for inguinal hernias (cover the hernial orifices and ask the patient to cough). At the end of an examination, the covers must be replaced and the patient thanked. In an OSCE, a student should state that they would go on to perform a digital rectal examination and an examination of the external genitalia.

Differences between the spleen and kidney on examination:
- the spleen moves down on inspiration but a kidney does not
- the spleen is dull to percussion while a kidney is resonant as loops of bowel overlie it
- the spleen has a palpable anterior notch
- a kidney is ballotable but the spleen is not
- it is possible to feel above a kidney but not above the spleen.

Disease indications from an examination

Causes of a distended abdomen can be remembered by the 5Fs: fat, fluid (ascites), faeces, flatus (air) and fetus.

Causes of ascites can be remembered by 3C + 1N (but are classified into transudates and exudates, Ch. 11):

- cirrhosis: leading to portal hypertension
- congestive cardiac failure
- cancer: ovarian in women, otherwise may be colonic or peritoneal metastases
- nephrotic syndrome: hypoalbuminaemia.

The causes of hepatomegaly, splenomegaly and hepato-splenomegaly can be found in a medical text book.

A gastrostomy/jejunostomy is used for feeding (a percutaneous endoscopic gastrostomy (PEG) tube)

A loop colostomy is used to rest a distal anastomosis

A bile drain (contains green bile) follows open cholecystectomy, where a T-tube is placed into the bile ducts to prevent leaks

Urine

Percutaneous nephrostomy drains the kidney in obstruction

Flat

A colostomy collects solid faeces

Surgical drain (the scar tissue is new and the bag contains blood, serous fluid, etc.)

Spout

Urinary catheter

An ileostomy would collect liquid stool. NB If the bag contains urine, this is an ileal conduit, which is a urinary diversion following bladder removal

Fig. 3.6.2 Stomas and drains.

7. Stomach disorders

Questions
■ What are the causes of dyspepsia?
■ What is gastro-oesophageal reflux disease and how is it treated?
■ What are the complications of peptic ulcers?

Dyspepsia

Dyspepsia is a broad term encompassing a range of symptoms: pain (epigastric or retrosternal), heartburn, acid regurgitation and bloating. Fig. 3.7.1 shows the causes of dyspepsia.

Management depends on the age and the presentation:

■ new-onset dyspepsia in anyone over 45 years of age should be investigated with endoscopy within 2 weeks to exclude cancer
■ a patient of any age with alarm symptoms (weight loss, haematemesis, malaena, dysphagia, anaemia) should be investigated with endoscopy promptly
■ those under 45 years of age should be tested and treated for *Helicobacter pylori* (see below) for 2 weeks; endoscopy is indicated if symptoms persist.

Gastro-oesophageal reflux disease

GORD is the most common upper gastrointestinal diagnosis. Reflux occurs when the lower oesophageal sphincter temporarily relaxes, and acid refluxes up the oesophagus. This in itself is a normal physiological mechanism but when inflammation of the oesophagus occurs (**oesphagitis**) it is known as GORD. It affects 7% of the population and obesity is a risk factor. A **hiatus hernia** may be present and contributing to symptoms.

Clinical features

Heartburn may be intermittent and is the most common presentation. Other presentations include dysphagia, dyspepsia, chest pain (mimicking angina), globus sensation (feeling a lump in the throat), wheezing and bronchitis (from aspiration) or odynophagia (painful swallowing).

Investigation

Endoscopy is the investigation of choice in those over 45 years (to exclude carcinoma and ulcer); it may identify a hiatus hernia. **Barrett's oesophagus** or **syndrome** (Ch. 9) may be found. Diagnosis of GORD is made objectively with pH studies (pH is < 4 for > 4% of a 24-hour period) and oesophageal mamometry (showing a hypotonic lower oesophageal sphincter).

Management

Management can be **conservative** (stop smoking, avoid alcohol and eating late, lose weight, raise head of bed (gravity)), **medical** (proton pump inhibitors (omeprazole) as first-line treatment) or **surgical**: fundoplication performed laparoscopically (part of the stomach is wrapped around the lower oesophagus) is effective in > 95% of patients. Surgery is used when medical therapies have failed or for patients who prefer not to take long-term medication.

Hiatus hernia

Hiatus hernia occurs when proximal stomach herniates through the diaphragmatic hiatus into the thorax (Fig. 3.7.2). They are common (50% of people over 50 years are affected) although only one-third of these will have symptoms of reflux.
There are two types (Fig. 3.7.2):

■ **sliding** (80%): the gastro-oesophageal junction slides into the chest and so these are frequently associated with reflux
■ **rolling** (20%): para-oesophageal hernias where only a bulge of stomach herniates up beside the oesophagus; the gastro-oesophageal junction remains in the abdomen and so reflux is uncommon; these are mostly asymptomatic.

Diagnosis is made by barium swallow or endoscopy. Para-oesophageal hernias are treated operatively with fundoplication. Sliding hernias may be initially managed conservatively (as for GORD); if there is no improvement of symptoms or as an alternative to long-term medication, surgery can be used.

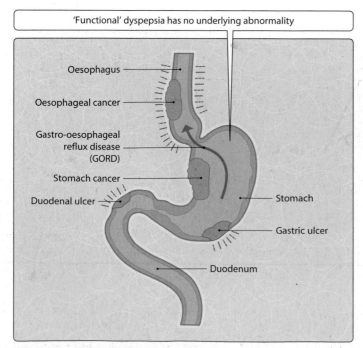

'Functional' dyspepsia has no underlying abnormality

Oesophagus

Oesophageal cancer

Gastro-oesophageal reflux disease (GORD)

Stomach cancer

Duodenal ulcer

Stomach

Gastric ulcer

Duodenum

Fig. 3.7.1 Causes of dyspepsia.

Peptic ulcer disease

A peptic ulcer is a break in the continuity of the epithelial surface of the stomach or duodenum and is common. Peptic ulcers are associated with:

- infection with *H. pylori*
- long-term (> 5 years) treatment with non-steroidal anti-inflammatory drugs (NSAIDs)
- treatment with steroids
- smoking, alcohol and stress (burns, major surgery, lifestyle) are contributory
- Zollinger–Ellison syndrome (rare): a peptic ulcer associated with a gastrin-secreting pancreatic adenoma and suspected in disease resistant to treatment.

Clinical features are dyspepsia, heartburn and epigastric pain: related to eating.

H. pylori has been implicated in formation of peptic ulcers, gastric cancer, atrophic gastritis and ischaemic heart disease. It is widely found, but most patients with *H. pylori* do not have a peptic ulcer, although 90% of patients with a duodenal ulcer have *H. pylori*. It can be tested for in three ways:

- serum test: only tells if patient has been infected at some point, not if they are currently affected
- breath test: good for identifying current infection; used 4 weeks after stopping treatment to assess success
- biopsy at endoscopy (CLO test: for campylobacter-like organisms) is the gold standard but is invasive.

Eradication of *H. pylori* is with the 'test and treat' principle. Eradication therapy is initiated immediately and adjusted when test results are available. Medical treatment for *H. pylori* is with triple therapy: a proton pump inhibitor (e.g. omeprazole, lansoprazole), amoxicillin and clarithromycin for 1 week (metronidzaole can be substituted for amoxicillin if there is no improvement). With triple therapy, 80% of patients improve. Eradication of *H. pylori* is important in reducing the risk of gastric carcinoma.

Complications of peptic ulcers

Chronic peptic ulcer can cause overt bleeds leading to melaena or iron-deficient anaemia, which may present as tiredness (assess with full blood count). The three classical complications are relatively common.

Haemorrhage. Bleeding may be massive, with marked haematemesis or malaena; treatment is to stabilize the patient (ABC) and then use endoscopy to identify and stop bleeding. Failure or rebleeding may necessitate surgery.

Perforation. The ulcer perforates through the wall. Patients are peritonitic and shocked. Erect chest radiograph shows free gas under the diaphragm. The perforation is closed with an omental plug at laparoscopy (or less commonly laparotomy).

Pyloric stenosis. Stenosis can occur following healing of chronic dudodenal ulcers, presenting with nausea, projectile vomiting and weight loss. Treatment is with endoscopic balloon dilatation or surgery (gastroenterostomy).

Investigations

Endoscopy is the investigation of choice, where biopsies can be taken to confirm diagnosis.

Management

Medical management. Medical treatment cures most patients. Triple therapy to eradicate *H. pylori* is effective in most patients. Conservative measures should also be advised: stop smoking and drinking, reduce stress, lose weight.

Surgical treatment. Medication treats most, so surgery is only required to treat complications (as above). Historical types of elective surgery are:

- vagotomy: a highly selective vagotomy (HSV) divides some local roots of the vagus nerve close to the stomach, thus selectively reducing acid production
- partial gastrectomy.

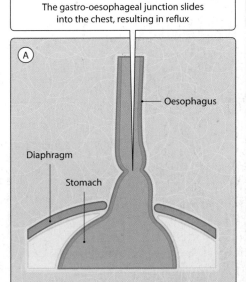
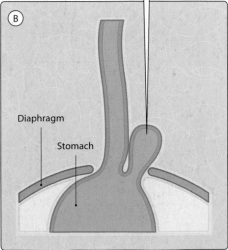

The gastro-oesophageal junction slides into the chest, resulting in reflux

The gastro-oesophageal junction stays below the diaphragm but part of the stomach rolls up alongside the oesophagus and herniates

Oesophagus

Diaphragm

Stomach

Diaphragm

Stomach

Fig. 3.7.2 Types of hiatus hernia: (A) sliding (80%); (B) rolling (paraoesophageal; 20%).

8. Upper gastrointestinal bleeding

Questions
- What are the causes of upper gastrointestinal bleeding?
- What is the initial management priority?
- What is variceal bleeding and how would you manage it?

Upper gastrointestinal bleeding (UGIB) is a medical emergency and may become a surgical emergency. It is associated with significant morbidity and mortality. These patients must be stabilized before endoscopy, which is the investigation of choice and also allows therapeutic intervention.

Aetiology
The causes of UGIB are shown in Fig. 3.8.1.

Clinical features
The most common presentations are:

- haematemesis: vomiting with bright red blood, dark clots or coffee grounds; this may be repeated minor episodes or it may be a large lethal episode where thick clots are passed and the airway becomes compromised
- malaena: black, sticky, smelly, tar-like stools; bleeding is from proximal to and including the caecum
- anaemia: chronic UGIB may present with tiredness, symptomatic of anaemia; the patient may not have noticed associated malaena
- collapse or shock: acute presentation with tachycardia, hypotension, urine output < 30 ml/h
- weakness

- sweating
- palpitations, postural syncope and dizziness.

Management
The first priority is resuscitation, with particular care to secure the airway, followed by measures to stop the bleeding. Once the patient is stable, endoscopy is diagnostic and often therapeutic; it should be performed within 12 h. In urgent cases, the on-call endoscopy team should be summoned.

Initial management:

- ABC: protect the airway, gain intravenous access (two large venflons in two large veins) and restore circulating volume using crystalloids, colloids, O-negative and cross-matched blood
- bloods: FBC (anaemia may be profound), U&E, glucose, liver function tests, clotting, cross-match 4–8 units; consider arterial blood gases; decreasing haemoglobin and increasing urea suggest a gastrointestinal bleed
- urine: pass a catheter to monitor urine output
- correct clotting: vitamin K, fresh frozen plasma, platelets.

Once these have been instituted, the cause can be sought:

- history: dyspepsia (ulcer, malignancy), alcohol (varices), NSAIDs and warfarin (ulcers), recent vomiting (Mallory–Weiss tear), ulcers, gastrointestinal surgery

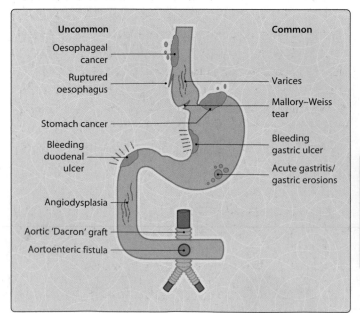

Fig. 3.8.1 Causes of upper gastrointestinal bleeding.

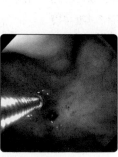

Fig. 3.8.2 Injection scleropathy around a bleeding blood vessel within an ulcer.

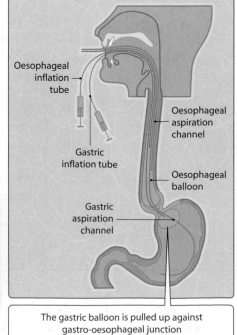

The gastric balloon is pulled up against gastro-oesophageal junction

Fig. 3.8.3 Balloon tamponade using a Sengstaken–Blakemore tube.

- examination: stigmata of chronic liver disease abdominal aortic aneurysm (palpation and auscultation for a bruit); rectal examination is vital
- endoscopy: oesophago-gastro-duodenoscopy (OGD) enables diagnosis and often treatment.

Specific management of bleeding

Specific measures to arrest the bleeding should *only* commence once the patient has been resuscitated and stabilized. The management will depend on the cause.

Haemorrhage from an acute peptic ulcer

Haemorrhage from an acute peptic ulcer is the most *common* cause of UGIB and the leading cause of death from peptic ulcer disease. Overall mortality is 10%. There may be frank haematemesis, or overt chronic bleeds presenting as melaena or iron-deficient anaemia. NSAIDs, steroids and warfarin may all be present in the history. **Endoscopy** is diagnostic and therapeutic. It allows the bleeding site to be visualized; treatment is with:

- injection of adrenaline (epinephrine) around the ulcer (Fig. 3.8.2)
- electrocoagulation
- laser coagulopathy.

For gastric ulcers, endoscopy is repeated at 6 weeks to check healing and to repeat biopsies (to exclude malignancy). **Surgery** may be required: a duodenal ulcer is oversewn to stop the bleeding; a gastric ulcer may require gastrectomy.

Variceal haemorrhage

Oesophageal and gastric varices develop as a result of **portal hypertension**, commonly secondary to alcohol use causing cirrhosis (but there are many other causes of chronic liver disease). Overall mortality is 30%. Managing these cases is important (initially it may be the responsibility of a house officer at midnight):

- assess with ABC and resuscitation; *secure an airway and intravenous access quickly*
- correct clotting
- active resuscitation is life saving: fluids, blood, fresh frozen plasma and/or platelets must be considered urgently
- the on-call endoscopy team is called.

Endoscopy is the treatment of choice and is diagnostic; it should be performed within 4 h. Bleeding is usually treated with **injection scleropathy**. **Band ligation** can be used if this fails or if there are technical difficulties. Other treatments include:

- terlipressin reduces portal pressure and may be used in conjunction with an intravenous proton pump inhibitor while awaiting emergency endoscopy

- if treatment is likely to be delayed, a **balloon tamponade** may be performed (Fig. 3.8.3), though only by experienced staff: a Sengstaken–Blakemore tube is inserted down the oesophagus; when the balloon is inflated, it compresses the varices and blocks off the bleeding source but should not be left in place for longer than 12 h
- emergency surgery may be required to reduce portal pressure if none of the above are successful: a transjugular intrahepatic portosystemic shunt (TIPS; see Fig. 3.11.2), an oesophageal transection (with gun-stapled reanastomosis) or a portosystemic shunt; elective TIPS can reduce the long-term portosystemic pressure.

Mallory–Weiss tear

A Mallory–Weiss tear occurs at the gastro-oesophageal junction and is caused by prolonged vomiting and/or retching, which most often follows large bouts of alcohol consumption. Vomit is initially normal but then bright red. Most stop bleeding spontaneously and surgery is only required in 10%.

Oesophagitis/erosive gastritis

Oesophagitis/erosive gastritis presents as relatively minor bleeds and is associated with NSAID and aspirin use. Proton pump inhibitors usually stop the bleeding but surgical resection may rarely be required.

Tumours

Leiomyoma of the oesophagus and stomach may bleed (the most common presentation). This benign tumour is excised. Malignant tumours, gastric adenocarcinoma or bleeding lymphoma, require subtotal or total gastrectomy.

Aortoenteric fistula

An aortoenteric fistula results from erosion of a chronically infected aortic graft (abdominal aortic aneurysm replacement) into the bowel lumen. Patients often present with a self-limiting 'herald UGIB', followed by a second massive gastrointestinal bleed. Endoscopy and intravenous enhanced CT scan are usually diagnostic. Laparotomy is required to excise the graft, debride and close the duodenum and to place a vascular bypass to vascularize the lower limbs (the option of placing an endovascular stent into the aorta is being assessed). Perioperative mortality is 25–90%.

Angiodysplasia

An abnormal collection of small blood vessels on the wall of the bowel (angiodysplasia) may bleed, causing UGIB or lower gastrointestinal haemorrhage. Diagnosis and treatment is with endoscopy and diathermy, or by surgical removal.

9. Oesophageal disorders

Questions
- What are the causes of dysphagia?
- What is the risk of cancer with Barrett's oesophagus?
- What is achalasia and how is it treated?

Dysphagia

Dysphagia, difficulty in swallowing (first solids, then liquids), requires urgent investigation with endoscopy. Progressive dysphagia and weight loss in the elderly is assumed to be oesophageal cancer until proved otherwise. Causes of dysphagia are illustrated in Fig. 3.9.1.

Oesophageal cancer

The incidence of oesophageal cancer and adenocarcinoma is rapidly rising. Certain aetiological factors have been identified:

- smoking and high alcohol intake
- Barrett's oesophagus (see below)
- long-standing achalasia, webs and strictures
- tylosis: a rare autosomal dominant condition leading inevitably to oesophageal cancer (hyperkeratosis of the palms and soles occurs)
- male sex: male to female ratio is 7:1.

Pathology. **Squamous cell carcinomas** tend to arise in the upper and middle oesophagus. **Adenocarcinomas** have a strong association with **Barrett's oesophagus**, a premalignant condition with 40% increased risk of adenocarcinoma. In 10% of patients with gastro oesophageal reflux disease (GORD) (Ch. 7), the squamous cells of the lower oesophagus are destroyed by acid stomach contents. They are replaced with tall columnar epithelium (which is more resistant to stomach acid). Some normal mucosa is visible around the top. Endoscopic surveillance monitors for malignant change (Fig. 3.9.2).

Clinical features. Dysphagia is typically the first symptom and is often subtle. It may be the only symptom, and so presentation is often also with metastases. Other symptoms are weight loss, haematemesis, oesophageal pain, lymphadenopathy and recurrent chest infections (aspiration pneumonia caused by oesophageal obstruction). Metastatic spread leads to hoarseness (recurrent laryngeal nerve invasion), chest pain and bronchial invasion.

Investigations. Investigation is by oesophago-gastro-duodenoscopy (OGD) with biopsy (Fig. 3.9.2), barium swallow and/or CT/MRI.

Surgical management. Thoracoscopic and laparoscopic surgery is developing. The aim is to obtain clear margins of excision 5 cm or greater. Only 40% of tumours are operable, as curative resection is contraindicated when there are metastases. Operative mortality is < 5% in specialist centres;

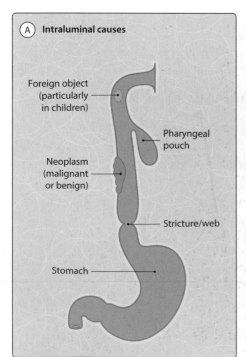

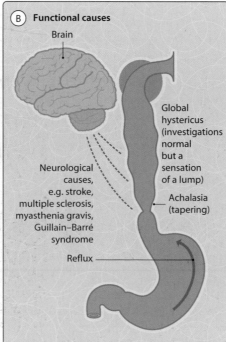

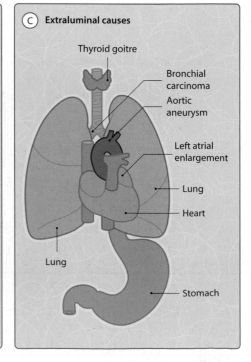

Fig. 3.9.1 Causes of dysphagia.

complications are common. Approaches for anastomoses in the week after oesophagectomy are thoracoabdominal, thoracic + abdominal (separate), abdominal + trans–hiatal, and abdominal + substernal.

Palliative treatment. **Endoscopic stenting** may relieve dysphagia or obstruction.

Prognosis. Tumours have often metastasized at presentation or spread locally to the great vessels; overall 5-year survival is 10%.

Achalasia

Achalasia (Fig. 3.9.3) is a failure of relaxation of the lower oesphageal sphincter and loss of peristalsis, leading to functional obstruction when swallowing. It is an idiopathic oesophageal motility disorder in which there is imbalance of the excitatory and inhibitory neurotransmission within the myenteric plexus. Dysphagia is the most common symptom, with regurgitation and aspiration. There is an increased risk of malignant change.

Investigations. These include:

- radiography with barium swallow: normally diagnostic
- oesophageal manometry
- OGD: biopsies are taken to exclude gastro-oesophageal carcinoma if the diagnosis is unclear.

Management:

- endoscopic balloon dilatation: the gold standard treatment, which relieves symptoms in 50%, although perforation occurs in 2%
- endoscopic injection of botulinum toxin: irreversible blockade of the neuromuscular junctions; best reserved for elderly patients

- Heller's cardiomyotomy: surgical division of the sphincter performed laparoscopically if balloon dilatation fails.

Oesophageal strictures

Strictures most commonly present with dysphagia. Diagnosis is with barium swallow and OGD to exclude carcinoma. Strictures may be caused by long-standing GORD, cancer, collagen disorders (e.g. scleroderma, systemic lupus erythematosus), radiotherapy or caustic ingestion (alkalis are worse than acids: **caustic strictures**). Complications are food impaction and consequences of **pulmonary aspiration** (chronic cough, asthma or pneumonia).

Treatment involves endoscopic dilatation (bougies or balloons), with medical therapy for reflux. Occasionally oesophageal replacement surgery is necessary.

Oesophageal perforation

Perforation of the oesophagus carries a high mortality and is either:

- spontaneous rupture following a violent bout of vomiting or retching (**Boerhaave syndrome**) is a full-thickness rupture and requires surgery (compared with a Mallory–Weiss tear (Ch. 8), which has the same pathogenesis but is partial thickness and rarely requires surgery)
- instrumentation (**iatrogenic**, e.g. endoscopy, dilatation of a stricture or carcinoma): most small leaks are treated conservatively (nil by mouth, total parenteral nutrition, antibiotics, chest drain); large leaks may require surgery.

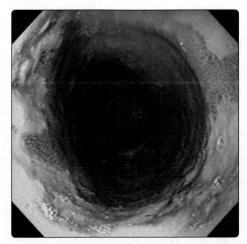

Fig. 3.9.2 A long segment of Barrett's oesophagus extending upwards from the oesophago-gastric junction (at bottom) shown by OGD.

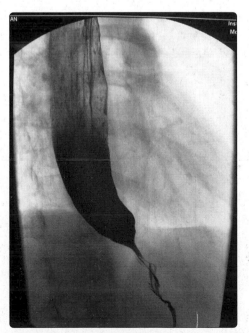

Fig. 3.9.3 A radiograph showing tapering of distal oesophagus ('bird's beak' deformity) in achalasia.

10. Stomach cancer

Questions
- What are the most common sites and type of stomach cancer?
- Does stomach cancer tend to present early or late?
- How is a suspected stomach cancer investigated?

Although the frequency of stomach cancer in the UK is falling, there is currently a sharp rise in the incidence of adeno-carcinoma of the gastro-oesophageal junction. Presentation is often late when cancer is advanced, so prognosis is very poor. Stomach cancer is the second most common cancer worldwide (particularly in China, Japan, Korea).

Aetiology
Stomach cancer is linked with:

- blood group A
- smoking
- male to female ratio of 2:1
- premalignant conditions: pernicious anaemia, intestinal metaplasia and dysplasia
- geographical variation
- diet: related to nitrosamines (fish, vegetables, low vitamin C, high salt)
- *Helicobacter pylori*: lifelong infection.

Pathology
The incidence of stomach cancer is rising. Most are **adenocarcinomas** and the most common location is within the body of the stomach or near the gastro-oesophageal junction.

Clinical features
Early stomach cancer is often asymptomatic, and so 90% of patients present with advanced disease. **Dyspepsia** is the first symptom and is often vague. All patients over 45 years of age with new-onset dyspepsia should be investigated with endoscopy before any treatment (e.g. if suspected peptic ulcer disease, antacids reduce symptoms and so the true diagnosis is missed). Signs of *advanced disease* are weight loss, anaemia (frequent bleeding from the tumour), epigastric pain and mass. Only at this stage are ascites and hepatomegaly detectable.

Spread of cancer occurs by:

- local invasion to spleen, colon, liver, pancreas, superior or mesenteric vessels, portal vein, coeliac axis

- lymphatic spread: a palpable lymph node in the left supraclavicular fossa is called **Virchow's node** (the first point of lymphatic drainage of the stomach) and if found is called **Troisier's sign**
- haematogenous spread to the liver
- transperitoneal: causing ascites, pleural effusions and ovarian metastases (**Krukenberg's deposits**).

Investigations
Endoscopy (oesophago-gastro-duodenoscopy) allows multiple biopsies (at least 10) to be taken. Staging is achieved using CT, endoscopic ultrasound and laparoscopy. Stage and prognosis are assessed with the TNM (tumour, node, metastasis) system (Table 3.10.1).

Management
Surgery provides the only chance of cure but is contraindicated when disease is advanced or there are metastases (70% of cases).

Curative surgery. Clear margins of excision of at least 5 cm are attempted. Either a total (Fig. 3.10.1) or a subtotal (Fig. 3.10.2) gastrectomy with or without the lower oesophagus

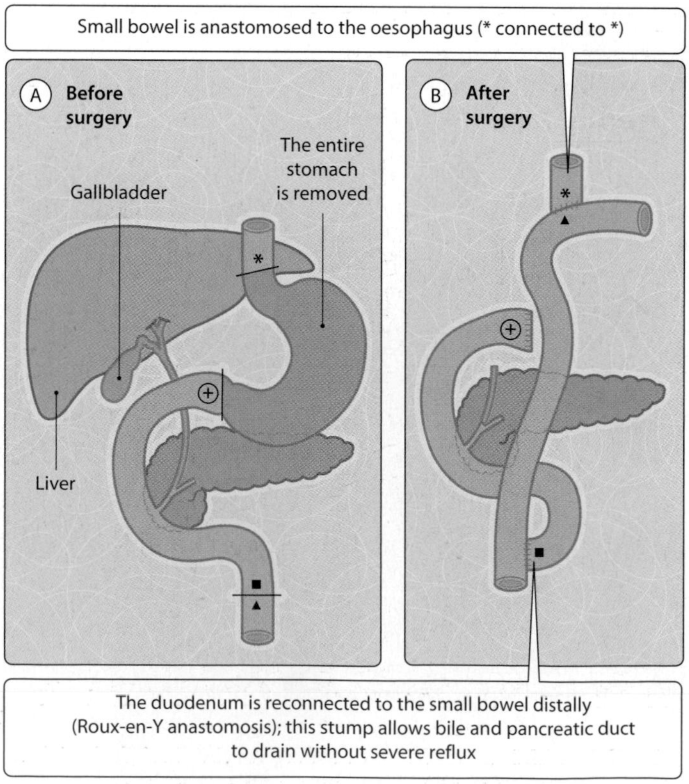

Small bowel is anastomosed to the oesophagus (* connected to *)

A Before surgery

Gallbladder

The entire stomach is removed

Liver

B After surgery

The duodenum is reconnected to the small bowel distally (Roux-en-Y anastomosis); this stump allows bile and pancreatic duct to drain without severe reflux

Fig. 3.10.1 Total gastrectomy with Roux-en-Y reconstruction (to prevent bile reflux and severe oesophagitis)

Table 3.10.1 STAGING STOMACH CANCER

Stage	Tumour	Classification Node[a]	Metastasis	Surviving at 5 years (%)
1	1, 2	0	0	80–90
2	1–4	1, 2	0	30
3	1–3	1–3	0	10
4	4	3	1	0

[a]Lymph node involvement.

depends on the location and extent of tumour. Lymph nodes are resected in either a **D1 resection** (regional perigastric nodes) or a **D2 resection** (perigastric and nodes around the caeliac axis). Loss of intrinsic factor leads to pernicious anaemia and vitamin B_{12} deficiency (lifelong injections are needed).

Palliative surgery. Total gastrectomy is to palliate chronic blood loss or obstruction; gastroduojeunostomy relieves inoperable lesions causing pyloric obstruction.

Prognosis

Overall, 5-year survival in the UK is 5–10%. When found early (uncommon in UK but common in Japan because of screening) prognosis is excellent.

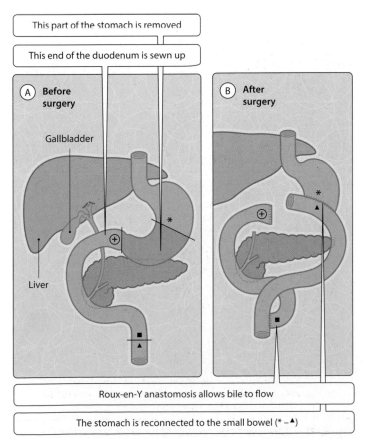

Fig. 3.10.2 Subtotal gastrectomy with Roux-en-Y reconstruction.

■ OTHER TUMOURS OF THE STOMACH AND SMALL BOWEL

Lymphomas. Lymphomas account for > 10% of stomach tumours and also occur in the small bowel. They are associated with *H. pylori* infection and tend to occur in children or young adults. Symptoms are similar to those of gastric carcinomas and they may present with bleeding or perforation. Treatment is with surgical resection and chemo- and radiotherapy.

Gastrointestinal stromal tumours. These are a rare type of soft tissue sarcoma (known as GIST) mostly occurring in the stomach and small bowel. They can be of *low* (< 2 cm, low metabolic activity) or *high* (> 2 cm, high metabolic activity) *malignant potential*. Wide surgical resection and chemotherapy are attempted for malignant tumours; imatinib (Glivec or STI 571) can be used if surgery is not possible.

Leiomyomas. These benign tumours may occur anywhere in the gastrointestinal tract but are most common in the stomach and oesophagus. They present with bleeding from surface ulceration and they can occasionally become malignant (leiomyosarcoma).

Carcinoid tumours. Carcinoid tumours arising from APUD (amine precursor uptake and decarboxylation) cells are commonly small and benign tumours found in the appendix (although they can occur anywhere in the gastrointestinal tract). If they metastasize to the liver, they may secrete catecholamines, resulting in **carcinoid syndrome** (hot flushes, hypertension, asthma and diarrhoea). Diagnosis is formed on raised 24-h collection of urinary 5-hydroxyindoleacetic acid (5-HIAA). Surgical resection with chemotherapy is curative.

Peutz–Jeghers syndrome. This rare inherited autosomal dominant disorder leads to multiple benign polyps in the small bowel. There is characteristic pigmentation of the lips, gums, hands and feet. The polyps may cause chronic bleeding and anaemia plus obstruction from intussusception; malignant transformation is uncommon.

11. The liver and spleen

Questions

- What is a TIPS procedure?
- What is the most common type of liver malignancy in the UK?
- What are the complications of splenectomy?

■ THE LIVER

The liver has a dual blood supply, from the **hepatic artery** (arterial blood) and the **hepatic portal vein** (splanchnic blood). The hepatic portal vein is formed from the splenic vein and the superior mesenteric vein. The common bile duct, hepatic artery and portal vein form the **portal triad**. Three main hepatic veins drain from the liver into the inferior vena cava.

Portal hypertension

Portal hypertension (Fig. 3.11.1) occurs when the outflow to the hepatic portal vein is blocked, causing backflow. The portal system has five sites of anastomoses with the systemic circulation (**portal systemic anastomoses**; Table 3.11.1). When portal hypertension occurs, portal blood flow through these sites increases and causes formation of **varices**. The most important site is the lower oesophagus, as these **oesophageal varices** may cause massive upper gastrointestinal haemorrhage and possibly death (Ch. 8). Portal hypertension can also cause ascites (below).

Management. The **transjugular intrahepatic portosystemic shunt** (TIPS; Fig. 3.11.2) may be used for long-term management. It is an interventional radiological procedure. A metallic stent creates a communication between the hepatic vein (low pressure) and the portal venous system (high pressure), allowing blood to flow into the inferior vena cava without passing through the liver.

Ascites

Ascites is the accumulation of free fluid within the peritoneal cavity (see Ch. 6). A **peritoneal tap** is diagnostic and should be sent for analysis of protein content, malignant cells, bacteria and biochemistry. Ascites can be classified by protein content:

- exudates: high protein content (> 30 g/dl (> 300 g/l)); peritonitis (infection), carcinoma

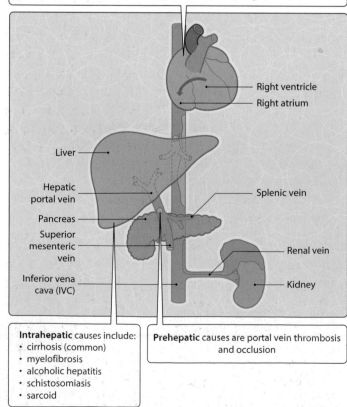

Posthepatic causes include:
- Budd–Chiari syndrome (thrombosis caused by blood clot or tumour)
- right heart failure (causing backflow of blood)
- veno-occlusive disease (including renal cancer invading the IVC)

Right ventricle
Right atrium
Liver
Hepatic portal vein
Splenic vein
Pancreas
Superior mesenteric vein
Renal vein
Inferior vena cava (IVC)
Kidney

Intrahepatic causes include:
- cirrhosis (common)
- myelofibrosis
- alcoholic hepatitis
- schistosomiasis
- sarcoid

Prehepatic causes are portal vein thrombosis and occlusion

Fig. 3.11.1 Causes of portal hypertension.

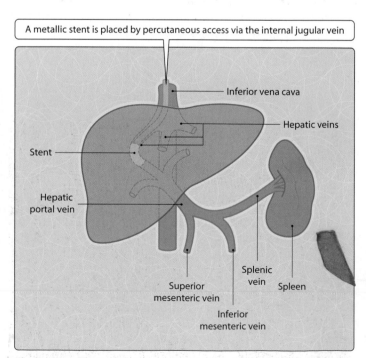

A metallic stent is placed by percutaneous access via the internal jugular vein

Inferior vena cava
Hepatic veins
Stent
Hepatic portal vein
Superior mesenteric vein
Splenic vein
Spleen
Inferior mesenteric vein

Fig. 3.11.2 The transjugular intrahepatic portosystemic shunt (TIPS) procedure.

■ transudate: low protein content (< 30 g/dl (< 300 g/l)); cardiac failure, portal hypertension and cirrhosis, Budd–Chiari syndrome, hyponatraemia (nephrotic syndrome).

Definitive management depends on the cause. Potassium-sparing diuretics and restriction of sodium and fluid intake should be started. Advanced ascites can be controlled with regular paracentesis (aspiration of ascites). A peritoneal–venous shunt may be placed surgically to drain the peritoneal cavity to the internal jugular vein.

Liver malignancy

Secondary liver tumours (metastases; Fig. 3.11.3) are much more common than primary tumours in the UK, although primary cancer is more common worldwide. Presentation is with weight loss, abdominal pain, upper abdominal mass and jaundice in 50%. The most common primary malignancy is **hepatic cell carcinoma**. It commonly arises in cirrhotic livers and may be multifocal.

> *Investigations.*   Liver function tests are not useful as they are non-specific. A suspected liver tumour is investigated by
> - ultrasound: differentiates solid masses and cysts
> - tumour markers: α-fetoprotein (AFP) may be raised.
> - MRI characterizes of solid liver masses
> - CT arterioportography: dye is injected into the hepatic artery and spiral CT gives an accurate image of the liver; positron emission tomography (PET) and CT may aid staging
> - liver biopsy: only if surgical resection is planned
> - laparoscopy: to identify a colonic primary or to clarify any doubt about diagnosis or staging.

The number and size of tumours and the degree of liver failure determines the procedure: surgical resection, chemo-embolization, radiofrequency ablation or liver transplantation. There is a 20% 5-year survival with surgical resection; otherwise, most die at 1 year.

Metastatic liver tumours

If there is no evidence of extrahepatic spread, the secondary liver tumours can be resected or treated by radiofrequency ablation. Prognosis after resection is irrespective of the number and size of liver metastases as long as there are clear margins and enough liver tissue (40%) to sustain life: the liver has the ability to regenerate completely. Tumours that commonly metastasize to the liver are colorectal, breast, prostate, lung, kidney and thyroid.

THE SPLEEN

The spleen lies in the left upper abdomen and is in contact with the left lower ribs. Elective **splenectomy** is performed in hereditary spherocytosis, autoimmune haemolytic anaemias, idiopathic thrombocytopenic purpura or as part of a wide resection for intra-abdominal tumours (e.g. radical gastrectomy).

Emergency splenectomy is required if the spleen is ruptured, often by blunt abdominal or lower left chest injury. The patient usually presents immediately after trauma and may be shocked, although they may present some weeks later from a late rupture and chronic haematoma. Bleeding can be significant and urgent action is required; urgent ultrasound or CT are usually diagnostic.

Short-term complications of splenectomy relate to a large increase in the white cell and platelet count in the early postoperative period, which can predispose to thrombosis; platelet count is monitored daily and prophylactic anticoagulation is used. In the long term there is a higher risk of sepsis, and so **pneumoccoal** and **influenza B vaccines** are given; long-term prophylaxis with oral penicillin is justified in high-risk patients.

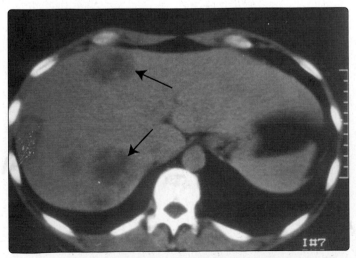

Fig. 3.11.3 A CT scan showing metastatic liver tumours.

Table 3.11.1 PORTOSYSTEMIC ANASTOMOSES

Area	Portal veins	Systemic veins
A Lower oesophagus	Left gastric	Azygos (via oesophageal veins)
B Rectum	Superior rectal into inferior mesenteric	Middle/inferior rectal into pudendal/internal iliac
C Bare area of liver	Hepatic	Inferior phrenic
D Periumbilical	Paraumbilical vein	Anterior abdominal wall
E Retroperitoneum	Colic and splenic	Lumbar

12. Pancreatic disorders

Questions
- What are the *common* causes of acute pancreatitis?
- How is the severity of acute pancreatitis assessed?
- What is the prognosis for pancreatic cancer?

Acute pancreatitis

Acute pancreatitis ranges from mild to severe and life-threatening; mortality is 5–10%. The incidence is rising, closely linked to increased alcohol consumption and gallstone disease (the main causes). Surgery is rarely required (unless as salvage for complications of haemorrhagic pancreatitis).

Pathology. Following insult to the pancreas, pancreatic enzymes leak into the pancreatic parenchyma. The **systemic inflammatory response syndrome** (SIRS) may be activated; the most severe complications of pancreatitis are **haemorrhagic pancreatic necrosis** and **infected pancreatic necrosis**. The causes of acute pancreatitis can be remembered by the acronym GET SMASHED: gallstones, ethanol, trauma, steroids, mumps, autoimmune, scorpion venom, hyperlipidaemia, endoscopic retrograde cholangio-pancreatography (ECRP), drugs (diuretics, immuno-suppressants). Gallstones and ethanol are common causes (80% of all cases); the rest are rare. After investigations, some cases remain idiopathic.

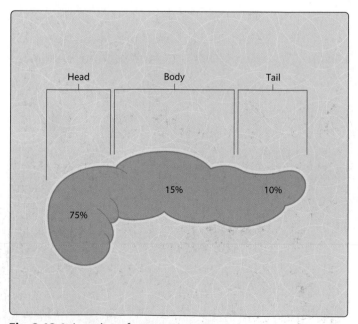

Fig. 3.12.1 Location of pancreatic tumours.

Clinical features. These are:
- pain: severe, constant epigastric pain that may radiate to the back; right upper quadrant, central abdominal or chest pain may also be present
- nausea and vomiting
- jaundice: may indicate gallstones or oedematous pancreatic head
- Grey–Turner's sign (bruising in the left flank) and Cullen's sign (periumbilical discolouration) may be found in haemorrhagic pancreatitis.

Differential diagnosis: **perforated peptic ulcer** and **mesenteric infarction**.

Investigations. Key investigations are:
- amylase: diagnostic when 3× upper limit of normal (although this may be normal and raised amylase levels are also seen in acute cholecystitis, peptic ulcer disease, aortic aneurysm and ectopic pregnancy); serum lipase is raised and more accurate but the test is less available
- ACRP > 210 at 96 h is the best predictor of acute, severe pancreatitis.
- liver function tests: may help to identify a biliary cause
- ultrasound: identifies gallstones; ERCP should be avoided in the acute setting
- radiography: abdominal radiograph may show an isolated loop of proximal jejunum caused by local ileus (a sentinel loop); chest radiograph may show a pleural effusion
- intravenous enhanced CT: if symptoms persist for longer than 7–10 days to identify areas of necrosis.

Early complications. Early complications are hypovolaemic shock, hypocalcaemia, diabetes mellitus, disseminated intravascular coagulation and respiratory and renal failure.

Late complications. These are an infected pancreatic necrosis, when severe sepsis develops, and pancreatic pseudocyst, a collection of pancreatic juices that escapes from a ruptured pancreatic duct. The pseudocyst has a non-epithelized wall formed from fibrous and granulation tissue. It presents several weeks after the initial attack, manifesting as severe epigastric pain, nausea and vomiting, an epigastric mass or systemic infection. A CT scan will show the cyst. Most resolve with conservative management, although surgical drainage is indicated if complications develop (e.g. symptoms, infection, rupture). Many scoring systems exist to assess severity and predict survival, such as the Ranson, Glasgow (see the clinical box) or APACHE-II.

Management. The initial management is supportive (which is still aggressive), where most cases resolve. Surgery is only indicated if the complications supersede. **Conservative management** involves:

- ABC with oxygen
- aggressive intravenous fluid replacement (and monitor urine output): to treat hypovolaemic shock
- initially nil by mouth, followed by early feeding
- analgesia.

Continuing management:

- monitor the prognostic factors (see the clinical box) daily
- prophylactic antibiotics in severe cases
- hypocalcaemia: correct with Calichew or may need parenteral supplementation in the acute stage
- transient diabetes may require insulin (sliding scale)
- management in intensive care (for severe cases and if respiratory or renal failure develop)
- ERCP to remove gallstones in selected patients.

Surgical management is to debride and washout areas of infected necrosis, and to drain pseudocysts.

Chronic pancreatitis

Chronic pancreatitis normally develops after repeated acute attacks, commonly from alcohol abuse (70%). Other causes include gallstones, cystic fibrosis, idiopathic and rare causes such as α_1-antitrypsin deficiency. Genetic mutations have been found in patients with unexplained pancreatitis. There is an increased risk of developing pancreatic carcinoma.

Clinical features. These are:

- epigastric pain and radiating to the back jaundice
- pancreatic insufficiency: diabetes mellitus, malabsorption (leading to weight loss) and steatorrhoea are late signs (90% of pancreatic function has been lost)

Conservative management. This is achieved for the majority of patients over long periods: pain management, pancreatic enzyme supplementation, diabetes mellitus control (insulin), stop alcohol intake and smoking.

Surgical management. Surgery is uncommon; it is mainly used to treat intractable pain, with pancreatic resection or drainage (**pancreaticojejunostomy**).

Pancreatic tumours

Pancreatic tumours often present late and have an extremely poor survival (Fig. 3.12.1). Most are adenocarcinomas in the head of the pancreas (75%). Those near the ampulla (10%) have better prognosis as they obstruct the common bile duct and so presentation with jaundice is earlier. Most pancreatic adenocarcinomas have either spread locally or have metastasized.

Clinical features. Patients present with:

- obstructive jaundice: **Courvoisier's law** states that, in the presence of jaundice, a palpable gallbladder is unlikely to

be caused by gallstones; carcinoma of the head of the pancreas or the lower biliary tree (blocking the gallbladder outflow) is more likely because the gallbladder with stones is usually chronically fibrosed and, therefore, incapable of enlargement

- marked weight loss
- intractable abdominal pain.

Investigations. Ultrasound, ERCP and spiral CT are used to identify patients who may have localized disease without evidence of widespread dissemination.

Management. **Surgical resection** is only used in 10% and only for tumours of the pancreatic head that are < 3 cm. Modern resection is with a modified Whipple's resection—**a pylorus-preserving proximal pancreatico-duodenectomy**. **Palliation** is by endoscopic stenting. ERCP is used to place a biliary stent to relieve jaundice. Opiate analgesia is used for pain. **Cholecystojejunostomy** connects the bile duct directly to the jejunum to relieve jaundice where ERCP fails.

Prognosis: 90% die in the first year.

Biliary tumours

Cholangiocarcinoma. These are tumours of the bile ducts and are associated with bile duct stones. Jaundice is the most common representing feature (90%). Biliary stenting relieves jaundice and pruritis; surgical resection is sometimes possible. The prognosis is usually poor.

Gallbladder tumours. These are uncommon and present with jaundice or a painful biliary mass, or are found during cholecystectomy for gallstones (70% coexist with gallstones; most are adenocarcinomas). Surgical resection is rarely possible and survival is extremely poor.

USING THE GLASGOW SCORE FOR ASSESSING SEVERITY OF ACUTE PANCREATITIS

Three or more of the following factors indicate severe acute pancreatitis:

- P: arterial oxygen partial pressure ↓ ($PaO_2 < 8$).
- A: age > 55 years
- N: neutrophils; white cell count ↑
- C: Ca^{2+} ↓ (most significant prognostic factor for death) albumin ↓
- R: raised enzymes lactate dehydrogenase (LDH) aspartate aminotransferase (AST) ↑
- E: elevated urea
- S: sugar; plasma glucose ↑

13. Colorectal cancer and polyps

Questions
- How does colorectal cancer present?
- How would you investigate suspected colorectal cancer?
- How is colorectal cancer staged, and what is the significance?

Colorectal carcinoma is the second most common cause of death from malignancy in developed countries (after lung cancer), and its incidence is increasing.

Aetiology
Factors linked to colorectal cancer are:

- polyps: sporadic polyps cause 80–90% of cancers
- genetic conditions with high-penetrance genes: cause 5% of colorectal cancers and occur particularly in the young; identified patients should be monitored with yearly colonoscopy and their families screened
  - **familial adenomatous polyps** (FAP): causes thousands of polyps in the colon and the risk of cancer is near 100%
  - **hereditary non-polypopis colorectal cancer**: involving an autosomal dominant gene, typically causing right-sided cancers in those under 50 years of age; family members often have a history of gynaecological malignancy

- family history: low-penetrance genes
- age: risk increases with age with colorectal cancer most common in those over 60 and maximal in those aged 70–75 years (> 5% in those under 30 years)
- ulcerative colitis: total colitis for > 10 years; 1% of cancers
- diet: low fibre causes slow transit times, which increases carcinogen contact time; red meat and animal fats increase risk (aspirin and NSAIDs are protective).

Pathology
The tumours can be polypoid, ulcerating, annular or infiltrative. Synchronous tumours are present in 3% of patients.

Colorectal polyps. Most colorectal tumours are adenocarcinomas that have evolved from polyps. The types of polyp are adenomas, tubulovillous adenomas and villous adenomas. The risk of cancer is increased with increasing size, the presence of tubulovillous adenomas and dysplasia. These polyps are removed by coloscopic polypectomy. Patients should be followed up with surveillance because of the high risk of recurrent polyps.

Clinical features
The presenting symptoms (Fig. 3.13.1) help to predict location but are not always present.

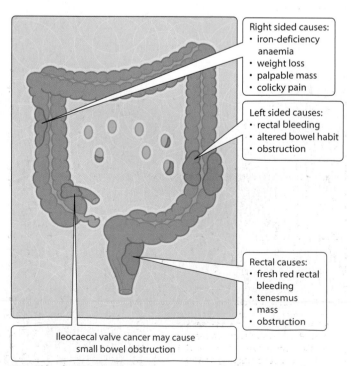

Right sided causes:
- iron-deficiency anaemia
- weight loss
- palpable mass
- colicky pain

Left sided causes:
- rectal bleeding
- altered bowel habit
- obstruction

Rectal causes:
- fresh red rectal bleeding
- tenesmus
- mass
- obstruction

Ileocaecal valve cancer may cause small bowel obstruction

Fig. 3.13.1 The presenting symptoms and distribution of colorectal cancer.

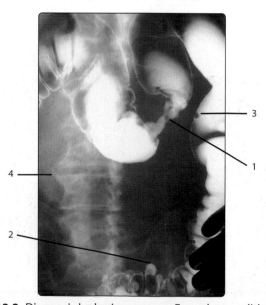

Fig. 3.13.2 Diagnosis by barium enema. Four abnormalities can be seen: (1) stenosing adenocarcinoma of the colon giving rise to an apple-core stricture and causing a mechanical large bowel obstruction; (2) diverticula in the sigmoid colon; (3) a polyp (descending colon); and (4) osteoarthritis of the spine (notice the marked 'lipping' of the vertebrae).

Table 3.13.1 STAGING COLORECTAL CANCER

Stage	Tumour(T)	Classification Node (N)	Metastasis(M)	Surviving at 5 years (%)
1	1–2	0	0	~90
2	3, 4	0	0	~60
3	1–4	1, 2	0	~30
4	Any	Any	1	~10

Primary tumour: T0, none; Tis, carcinoma in situ (mucosa only); T1, submucosa; T2, muscularis propria; T3, subserosa but not neighbouring organs; T4, local tissues or organs.

Node: N0, no lymph node involvement; N1, 1–3 regional nodes; N2, 4 or more regional nodes; N3, paraaortic nodes.

Metastases: M0, none; M1, distant metastases.

Approximately 30% of patients present as an emergency with obstruction (80%), perforation (15%) or haemorrhage (5%), which have a four-fold increased mortality. Two-thirds of colorectal cancer is on the left.

Investigations

Patients with suspicious features should be rapidly assessed in cancer clinics with a 2-week referral time:

- sigmoidoscopy: best for rectal and left-sided carcinomas: rigid sigmoidoscopy views up to 25 cm of bowel and 50% of carcinomas; flexible sigmoidoscopy views up to 60 cm and 75% of tumours
- colonoscopy: visualizes the entire inner surface of the large bowel, with biopsy of any lesions found; complete removal of polyps reduces the risk of cancer by 75%
- barium enema: outlines and views the entire colon and most cancers and polyps (Fig. 3.13.2); it is complementary to colonoscopy.

If a tumour is found, further tests are:

- carcinoembryonic antigen (CEA): a non-specific marker
- CT, MRI and liver ultrasound for spread and staging (liver function tests are non-specific.

Modern staging is with the TNM system (Table 3.13.1). The **Duke's staging system** is being phased out.

Management

Surgical management

Attempted curative surgical resection is appropriate in 80% of patients. Operative mortality is 2–5% electively and 15–20% for emergency resection. Palliative surgery has a place for symptom relief, especially to relieve obstruction. The type of operation varies according to the location of the tumour (Fig. 3.13.3). Distal rectal cancer requires removal of the entire rectum and anal canal (via abdominal and perineal incisions), with formation of a permanent end-colostomy. Proximal rectal cancer requires removal of the rectum and sigmoid colon with sphincter preservation; reanastomosis of the colon to the remaining anorectum avoids the need for a permanent end-colostomy but often a covering stoma is used (loop colostomy or ileostomy).

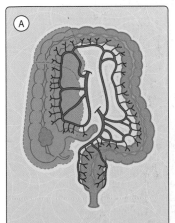
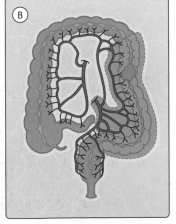
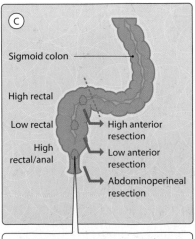
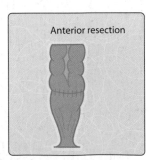
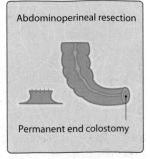

Fig. 3.13.3 Operational procedures. (A) Right hemicolectomy for right colon cancer (no bowel preparation); can be extended for transcolon or upper descending cancer (bowel preparation); (B) left hemicolectomy; (C) low anterior resection or abdominoperineal resection for rectal cancer or obstructing or perforating colon cancer.

Sigmoid colon

High rectal

Low rectal

High rectal/anal

High anterior resection

Low anterior resection

Abdominoperineal resection

A low anterior resection is carried out more often than an abdominoperineal resection now because of the availability of circular rectal stapling devices, which makes the former easier

Anterior resection

Abdominoperineal resection

Permanent end colostomy

14. Bowel obstruction

Questions
■ What are the common causes of bowel obstruction?
■ What are the key initial investigations?
■ When is surgical intervention indicated?

Bowel obstruction can be broadly classified as being *mechanical* or *functional* and affecting the *small* or *large* bowel.

Mechanical obstruction

Figure 3.14.1 shows areas of potential mechanical obstruction. Sigmoid volvulus appears as an 'inverted U' or 'rugby ball' on abdominal radiograph; if a flatus tube cannot decompress the obstruction, surgery is indicated. In a **closed loop obstruction** (Fig. 3.14.1D), the large bowel contents distend the thin-walled caecum because a *competent* ileocaecal valve prevents reflux. The risk of perforation is very high. Right iliac fossa tenderness becomes constant or localized if perforation is imminent. An incompetent valve allows reflux (20% of cases), causing vomiting. **Strangulation** occurs in unresolved bowel obstruction; occlusion of venous return will later block arterial supply to the affected loop, leading to infarction and perforation, and subsequent **peritonitis**. It is commonly caused by an **obstructed hernia** (check the hernial orifices) or **volvulus**. Signs of strangulation are rapid worsening in general condition, sharp and constant pain, increasing fever and heart rate, worsening peritonitis and a raised white cell count.

Clinical features

The key features of obstruction are (CAVA), <u>c</u>olicky abdominal pain, <u>a</u>bdominal distension, <u>v</u>omiting (the more proximal the obstruction, the earlier it occurs), <u>a</u>bsolute constipation (no passage of faeces or flatus).

Other features are 'tinkling' (high-pitched) bowel sounds (a 'sloshing' sound may be heard because of fluid accumulation), dehydration and strangulated hernias.

Investigations:

■ bloods: FBC and U&E to identify electrolyte imbalance
■ plain abdominal radiograph: *the key investigation* (Table 3.14.1 and Fig. 3.14.1C,D)

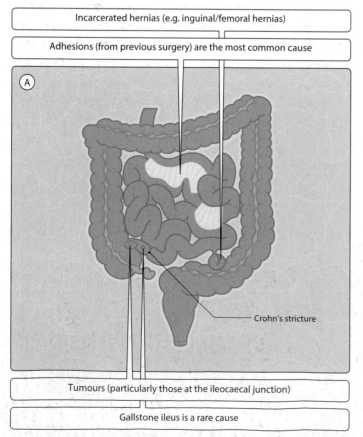

Incarcerated hernias (e.g. inguinal/femoral hernias)

Adhesions (from previous surgery) are the most common cause

A

Crohn's stricture

Tumours (particularly those at the ileocaecal junction)

Gallstone ileus is a rare cause

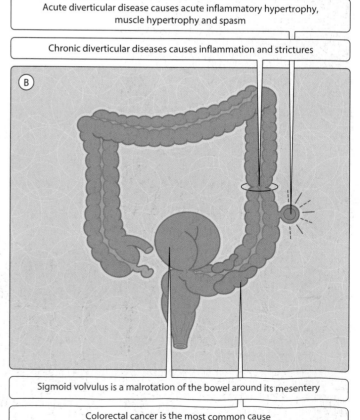

Acute diverticular disease causes acute inflammatory hypertrophy, muscle hypertrophy and spasm

Chronic diverticular diseases causes inflammation and strictures

B

Sigmoid volvulus is a malrotation of the bowel around its mesentery

Colorectal cancer is the most common cause

Fig. 3.14.1 Bowel obstruction. (A,C) small; (B,D) large. Table 3.14.1 lists the features that can be identified in (C) and (D).

- gentle contrast studies: using a water-soluble contrast medium (e.g. gastrograffin), as it is not as dangerous as barium if leakage occurs, and without bowel preparation to minimize the risk of perforation.

CT confirms the nature and site of obstruction (especially to stage tumours) and identifies other details (e.g. abscesses).

Management

Conservative management is a 'drip and suck' regimen for 48–72 h: nil-by-mouth; nasogastric tube to decompress the stomach—aspiration of contents removes swallowed air, decreases nausea and vomiting and prevents aspiration; and fluid resuscitation.

Improvement is indicated by decreasing nasogastric aspirates, decreasing pain and passage of flatus. Intussusception is sometimes successfully treated by air enema to 'push back' the telescoped bowel.

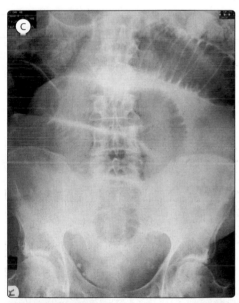

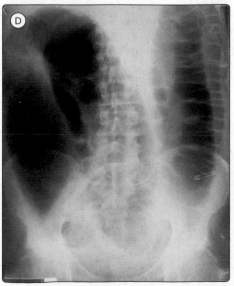

Surgery is indicated if symptoms persist and in specific situations. Often treatment merely involves division of adhesions or reduction and reposition of a hernia. If there is evidence of peritonitis and the bowel is involved (and often not prepared), a two-stage Hartmann's procedure may be used to resect affected bowel (Ch. 15). Indications for surgical resection are:

- failure of conservative therapy
- strangulation: urgent surgery (within 1 h) is needed for a tender, irreducible hernial mass to avoid infarction
- tumour: most right-sided tumours can be dealt with by resection and primary anastomosis, although some, usually left sided, may require a Hartmann's procedure (Ch. 15).
- Large-bowel obstruction is more likely to need surgical intervention than small-bowel, as gross or worsening dilatation is indicative of perforation.

Functional obstruction

Functional obstruction can occur after surgery (paralytic ileus) or from metabolic disorders (peseudo-obstruction). **Paralytic ileus** can result from peritonitis, blood in the abdomen, opiates, handling of the bowel during surgery or electrolyte imbalance (especially hypokalaemia); it is resolved by treating the primary cause. **Pseudo-obstruction** can be caused by anti-cholinergic and anti-parkinsonism drugs, renal failure, trauma (spinal fracture, hip or pelvic fracture), orthopaedic procedures and a variety of metabolic disorders. Functional obstruction commonly mimics mechanical obstruction. Bowels sounds are diagnostically absent as there is no peristalsis. Treatment is conservative. The underlying cause is treated; fluid and electrolyte balance corrected and a nasogastric tube passed. A decompressing sigmoidoscopy may be indicated in pseudo-obstruction. Laparotomy should be avoided unless there is sepsis.

Table 3.14.1 RADIOLOGICAL FEATURES OF INTESTINAL OBSTRUCTION

Feature	Small bowel (Fig. 3.14.1C)	Large bowel (Fig. 3.14.1D)
Diameter (cm)	> 3	> 8
Bowel markings	Valvulae conniventes (crossing all the way across the bowel wall)	Haustra (tenaei coli: pass a third of the way around the wall)
Dilated loops	Central	Peripheral
Gas	None in the large bowel	None in the small bowel unless the ileocaecal valve is incompetent
Fluid levels	Short and many	Long and few

15. Diverticular disease

Questions
- What is the difference between diverticular disease and acute diverticulitis?
- What are the complications of diverticular disease?
- What is a Hartmann's procedure?

Diverticular disease is a very common disorder in the West; 5% of those affected are in their fifties and 50% of people are over 70 years of age; 80% of diverticula are asymptomatic.

Pathology
A low-fibre diet leads to high luminal pressures, causing mucosa to herniate through the muscle layers to form pouches, called diverticula. Diverticula tend to occur in rows, commonly in the sigmoid colon (> 90%):

- **diverticulosis**: symptomless diverticula
- **diverticular disease**: diverticula cause symptoms in 10–25% of people, such as altered bowel habit or low-grade grumbling bowel pain; smoking and NSAIDs have been implicated in exacerbating complicated disease
- **acute diverticulitis**: if the diverticula become infected, secondary to occlusion of the orifice (as in appendicitis), the patient may present with severe abdominal pain, fever and localized or generalized abdominal sepsis

Clinical features
There is a wide variety of presentations:

- asymptomatic: only 20% are symptomatic; diverticula are identified on colonoscopic or barium examination

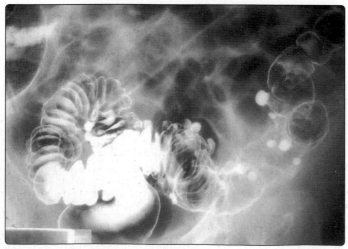

Fig. 3.15.1 Barium enema showing multiple diverticula of the sigmoid colon.

- abdominal pain: chronic, progressive lower abdominal or left iliac fossa pain is a common chronic presentation
- altered bowel habit: exclude colorectal cancer
- rectal bleeding (rare)
- pneumaturia: **frothy urine**, which is caused by colovesical fistula allowing air from the bowel to enter the bladder
- faeces per vaginum: usually after a previous hysterectomy forming a colovaginal fistula
- acute diverticulitis: see Complications.

Investigations
The symptoms of uncomplicated disease can be impossible to differentiate from colorectal cancer, and investigations are needed:

- rectal examination: a sigmoid mass may be detectable, although this may be a diverticula abscess or a carcinoma
- barium enema (Fig. 3.15.1): diverticula are usually more obvious than on colonoscopy
- colonoscopy to exclude colorectal cancer.

If the presentation is of acute diverticulitis, barium enema and colonoscopy are contraindicated as they may cause perforation.

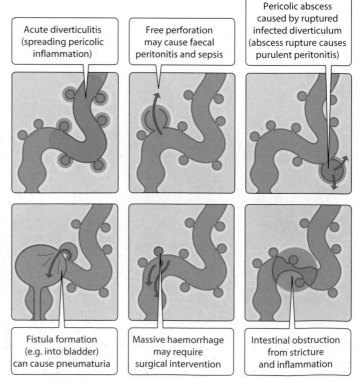

Fig. 3.15.2 Complications of diverticula.

CT is the investigation of choice in acute disease; it confirms the diagnosis and identifies any abscess or perforation.

Complications of diverticular disease

Potential complications of diverticular disease (Fig. 3.15.2) include:

- **acute diverticulitis**: infection of a diverticulum causes acute left iliac fossa pain, tender mass, local peritonism, which is often recurrent and periodic; systemic sepsis only occurs if there is a perforated abscess or bowel perforation
- **bowel perforation**: causes faecal peritonitis and has a high mortaility; urgent laparotomy, after resuscitation, with a Hartmann's procedure is the only safe treatment
- **pericolic abscess** (ruptured infected diverticulum): identifiable on plain abdominal radiograph, when the bowel wall is more pronounced as it is lined by gas on its interior and exterior surface (**Rigler's sign**); there is a swinging fever and a painful mass and it may burst causing purulent peritonitis, form a fistula or resolve
- **fistula**: these can be colovesical (into the bladder causing pneumaturia or recurrent urinary tract infections), colovaginal or to the abdominal wall
- **massive haemorrhage**: often painless; many patients improve with bed-rest, although blood transfusion and surgical intervention (embolization or colonic resection) may be required
- **inflammatory stricture**: causing obstruction.

Management

Conservative management. Mild attacks can be managed at home with fluids and antibiotics. Attacks are reduced by a high-fibre diet with lots of clear fluids (water), by exercise and by weight loss.

Medical management. Patients with acute diverticulitis need appropriate resuscitation as an emergency if there is sepsis, after which management is surgical or conservative. The patient should be given nil by mouth (bowel rest) with intravenous fluids, antibiotics and analgesia. CT-guided percutaneous drainage of an abscess may avoid emergency surgery. Surgical intervention is indicated for peritonitis, unresolved sepsis or, at a later date, a fistula.

Acute surgical management. A Hartmann's procedure (below) is indicated for a patient with an acute attack who develops peritonitis (perforation). Obstruction or fistulae can usually be managed with a resection and primary anastomosis.

Elective surgery. Resection and primary (immediate) anastomosis is performed for recurrent attacks.

Hartmann's procedure. This is an emergency two-stage procedure (Fig. 3.15.3) used when the bowel is unprepared or peritonitis is present and the risk of infection and anastomosis breakdown is too high for primary anastomosis. Initial resection is followed later by reanastomosis once signs of infection have resolved for ≥ 3 months (temperature, white cell count, erythrocyte sedimentation rate (ESR), C-reactive protein (CRP)). A temporary loop ileostomy or colostomy may be used to protect the colorectal anastomosis (Ch. 16). Note that only 70% proceed to a two-stage procedure because of comorbidity.

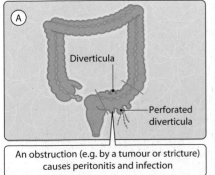

An obstruction (e.g. by a tumour or stricture) causes peritonitis and infection

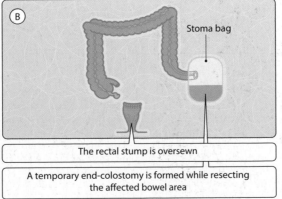

The rectal stump is oversewn

A temporary end-colostomy is formed while resecting the affected bowel area

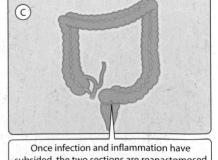

Once infection and inflammation have subsided, the two sections are reanastomosed in some patients, possibly with a covering loop ileostomy

Fig. 3.15.3 Hartmann's procedure. (A) Obstruction from a mass, with peritonitis and infection. (B) The affected bowel is resected and a temporary end-colostomy is formed. The rectal stump is tied off, allowing the bowel to 'rest'. (C) Reanastomosis is performed in a second procedure once infection and inflammation have died down, improving the chance that the anastomosis will not leak and break down.

16. Stomas

Questions
- What are the different types of stoma?
- What are differences between a colostomy and an ileostomy?
- What are the complications of stomas?

A stoma is a surgically created opening in the body between the skin and a hollow viscus (*stoma* is Greek for mouth).

Intestinal stomas

The common abdominal stomas (Fig. 3.16.1) are used to divert faeces outside the body, either from the colon (large bowel; **colostomy**) or from the ileum (small bowel; **ileostomy**), where it is collected in a bag at the skin. The stoma is either *permanent* or *temporary*. The majority of stomas are required after operations for tumours, although they are also used for diverticulitis and inflammatory bowel disease.

In an OSCE station, a student should be able to identify the type of stoma, explaining what features identify it, and the likely operation. If asked to inspect the stoma, the patient should be asked first if the bag contents can be inspected: full faeces, liquid faeces, urine (urostomy).

Colostomy

A colostomy is formed from the large bowel and is usually located in the left iliac fossa (Fig. 3.16.2). Since the large bowel has had time to absorb water from the faeces, the contents are solid. The contents contain fewer enzymes, are more solid and less alkali than ileal contents, are not toxic and will not damage the skin. Consequently, no spout is needed and the colostomy is flat against the skin. Typically one motion per day is passed after breakfast. A high-fibre diet helps to maintain motions.

Permanent end-colostomy. A permanent end-colostomy is used following abdominoperineal resection for low anorectal cancer. The large bowel is brought to the skin and faeces are collected into a bag. Although the surgeon should always attempt to save the anal sphincter, cancers that are < 5 cm from the anal verge mean that the entire rectum must be removed, so normal defecation is no longer possible. The remaining end of the colon is brought to the skin, forming an end-colostomy.

Temporary end-colostomy. A temporary end-colostomy is used during two-stage resections (Hartmann's procedure; Ch. 15) as a means to rest the bowel following a difficult or emergency resection (e.g. acute diverticulitis, obstruction by a tumour). This is identical to a permanent colostomy but it can be removed at a later date and the bowel segments reanastomosed.

Loop colostomy. A loop colostomy is a temporary colostomy to protect distal anastomoses. A **defunctioning loop colostomy** is formed in a position proximal to the anastmosis, commonly in the transverse colon (for a left-sided anastomoses). A loop of bowel is brought to the skin and half opened. This enables faecal matter from the proximal pole to drain into the colostomy, thus preventing faeces reaching the distal anastomoses, without the need for a full colostomy. A supporting rod is used to hold the loop onto the surface of the abdominal wall. When the distal anastomoses have had time to heal, the surgeon can remove the rod and close the loop, simply reverting the bowel to normal. Examples of use are following a difficult left/sigmoid hemicolectomy or an anterior resection (Ch. 16).

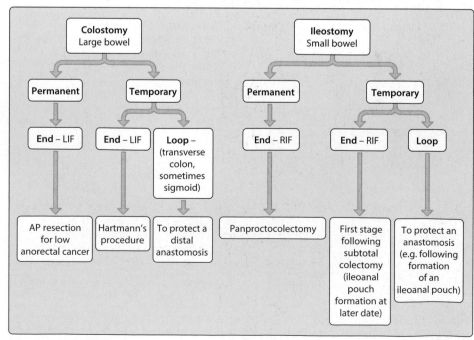

Fig. 3.16.1 Different types of abdominal stoma. RIF, right iliac fossa; LIF, left iliac fossa; AP, abdominoperineal.

Ileostomy

An ileostomy is formed from the small bowel and so is usually located in the right iliac fossa (Fig. 3.16.3). The small bowel does not absorb as much water as the large bowel, so the contents of an ileostomy are more liquid and lighter in colour than for colostomies. The high enzyme contents of the liquid are toxic to the skin and should not come into contact with it. Therefore, a spout is required to allow faecal matter to drain into the bag without damaging the skin. An ileostomy may be permanent, as following a panproctocolectomy (removal of the anus, rectum and colon), or temporary, as in an emergency subtotal colectomy before construction of an ileoanal pouch.

Permanent end-ileostomy. A permanent end-ileostomy is fashioned following **panproctocolectomy** for ulcerative colitis (Ch. 17) or familial adenomatous polyposis. This procedure involves removal of the anorectum and the entire colon to prevent malignancy change. The remaining end of the small bowel is brought to the skin, and a permanent ileostomy formed. Permanent end-ileostomy for ulcerative colitis or familial adenomatous polyposis has become much less common as ileoanal pouch formation is increasing.

Temporary ileostomy (end or loop). The loop ileostomy is very common and is used temporarily to protect a distal anastomosis that might leak. It is closed as a local procedure around the stoma (no laparotomy). An end-ileostomy may be temporary after an emergency bowel resection such as a right hemicolectomy, when it is considered unsafe to perform an anastomosis (sepsis, hypotension, bleeding, steroids, malnutrition). Closure involves a laparotomy to rejoin the bowel ends when the patient is fit and well (6–12 months).

Other types of stoma

Jejunostomy. A tube is inserted into the jejunum to aid feeding in those who cannot feed orally.

Gastrostomy. A tube into the stomach to aid feeding.

Percutaneous endoscopic gastrostomy (PEG). A tube is placed endoscopically to allow feeding directly into the stomach (Fig. 3.16.2).

Urostomy (an ileal conduit). Following cystectomy (removal of the bladder; Ch. 34), an ileal conduit is the preferred method to drain urine (Fig. 3.16.4). Once the bladder has been removed, a small piece of ileum is resected; the ureters are attached to one end and the other end is everted and attached to the skin. The ureters drain urine via the piece of bowel into a stoma bag at the skin. It is sited in the right iliac fossa and is therefore identical to an ileostomy except that the stoma bag drains urine.

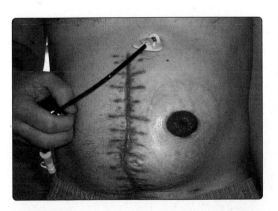

Fig. 3.16.2 A colostomy. It is flat and is in the left iliac fossa. The patient has had repeated laparatomies, leaving a large scar. There is also a percutaneous endoscopic gastrostomy (PEG) tube.

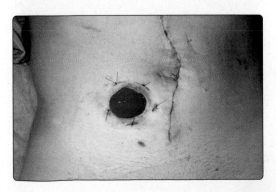

Fig. 3.16.3 An ileostomy. It has a spout and is in the right iliac fossa. It is recently fashioned; notice the sutures and recent laparotomy scar.

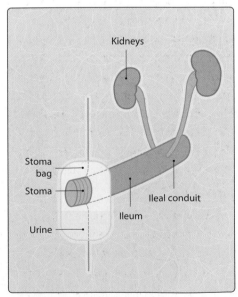

Fig. 3.16.4 An ileal conduit for an urostomy has the external appearance of an ileostomy, but the draining bag contains urine.

17. Ulcerative colitis

Questions
- What are the main pathological features of ulcerative colitis?
- What features would you see on a barium enema?
- What is the main long-term complication and how can you prevent it?

Ulcerative colitis is a chronic relapsing and remitting inflammatory bowel disease that causes inflammation of the **mucosa** and **submucosa** of the large bowel only. It affects both sexes equally and is most common in those aged 20–40 years. The cause of ulcerative colitis is not known, although the following associations exist: genetic (family members have a 10–15% increased risk; association with HLA-B27), environmental/dietary (low-fibre diet, additives, viral or bacterial pathogens), stress (can cause relapses). Smoking is *protective*.

Pathology

Ulcerative colitis *starts in the rectum and extends continuosly proximally,* without leaving normal patches of mucosa. **Pancolitis** affects the whole colon, **proctitis** only the rectum. Rarely it affects the terminal ileum when 'back wash' occurs at the ileocaecal valve (**backwash ileitis**). Infiltration of lymphocytes and neutrophils into the colonic glands (crypts of Lieberkühn) gives rise to crypt abscesses. **Psuedopolyps** are intact islands of normal muscosa. See Fig. 3.18.1 for a comparison with Crohn's disease.

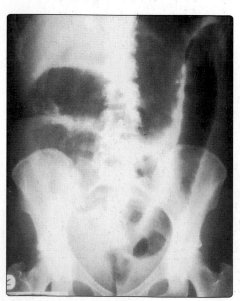

Fig. 3.17.1 Plain radiograph showing toxic megacolon (notice the uneven mucosal surfaces).

Clinical features

Presentation is commonly with a triad of gradual-onset diarrhoea (with blood and mucus), abdominal pain and weight loss.

Early or limited disease. Anaemia, anorexia and crampy lower abdominal pain (relieved by defecation) may be present.

Acute disease. There may be signs of peritonitis, septicaemia, severe bleeding and weight loss; this may be **toxic dilatation** (below).

Extracolonic manifestation of inflammatory bowel disease (HLA-B27 associations): eyes (iritis, conjunctivitis), joints (arthralgia, ankylosing spondylitis, sacroiliitis), skin (pyoderma gangrenosum, erythema nodosum) and liver (chronic active hepatitis, primary sclerosing cholangitis).

Investigations

CRP/ESR. These are inflammatory markers and are good indicators of disease progress. FBC may show microcytic anaemia and increased platelet count.

Barium enema. This will show a **lead pipe colon** (owing to loss of haustrations) and pseudopolyps or complications such as strictures.

Colonoscopy. This is the investigation of choice as it allows for diagnostic biopsy and reveals the extent of disease. Early disease may show an uneven surface because of ulceration and inflammation, with pseudopolyps. Mucosal destruction and a loss of haustrations result in a smooth, narrow colon.

Complications

Toxic dilatation (megacolon). This is a surgical emergency. It occurs when severe inflammation causes gross dilatation of the large bowel (to >8–10 cm), and perforation is imminent. This is a low-pressure dilatation that stretches the bowel wall and compromises blood supply, leading to a loss of mucosal integrity and subsequent perforation. Plain abdominal radiograph (Fig. 3.17.1) is the key investigation (contrast studies would risk perforation). If there is not a prompt response to rehydration, antibiotics and steroids, emergency surgery is required: subtotal colectomy (removal of the affected colon, oversewing of the rectum and temporary ileostomy (Hartmann's procedure, Ch. 15)) prevents imminent perforation. In very sick patients, the rectal stump is brought out to the skin surface as a mucus fistula.

Massive haemorrhage. Rare but transfusion may be required (small, chronic haemorrhage is common).

Malignant change. With early-onset (age < 30 years) or long-standing (> 10 years) disease in patients with total colitis, colorectal adenocarcinoma may develop in 10–20%. Colonoscopy for features of dysplasia every year is advisable, leading up to prophylactic panproctocolectomy for severe dysplasia or early cancer.

Management

Medical management

Most patients are managed medically, unless complications are too severe and require surgical intervention.

Maintenance therapy or mild acute disease. The amino-salicylates (e.g. 5-aminosalicylic acid (mesalazine)) are of great value in maintaining remission. Oral prednisolone can be added for acute attacks and both drugs used as suppositories for acute proctitis.

Severe acute disease. This is defined as 6–20 bloody bowel motions per day, fever, dehydration, electrolyte imbalance, raised CRP/ESR. Hospital admission is required and the patient is treated with 5-aminosalicylic acid, intravenous hydrocortisone ± immunosuppressants (azothioprine ± ciclosporin), and with surgery if no response. Anti-diarrhoeal and anti-cholinergic drugs should not be given as they can precipitate ileus and megacolon. A clinical response—decreasing diarrhoea, pain and bleeding—should occur by day 5; no response is an indication for surgery.

Surgical management

Indications for surgery are acute fulminating colitis that does not respond to medication by day 5; chronic ulcerative colitis uncontrolled by medication; toxic megacolon, perforation or massive haemorrhage or *prophylactic* removal to prevent malignant change.

Panproctocolectomy with permanent end ileostomy. The entire colon, rectum and anus are resected.

Restorative proctocolectomy with ileoanal pouch formation. This is used to avoid permanent ileostomies (particularly in younger patients); the entire colon and rectum are resected, but the anus is left in place (Fig. 3.17.2). The first phase is a subtotal colectomy and temporary end-ileostomy; the rectal stump is oversewn. Phase II occurs once the patient has recovered. The rectum is removed leaving the anus; the ileostomy is taken down and the ileum anastomosed to the anal stump, with formation of an ileoanal pouch. This allows normal stool to be formed and passed. The pouch is often protected with a defunctioning loop ileostomy for 2–3 months, which is later closed. (The ileoanal pouch may be formed in a one-stage operation, especially for young, fit patients.)

Pouches. The main two types of pouch are the J and the W pouches. Inflammation of the pouch (**pouchitis**) is the main complication.

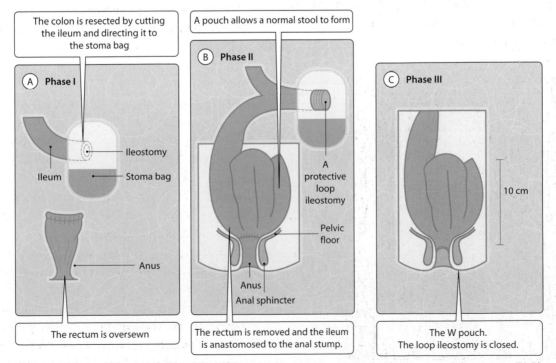

Fig. 3.17.2 Subtotal colectomy with ileoanal pouch formation. (A) Phase I is a subtotal colectomy and ileostomy. (B) Phase II is rectal excision and pouch formation. (C) Pouch formation.

18. Crohn's disease

Questions

- What area is affected by Crohn's disease?
- What are the differences between Crohn's disease and ulcerative colitis?
- What are the features found on small-bowel barium enema?

Crohn's disease is a *chronic transmural inflammatory disease* that can affect *any part of the gastrointestinal tract from mouth to anus*. The incidence is equal in males and females and it typically affects adults aged 20–40 years. It is a transmural process, where inflammation affects the whole thickness of the bowel wall.

Aetiology

The causes of Crohn's disease are unknown, although possible associations are:

- genetic: twin studies have identified the gene *NOD2*
- infection: some current thought implicates a bacterial infection (*Mycobacterium avium paratuberculosis*)
- environmental: cigarette smoking increases risk three times (opposite for ulcerative colitis); diets high in sugar and low in fibre are implicated.

Pathology

The small bowel (terminal ileum) is the most commonly affected site, followed by the perineum (resulting in anal sepsis) and then the colon (**Crohn's colitis**):

- transmural inflammation: may cause fistulae
- skip lesions are common
- mucosal oedema and fibrosis (which follows healing) can cause strictures and then small-bowel obstruction
- non-caseating granulomas are pathognomonic (although not always present).

Figure 3.18.1 shows the distribution and micropathology of Crohn's disease and ulcerative colitis.

Clinical features

Presentation in infants may be as failure to thrive (growth retardation). Features are:

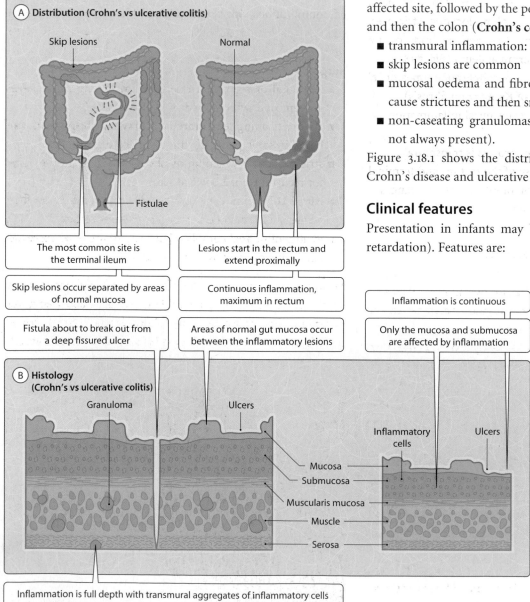

Fig. 3.18.1 Crohn's disease and ulcerative colitis (UC) showing the distribution (A) and the micropathology (B).

- general: triad of recurrent diarrhoea, colicky abdominal pain and weight loss
- acute: pain, diarrhoea, an inflammatory mass in the right iliac fossa
- chronic: clubbing, anal sepsis, mouth ulcers, ill-health, anaemia, wasting (malabsorption with steatorrhoea)
- complications: 5% present with recurrent anal complications (below).

Extracolonic manifestations.   Extracolonic manifestations are similar to those with ulcerative colitis (Ch. 17).

Investigations
Investigations are:

- CRP/ESR: acute-phase proteins are good indicators of disease activity; FBC may show microcytic anaemia
- barium follow-through visualizes the small bowel and a barium enema visualizes the colon, locating strictures, fistulae and disease position; characteristic findings are found especially around the terminal ileum (Fig. 3.18.2):
  — ulceration and oedema giving a 'cobblestone appearance'
  — multiple strictures (**string of Kantor** and fibrosis)
  — rosethorn ulcers caused by transmural inflammation
  — skip lesions
  — fistulae as the inflammation process is transmural
- colonoscopy: allows for biopsy of the rectum and terminal ileum and is good for detection of inflammatory changes
- stool culture to exclude infection.

Complications
The complications of Crohn's disease are:

- small-bowel obstruction by strictures
- abscess adjacent to the bowel caused by panmural disease
- fistulae: enterocutaneous, enterovaginal, enterovesical or enteroenteric (perforation uncommon)
- gallstones from ileal disease or following ileocaecal resection
- anal complications: anal abscess and fistula (present in 15–20% of patients), skin tags, fissure, ulcers and strictures.

Management

Medical management
Most acute exacerbations of disease are managed medically.

Mild disease.   5-Aminosalicylic acid is used, with anti-diarrhoeal drugs if there are no signs of obstruction.

Acute disease.   5-Aminosalicylic acid plus corticosteroids; oral prednisolone is used for symptoms and hydrocortisone enemas for rectal disease.

Extensive/severe acute disease.   This requires hospital admission and treatment with intravenous hydrocortisone and immunosuppressants (azathioprine or ciclosporin). Metronidazole controls active disease and perianal sepsis.

Severe active refractory disease.   Infliximab (suppresses tumour necrosis factor) can be used for disease refractory to steroids and inmmunosuppression, and for refractory intestinal fistulae.

Maintaining remission.   Azathipoprine, methotrexate and infliximab may have a role in maintaining remission (5-aminosalicylic acid is only of use if the colon is affected).

Dietary management
In the acute phase, patients may require total bowel rest. New diets deliver foods (e.g. fatty acids, amino acids and sugars) avoiding complex substances and antigen-related reactions, thus improving recuperation.

Surgical management
Surgery should be as conservative as possible to avoid the metabolic sequelae of extensive small-bowel resection: for relief of complications, for acute colonic disease unresponsive to steroids and for intolerable long-term symptoms and medical side-effects.

Surgery involves:

- ileocaecal or segmental resection: small sections of bowel are removed, with immediate reanastomosis
- a defunctioning temporary ileostomy may help to rest the bowel in some patients with severe acute disease
- stricturoplasty: widening of obstructing strictures, usually for recurrent small bowel disease
- partial colectomy, total colectomy or proctocolectomy may be needed for colonic or recurrent colonic disease
- treatment of anal complications (e.g. drainage of abscesses and laying open of fistulae; see Ch. 20).

Recurrence is common (50% require further surgery 10 years later). **Short bowel syndrome** (diarrhoea, fluid and electrolyte disturbance and malabsorption) follows extensive small-bowel resection and is worsened when the ileocaecal valve is removed.

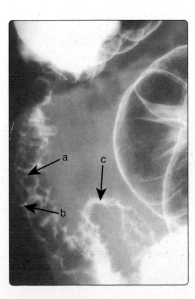

Fig. 3.18.2 Barium follow-through showing the features of Crohn's disease: (a) cobblestone mucosa, (b) rosethorn ulcers and (c) a stricture.

19. Rectal bleeding and rectal conditions

Questions
- What are the causes of rectal bleeding?
- What are the causes of haemorrhoids?
- What management options would you offer a patient with haemorrhoids?

Rectal bleeding

Rectal bleeding is a common presentation; bright red blood is passed around or with the stool or found on the paper.

Clinical features

'Red flag' features are change of bowel habit, weight loss and rectal bleeding. Causes of rectal bleeding (Fig. 3.19.1):

- common
  - haemorrhoids: their presence does not exclude other concurrent causes (e.g. cancer), especially in the elderly
  - rectal polyps: bleeding may be the only symptom
  - anal fissure: painful with bright red blood
  - colorectal polyps and cancer: must be excluded in those over 50 years; rectal cancer presents with bleeding more commonly than colon cancer
- occasional
  - irritable bowel disease (Crohn's disease ulcerative colitis)
  - acute diverticulitis: more common in patients > 60 years
  - trauma (maybe non-accidental injury in children)
- rare
  - blood clotting disorders
  - anal varices (portal hypertension)
  - angiodysplasia: acquired malformation of intestinal blood vessels, often elderly patients
  - intussusception: recurrent like jelly, in infants.

Investigations

Initial investigations include:

- rectal examination: to detect rectal masses; haemorrhoids are not palpable
- FBC: associated anaemia
- protoscopy: to visualize perianal condition
- sigmoidoscopy: to exclude rectal cancer
- colonoscopy: the investigation of choice for diagnosis, biopsy and treatment of rectal bleeding.

Management

Management is initially with ABC principles; the patient may be hypovolaemic and need resuscitation. Patients with chronic stable disease require investigation to establish cause and exclude serious pathology.

Haemorrhoids

Haemorrhoids (piles) are swollen displacements of the venous anal cushions, not varicose veins (Fig. 3.19.2). They are a very common benign condition affecting 50–90% of people at some point, although are uncommon in those < 20 years.

Pathology

Straining to pass hard stools causes the **anal cushions** (three gatherings of anal mucosa and the underlying venous plexus at the 3, 7 and 11 o'clock positions) to slide downwards into the anal canal. When they are torn, they bleed into the rectum, often upon defecation with straining. There is a genetic predisposition. Secondary rare causes include an underlying pathology that blocks venous return, resulting in raised venous pressure and engorging of the venous plexus (e.g. rectal cancer, pregnancy or an enlarged prostate causing straining). Secondary haemorrhoids occur in portal hypertension.

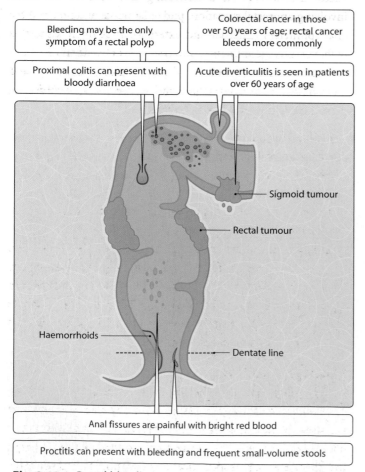

Bleeding may be the only symptom of a rectal polyp

Colorectal cancer in those over 50 years of age; rectal cancer bleeds more commonly

Proximal colitis can present with bloody diarrhoea

Acute diverticulitis is seen in patients over 60 years of age

Sigmoid tumour

Rectal tumour

Haemorrhoids

Dentate line

Anal fissures are painful with bright red blood

Proctitis can present with bleeding and frequent small-volume stools

Fig. 3.19.1 Rectal bleeding.

Clinical features

Haemorrhoids present with:

- rectal bleeding: the most common symptom; the blood should not be mixed with the stool (indicates possible colorectal cancer)
- prolapse: the patient may feel the prolapsed haemorrhoid
- anal irritation (*pruritus ani*) and discomfort
- thrombosed pile: the venous return of a prolapsed external haemorrhoid may become obstructed by the external sphincter, which can lead to thrombosis and strangulation; it is extremely painful and appears purple or black.

Investigations

Investigations are as for rectal bleeding. Internal haemorrhoids cannot be felt as they empty when pressed, and are not painful.

Management

The dentate line is an important landmark in the anal canal mucosa for applying treatments, above which the nervous supply is autonomic and painless, and below which is somatic from spinal neurons and, therefore, very sensitive.

Conservative management is suitable for first- and second-degree haemorrhoids: avoid straining, take a high-fibre diet/plenty of water.

Non-operative treatments are suitable for first- and second-degree haemorrhoids that continue to bleed.

Rubber band ligation.   A rubber band is slipped over a pedicle of mucosa above the haemorrhoid, above the dentate line or severe pain occurs. This causes painless strangulation, and the haemorrhoid drops off painlessly in a few days.

Injection sclerotherapy.   A 5% phenol solution is injected just above each haemorrhoid (above the dentate line).

Infrared coagulation.

Operative treatments are required for only 10% of patients and are suitable for persistently prolapsing third-degree and all fourth-degree haemorrhoids, and when the non-operative treatments fail:

- conventional haemorrhoidectomy: excising the skin and haemorrhoidal tissue at the usual primary sites
- circular stapled haemorrhoidectomy (performed as day-surgery): a circular strip of anal mucosa is excised from above the haemorrhoid, which interrupts the blood supply, reducing the haemorrhoids size and preventing prolapse.

Faecal incontinence

Faecal incontinence is a distressing and complex condition involving anorectal sensation, pudendal nerve function and the anal sphincters (internal and external). It is often associated with urinary incontinence. Internal sphincter damage causes soiling; external sphincter damage causes urgency and neuropathy, poor contraction and sensory loss, resulting in passive incontinence. Causes include:

- traumatic: direct, obstetric or surgical injury
- neurological: stroke, dementia, diabetes
- rectal prolapse (see below)
- faecal impaction
- severe diarrhoea: irritable bowel disease, dysentery
- idiopathic.

Management.   Conservative management is with diet, bulking agents, anti-diarrhoeal drugs, laxatives, pelvic floor exercises and enemas. Surgical management is suitable to repair local sphincter damage. Other procedures include formation of neosphincters and artificial sphincters, and colostomies for intractable problems.

Rectal prolapse

Rectal prolapse can be either complete or incomplete and can occur in the very young or elderly (typically elderly women). It is caused by intussusception of the rectum, chronic straining or poor fascial support to the rectum (starvation, the elderly). Investigations include identification of circumferential prolapse, visualized on straining and protography.

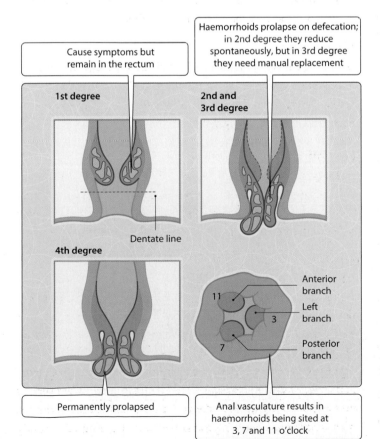

Cause symptoms but remain in the rectum

Haemorrhoids prolapse on defecation; in 2nd degree they reduce spontaneously, but in 3rd degree they need manual replacement

1st degree

2nd and 3rd degree

Dentate line

4th degree

Anterior branch

11

Left branch

3

7

Posterior branch

Permanently prolapsed

Anal vasculature results in haemorrhoids being sited at 3, 7 and 11 o'clock

Fig. 3.19.2 Haemorrhoids occur in the anus not the rectum.

20. Around the anus

Questions
- What are the conditions that affect the perianal region?
- What is the difference between a fistula and a sinus?
- What might you suspect if someone presents with recurrent fistulae and abscesses?

The conditions that occur around the anus are very common but are very distressing for the patient.

Abscesses

Perianal abscesses are common surgical emergencies. They are acute infections of an anal gland, and present with severe perianal pain and swelling, often with a painful mass (Fig. 3.20.1A). A fistula may form after drainage. Initial treatment is with surgical incision and drainage under general anaesthesia. Large abscesses should be packed while granulation tissue fills the defect.

Fistulae

A fistula is an abnormal communication between two epithelial surfaces (Fig. 3.20.1B). It presents as a painful discharging opening onto the skin. **Fistula-in-ano** can be classified by site: intersphincteric (70%; low), transphincteric (25%; low or high), suprasphincteric (5%; high) and extrasphincteric (<1%; supra-levator, high). The fistula may be carefully probed to identify the tract, and MRI provides detail in complicated cases. Fistulae can also be classified by *type,* using the 'surgical sieve' (p. 16):

- congenital: e.g. anorectal agenesis
- acquired:
  — traumatic: postoperative, foreign body
  — autoimmune: sarcoid, AIDS
  — ischaemic: sepsis, radiotherapy
  — inflammatory: Crohn's disease, diverticular disease, ulcerative colitis
  — infective, acute: cryptoglandular (anal gland infection, 90%), hidradenitis suppurativa, Bartholin's sepsis, pilonidal sepsis
  — infective, chronic: tuberculosis, actinomycosis
  — benign neoplasm: e.g. operations for disease such as fibroids
  — primary malignant neoplasm: carcinoma/lymphoma
  — secondary malignant neoplasm: local adenocarcinoma recurrence.

Management

The principles of surgery are to eliminate the fistula, prevent recurrence and preserve sphincter function.

Lay open method. This is the standard method; the fistula track is cut open and allowed to heal with granulation tissue (secondary intention). It is only suitable for simple low fistulae (avoid in women with an anterior fistula).

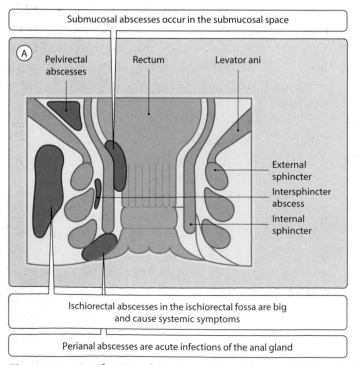

Submucosal abscesses occur in the submucosal space

(A) Pelvirectal abscesses — Rectum — Levator ani — External sphincter — Intersphincter abscess — Internal sphincter

Ischiorectal abscesses in the ischiorectal fossa are big and cause systemic symptoms

Perianal abscesses are acute infections of the anal gland

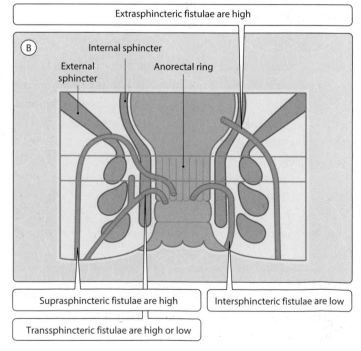

Extrasphincteric fistulae are high

(B) External sphincter — Internal sphincter — Anorectal ring

Suprasphincteric fistulae are high

Transsphincteric fistulae are high or low

Intersphincteric fistulae are low

Fig. 3.20.1 Classification of abscesses (A) and fistulae (B); high fistulae open into the anal canal at or above the anorectal ring.

A Seton suture or flap.   The lay open method may cause incontinence if large portions of the sphincter muscle are divided in a high fistula. The Seton sling passes through the fistula and stays in place. It can be a cutting type that slowly cuts the muscle allowing healing to proceed in stages or it can be a loose type that prevents recurrent sepsis. The fistula can be excised (fistulectomy) and the internal opening closed with an anorectal flap.

Pilonidal sinus

The **difference between a fistula and a sinus** is:

- a fistula is an abnormal communication between two epithelial surfaces
- a sinus is a blind-ending pouch that opens onto an epithelial surface.

Pilonidal sinuses occur when ingrowth of a hair leads to a subcutaneous sinus. They usually occur in the **natal cleft**, at the base of the coccyx (but are also found on the face or between the digits). They most often occur in young, hirsute men and present with pain, swelling and discharge. The two main theories of development are (a) hair penetrating the skin causing a local inflammatory reaction and (b) a developmental abnormality.

Management

Initial management is conservative (analgesia, local dressings and antibiotics) although if this fails, surgical management is indicated. Excision of the sinus and removal of all hair particles and tracts is followed by healing by either secondary (wound left open) or primary (wound closed) intention.

Anal fissure

An anal fissure is a split in the lining of the anal canal. A hard faecal mass tears the mucosa either acutely or chronically, most commonly in the midline of the posterior anal wall. A **sentinel pile** (inside) and a skin tag (outside) is associated with a chronic fissure. The typical presentation is of a young adult with sudden-onset pain after defaecation, and blood on the paper; it also occurs after childbirth. Fear of future defecation often worsens the existing constipation. Rectal examination is often too painful but the fissure can be visualized by gentle parting of the buttocks, which reveals a boat-shaped ulcer with a small skin tag.

Management

Conservative management.   High-fibre diets and stool softeners resolve many acute fissures. Chronic fissures frequently require further treatment:

Chemical sphincterotomy.   Most fissures are now managed medically without the need for surgery, using glyceryl trinitrate or diltiazem creams or botulinum toxin injections.

Surgical management.   Lateral internal sphincterotomy is the operation of choice (the lower fibres of the internal sphincter are divided). **Anal stretch** is uncontrolled and risks damaging the anal sphincters, it should not be performed.

Other conditions

Hidradenitis suppurativa.   This is a form of acne involving the apocrine glands and causing sepsis, sinuses and fistulae around the anus, the groin and axillae. Treatment is with antibiotics and drainage or excision. There are long remissions but recurrence is usual.

Perianal haematoma.   A thrombosed blood vessel of the external venous plexus of the anal mucosa presents with a small, blue spherical lump near the anal margin, which is extremely painful. It is *not* a thrombosed haemorrhoid. Management is either conservative with pain relief, allowing the haematoma to subside, or incision and drainage under anaesthesia.

Anal warts.   Anal warts are caused by the human papilloma virus (HPV), which is sexually transmitted. Topical podophyllin is effective for small numbers of warts, but multiple warts require surgical excision under general anaesthesia. Anal warts predispose to anal cancer.

Anal cancer.   These squamous cell carcinomas of the anus are rare and are associated with HPV infection (some anal warts are precancerous). Males with anoreceptive sex are at higher risk. They present with bleeding, discharge, pain or pruritis ani. Protoscopy with biopsy is diagnostic. Spread is to inguinal lymph nodes, distant metastases occurring in the liver. Chemo- and radiotherapy (mitomycin C, 5-fluorouracil and radiotherapy 50 grays) is first-line treatment, and abdominoperineal resection (Chs 13 and 16) is performed for resistant or recurrent disease. Perianal lesions have a good prognosis and can be treated by local excision. Anal lesions have a poor prognosis and may require salvage abdominoperineal resection.

Recurrent perianal disease.   Patients who present with recurrent perianal sepsis should be investigated for an underlying cause, most commonly Crohn's disease and diabetes mellitus (rarely AIDS, where disease is often severe). Always exclude tuberculosis or malignancy.

Crohn's disease.   See Ch. 18.

21. Varicose veins

Questions
- Which are the main veins that are affected?
- What are the signs and symptoms of varicose veins?
- What treatment options would you offer?

Varicose veins are tortuous dilatation of veins, commonly affecting the lower limbs. They are an extremely common disorder in the Western countries.

Aetiology
Varicose veins are classified as:

- primary: the majority are idiopathic, caused by an underlying primary valve defect
- secondary: only a minority have an underlying cause:
  — pelvic mass occluding venous return (pregnancy, fibroids, ovarian tumour, colorectal cancer, testicular tumour)
  — previous deep vein thrombosis (DVT)
  — arteriovenous fistulae
  — Klippel–Trénaunay syndrome (a venous abnormality giving rise to large varicose veins, port-wine stains and limb overgrowth).

Risk factors include female (×5), age, pregnancy, occupation, obesity, smoking.

Anatomy
There are two venous drainage systems of the lower limb:

- superficial: drains the skin and subcutaneous tissues and is formed from the *long* and *short* **saphenous veins**
- deep: lies within the deep fascia and drains the muscles.

The superficial system drains into the deep system and numerous small **perforator vessels** (*perforating* the deep fascia) connect the two systems. The main points of drainage of the superficial system into the deep system are at the **saphenofemoral** and **saphenopopliteal junctions**. Varicose veins occur commonly in the **long saphenous vein** and less commonly in the **short saphenous vein** (see Ch. 23).

Pathology
Competent valves and the calf muscle pump normally prevent backflow of venous blood (Fig. 3.21.1). **Superficial venous insufficiency** is caused by a failure of the valves in superficial and perforator veins, resulting in venous pooling and **chronic venous hypertension**, which leads to dilatation of the vessels (**varicosities**). **Deep venous insufficiency** occurs when the deep

valves fail (usually secondary to a previous DVT), which may cause backflow into the superficial system and thus varicose veins and swelling of the legs.

Clinical features
The main features are:

- varicosities: dilated, tortuous veins can be seen; these may be the only 'symptom'
- symptoms of heaviness, tension, aching, itching, which occur more commonly after standing; pain is not normally present unless **thrombophlebitis** is present
- saphena varix (Fig. 3.21.2A): dilatation of the saphenofemoral junction; it characteristically disappears on lying down and has a blueish tint (and can be confused with a femoral hernia because of its positive cough impulse).

Complications
Some of the following may occur:

- **thrombophlebitis**: inflammation of a superficial vein caused by venous stasis, causing pain
- **haemorrhage**: may be minor into subcutaneous tissue or major from a saphena varinx at high pressure

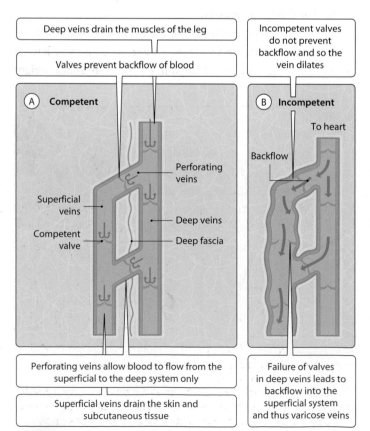

Fig. 3.21.1 Pathology of failing valves.

- **lipodermatosclerosis**: venous pooling causes chronic venous hypertension and leakage of red blood cells, which break down and cause brown **haemosiderin** deposition in the tissues; chronic deposition with fibrosis (caused by fibrin) leads to an inverted 'champagne bottle' shape to the calf (Fig. 3.21.2B).
- **venous ulcers and oedema**: these are chronic signs (see Ch. 28 for venous ulcers)
- **varicose eczema**: itching, scaling and rash, especially around ankles
- **chronic venous insufficiency**: caused by superficial and/or deep venous insufficiency and characterized by the insidious and chronic onset of long-standing varicose veins, ulcers, dependent oedema, lipodermatosclerosis, oedema and leg pain; this is difficult to treat

Investigations

Handheld Doppler ultrasound identifies backward reflux of blood (normally stopped by competent valves, Ch. 22). Colour duplex scan using B mode ultrasound and Doppler ultrasound produces a colour picture illustrating the direction of blood flow (blue forward, red back) and thus the presence of valvular incompetence.

Management

The management principles are to offer the patient *conservative*, *medical* and *surgical* options.

Conservative approaches are suitable for mild symptoms, the elderly, pregnant and unfit, and when deep venous insufficiency is present. Reassurance accompanies education about weight loss, regular walking and avoiding prolonged standing. Graded compression bandaging is used to treat venous ulcers and compression hosiery is used following healing.

Medical management is with **injection scleropathy**, which is mostly useful for small varicosities below the knee. Sclerosant is injected at sites of perforator incompetence in order to produce inflammation, thrombosis and subsequent closure of the vein.

Surgery can be performed under local anaesthesia as a day-case. The vein is identified with Doppler ultrasound and marked clearly with a pen.

Saphenofemoral ligation. The long saphenous vein and its tributaries are ligated and divided as it drains into the femoral vein to reduce recurrence (usually performed together with stripping of the long saphenous vein).

Below knee saphenous vein stripping, 'high, tie and strip'. A wire stripper is passed down the long saphenous vein and is retrieved below the knee. The stripper is tied to the long saphenous vein in the groin and pulled to 'strip out' the vein and incompetent perforators. A truly varicose vein will not be of any use as a conduit for future bypass surgery and can be safely removed.

Multiple avulsions. This technique is suitable for short or below knee saphenous varicose veins. Very small incisions are made along the course of the varicosities, and affected sections are removed. There is a high risk of recurrence when performed alone.

Specific complications of surgery:

- **haemorrhage**: normally, this is venous bleeding and can be controlled with elevation and compression of the limb until the bleeding stops
- **recurrence** < 5% if the saphofemoral junction is meticulously treated, > 20% if treatment is inadequate
- **venous thromboembolism**: a rare but potentially very serious complication
- **neuropraxia**: temporary or permanent injury to the saphenous, sural, popliteal or common peroneal nerves.

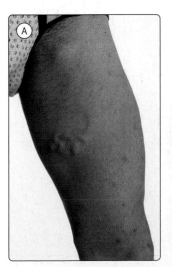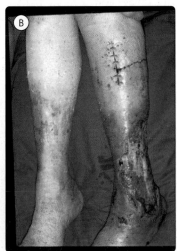

Fig. 3.21.2 (A) A modest varicose vein of the long saphenous vein with a saphena varinx. (B) Chronic venous insufficiency. There is lipodermatosclerosis with an inverted champagne bottle leg. The large venous ulcer is on the lateral side of the gaiter area (although they are more commonly found on the medial side), and there is poor quality, flaky skin.

22. Examination of varicose veins

Questions
■ What is the distribution of varicose veins?
■ What are the signs of chronic venous insufficiency?
■ What pulses would you feel in an arterial examination?

Introduction

The type of examination may not be immediately obvious if an examiner asks a student to 'examine this patient's legs'. The patient may be lying, sitting or standing. Once both the patient's legs are fully exposed, they should be examined for signs of varicose veins and chronic venous insufficiency (below), arterial ulcers and gangrene (Ch. 28), swollen/deformed joints (Charcot's joints; Ch. 28) and wasting (neurological, a medical issue).

Inspection

You may be asked only to make a visual inspection and talk about what you see, and not necessarily touch the limb. For varicose veins, it is necessary to identify *which vein is affected* and where the *level of incompetence* is. Inspect the legs while the patient is standing up with both legs fully exposed. Varicose veins have a dilated, tortuous course and this should be described (Fig. 3.22.1). The **long saphenous vein** is involved in most cases; it runs anterior to the medial malleolus and up the medial aspect of the calf, knee and thigh to drain into the saphenofemoral junction. The **short saphenous vein** is involved less often; it runs from the lateral aspect of the calf and into the popliteal fossa, to drain into the saphenopopliteal junction. Other features (Fig. 3.22.1A) can be remembered by the acronym VVV LAPS: varicose veins, venous ulcers, venous stars, lipodermatosclerosis, atrophy blanche, pitting oedema and scars (both groins and both legs may have scars of previous operations). Patients may have simple and solitary varicose veins, some of the features of chronic venous insufficiency or all of the features (indicating severe disease).

In **chronic venous insufficiency**, these features are long standing and the quality of the limb is poor; often there will be lipodermatosclerosis, varicose veins, ulcers, oedema.

Atrophy blanche are white areas of skin where underlying veins have been lost

Varicose vein

Venous stars are small intradermal dilated veins surrounded by micro-venuoles

Venous ulcers often occur in the medial gaiter area

Lipodermatosclerosis is thickened fibrosed scaly skin, causing an 'inverted champagne bottle' shape to the leg

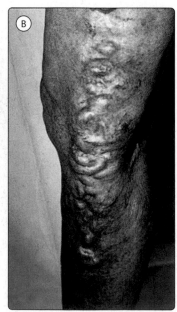

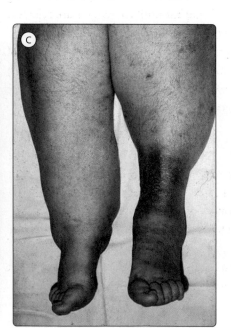

Fig. 3.22.1 Varicose veins. (A) Features; (B) a huge varicose long saphenous vein; (C) brown fibrosed haemosiderin and 'inverted champagne bottle' leg.

Lipodermatosclerosis
There are two phases.

Acute phase. Venous pooling in the varicose veins leads to chronic venous hypertension, forcing red bloods cells into the surrounding tissues. Haemoglobin is broken down into brown haemosiderin.

Chronic phase. Chronic haemosiderin formation leads to fibrin deposition and causes the skin to become thickened and shiny. The skin around the ankle constricts and the inverted champagne-bottle shape is seen (Fig. 3.22.1C).

Palpation

Temperature. Feel the limb with the back of the hand; it should feel warm; if it is cold, arterial disease may coexist.

Palpate the vein. This allows the course to be felt. Ankle tissues are checked for thickening.

Cough impulse. Place three fingers over the saphenofemoral junction. Ask the patient to cough; incompetent valves allow transmission of a *cough impulse* to the junction. Note that if the saphenofemoral junction is affected, it may dilate and show a blueish discolouration: this is a **saphena varinx** and is one of the causes of a groin lump. It has a cough impulse and can be confused with a femoral hernia, which also is seen with a cough impulse.

Trendelenburg test. This assesses the competence of the saphenofemoral junction. The patient lies flat and then the examiner elevates the leg until the varicose vein has emptied. Three fingers are placed over the saphenofemoral junction and the patient stands up.

- if the saphenofemoral junction is incompetent, the long saphenous vein will not fill until the fingers are released, when the vein will fill rapidly
- if the veins below the fingers fill slowly, then there are sites of incompetence below the junction usually in the perforators; this filling is increased by calf muscle contraction when the individual stands on their toes several times.

Percussion

Tap test (Fig. 3.22.2). Place a finger at any point on a varicose vein, and tap the vein proximally (above the finger). Incompetent valves allow transmission of a fluid thrill to the finger below, although this is unreliable.

Direction test. Empty a short section of the vein (place one finger on the vein and slide another finger firmly upwards). If the valves are incompetent, the vein will refill when you release the top finger.

Auscultation

Auscultation over large groups of veins may indicate a bruit (rare; indicating underlying arteriovenous malformation).

Special tests

Doppler ultrasound. Occasionally a Doppler ultrasound may occur as an OSCE station. This technique is used to mark the vein and the level of incompetence (with a black marker pen). The procedure is:
1. Place the Doppler probe (with jelly) on the vein at the ankle, and then switch it on
2. Squeeze the calf: blood is heard pulsing past the probe
3. Release the calf; if the valves are incompetent, the blood is heard refluxing back down past the probe
4. Repeat moving up the vein until no reflux is heard; this is the point of incompetence.

Tourniquet test. A student is unlikely to be asked to perform the tourniquet test, which assesses for incompetent perforators veins. The leg is elevated and emptied and a tourniquet is placed below the saphenopopliteal junction. The patient then stands up. If the veins fill, then the incompetence is below the point of the tourniquet. It is repeated with the tourniquet lower until veins stop filling; this is the level of incompetence.

Concluding the examination

In an OSCE, the student should state which vein is affected and whether there are signs of chronic venous insufficiency and that examination for secondary causes of varicose veins (abdomen with rectal, vaginal/testicular examination to exclude a mass that is obstructing venous return) should follow.

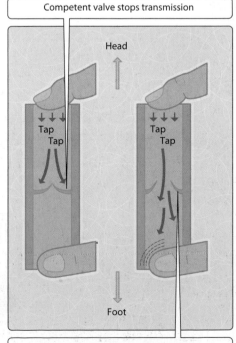

Fig. 3.22.2 The tap test.

23. Peripheral vascular disease

Questions
- Define intermittent claudication, and critical limb ischaemia
- What treatments are appropriate for intermittent claudication?
- What surgical options exist for critical limb ischaemia?

Peripheral vascular disease (PVD) occurs when there is narrowing of the arteries. It is almost always caused by atherosclerosis but may occur secondary to thromboembolism or inflammation (Fig. 3.23.1). Overall mortality after a diagnosis of PVD is 30% at 5 years and 70% after 15 years. Coronary heart disease is the major cause of death in people with PVD of the legs.

Aetiology

Risk factors should be elicited from the history:

- the four factors with strong association: hypertension, hyperlipidaemia, diabetes and smoking
- the three factors with weak association: stress, obesity and lack of exercise
- male sex
- age: particularly over 50 years.

Clinical features

Pain is the most prominent feature: claudication, rest pain, night pain, abdominal and back pain.

Intermittent claudication

Intermittent claudication (Fig. 3.23.2) is a *cramp-like* pain that occurs in a *group of muscles* upon exercise and is relieved by rest. The **superficial femoral artery** is most commonly affected where it passes through the **adductor hiatus** to become the **popliteal artery**. Stenosis or occlusion at this level may manifest as calf claudication. The **absolute claudication distance** is the distance of walking before the pain starts. Symptoms are stable in most patients for 5 to 10 years but are progressive in 15% and result in critical limb ischaemia.

Critical limb ischaemia

Critical limb ischaemia is rest pain, ulceration and/or gangrene that has been present for 2 weeks or more and requires strong analgesia. The pain is worse at night as lying flat distributes blood away from the legs and sleeping decreases blood pressure; pain progressively worsens. Disease is usually multilevel and tissue ischaemia leads to arterial ulcers and gangrene (p. 8). Pulses are rarely present, the peripheries are cold and Buerger's test is positive (Ch. 24). There is reduced sensation and movement in the foot, caused by ischaemia of the nerves, and calf or forefoot tenderness may also be present. The leg may be lost without intervention (70% require surgery). Table 3.23.1 shows how the level of disease affects the symptoms.

Investigations

Bloods. Measurements include FBC (anaemia, polycythaemia), ESR/CRP (underlying inflammatory disease), U&E (renal impairment), glucose (diabetes), cholesterol.

Ankle brachial pressure index. A pressure cuff is inflated around the limb above the malleoli and a Doppler probe used to measure the occlusion pressure in all three calf vessels (posterior tibial, dorsalis pedis and peroneal arteries) at the ankle and in the brachial artery (arm). In diabetics, arterial calcification gives an artificially high pressure. The ankle pressure is divided by the brachial pressure to give an index: normal, ≥ 1, intermittent claudication, < 0.9 and critical limb ischaemia, < 0.5.

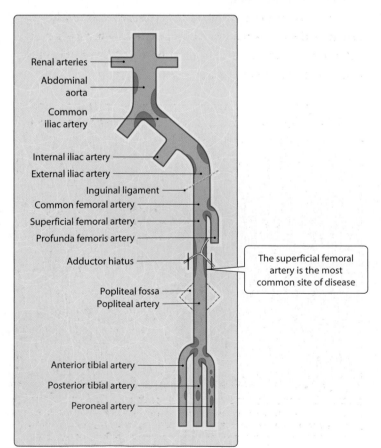

Renal arteries
Abdominal aorta
Common iliac artery
Internal iliac artery
External iliac artery
Inguinal ligament
Common femoral artery
Superficial femoral artery
Profunda femoris artery
Adductor hiatus

The superficial femoral artery is the most common site of disease

Popliteal fossa
Popliteal artery

Anterior tibial artery
Posterior tibial artery
Peroneal artery

Fig. 3.23.1 The anatomy of the lower limb vascular tree with the common sites of disease.

Duplex scan. This is a non-invasive test that demonstrates increased flow velocity at sites of stenosis.

Digital subtraction angiography. This is performed when surgical or endovascular intervention is planned.

Management

Conservative measures include stopping smoking immediately, exercise, weight loss, management of hypertension and cholesterol, diabetic management, aspirin (75 mg once daily) and pain relief. With conservative measures alone for intermittent claudication, one-third improve, one-third remain the same and one-third require further treatment. Conservative measures are the only measure in 10% of patients with critical limb ischaemia, although they should be instigated in all patients undergoing surgery. **Surgical management** depends on the disease and the history.

In **percutaneous transluminal angioplasty**, a catheter is passed into the femoral artery at the groin and then under radiograph guidance to the area affected. A balloon is inflated to dilate the diseased segment and a metal intraluminal stent may be placed. This is suitable for **stenosis** or **short occlusions** and best for iliac and superficial femoral vessels. Consequently, it is good for intermittent claudication.

Bypass surgery is best for **multilevel disease** and **long occlusions**, where the affected segment is bypassed using a synthetic graft or the long saphenous vein. The type of bypass depends on the level of obstruction (Fig. 3.23.3). Indications are rest pain and life-limiting intermittent claudication

Table 3.23.1 SYMPTOMS AND THE LEVEL OF DISEASE

Level of disease	Pulses	Symptomatic area
Aortoiliac	Bilateral loss of femoral, popliteal and foot pulses	Buttock, thigh, calf, foot; Leriche's syndrome (buttock pain and impotence)
Common iliac	Unilateral loss of femoral, popliteal and foot pulses	Buttock, thigh, calf, foot
Superficial femoral artery	Unilateral loss of popliteal and foot pulses	Calf

(uncommon). There are three types of bypass used. The **arterobifemoral bypass** for aorto-iliac artery disease is performed with a prosthetic 'trouser' graft (polyester dacron). Long-term patency exceeds 90%, but mortality is up to 5%. Complications include myocardial infarction, chest infection, renal failure, bowel ischaemia, graft infection and postoperative impotence. The **femoropopliteal bypass** for femoropopliteal artery disease uses the long saphenous vein, polyester or gortex grafts. The **femorodistal graft** for infrapopliteal artery disease uses the saphenous vein.

Unreconstructable PVD, fixed flexion deformities or extensive tissue loss require a major **amputation**, which is the definitive treatment in 10% of patients (PVD is the most common cause of amputation).

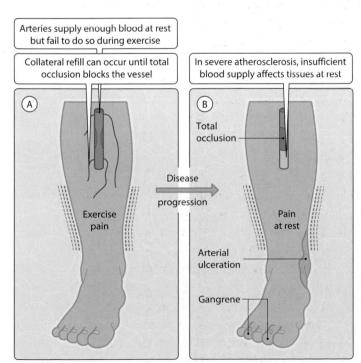

Fig. 3.23.2 Symptoms of intermittent claudication (A) and critical limb ischaemia (B).

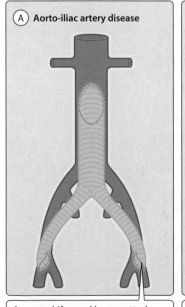
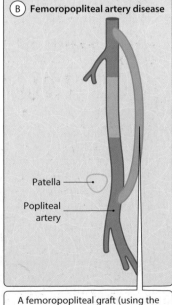
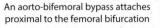

Fig. 3.23.3 Bypass surgery. (A) Arterobifemoral bypass. (B) Femoropopliteal bypass.

24. The peripheral vascular system: examination of pulses

Questions
- Which pulses would you feel?
- What is Buerger's test?
- If the popliteal and foot pulses are absent on the left side only, where is the occlusion?

An OSCE might comprise intermittent claudication, critical limb ischaemia, abdominal aortic aneurysm, postoperative patient (abdominal aortic aneurysm repair (laparotomy) or bypass graft), amputation, diabetic foot or ulcer.

Introduction

For examining the leg pulses, the patient should be lying flat, both legs fully exposed. It is essential to ask if the patient is in pain (this provides a clue to the presence of critical limb ischaemia).

Look

A number of features can be identified just by looking from the end of the bed:

- trophic changes: thin poor shiny skin, hair loss, gangrene, ulcers
- colour: the legs are pale (pallor)
- pressure points: look at the toes and then specifically between the toes and underneath the heel for gangrene and arterial ulcers
  — gangrene: black tissue, often starting at the tips of the toes; *dry* gangrene is non-infected and *wet* gangrene is infected
  — ulcers: arterial ulcers are found on the toes and forefoot; they are 'punched out' and painful (Ch. 28)
- scars: into the groins: these are evidence of previous bypass surgery; a laparotomy may indicate abdominal aortic surgery (grafting)
- an epigastric pulsation may indicate an abdominal aortic aneurysm (this pulsation may be normal!)
- patients may prefer to sit with their legs hanging over the side of the bed: in critical limb ischaemia, this improves the arterial blood flow with the aid of gravity
- amputation: peripheral vascular disease is the most common cause of amputation; the amputation may be above or below the knee
- any signs of infection or contractures in amputees.

Feel

Always ask if there is any pain or tenderness first:

- temperature: the limb may be cold; note the level of a temperature change
- sensation: ask the patient if there is any change in sensation (associated diabetic neuropathy)
- capillary refill time: press the big toenail for 2 seconds until it turns white; the capillaries should refill within 2 seconds (prolonged with arterial disease)
- pulses: assessing the pulses is the *main* part of the examination.

Pulses

In an OSCE, you may be asked to examine all the pulses (1–6), the abdominal and leg pulses (2–6), or the leg pulses only (3–6). The pulses that can be felt give an indication of the level of disease (Table 3.23.1).

1. Start by examining the **radial**, **brachial** and **carotid pulses**.
2. The **abdominal aorta** is examined by placing the hands on opposite sides of the abdomen and palpating inwards with the fingertips (like kneading bread). An expansile, pulsatile, abdominal mass indicates an abdominal aortic aneurysm. The size can be estimated by the distance between your fingers (less 1 cm for skin and fat, adjusting for the patient's size); this should correspond with the angiogram.
3. The **femoral pulse** is below the mid-inguinal point (half way between the pubic symphysis (*not* tubercle) and the anterior superior iliac spines (ASIS); Fig. 3.24.1). Make sure you know the difference between the mid-inguinal point and the mid-point of the inguinal *ligament*.

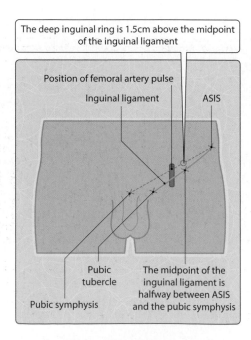

The deep inguinal ring is 1.5cm above the midpoint of the inguinal ligament

Position of femoral artery pulse

Inguinal ligament

ASIS

Pubic tubercle

Pubic symphysis

The midpoint of the inguinal ligament is halfway between ASIS and the pubic symphysis

Fig. 3.24.1 The landmarks of the femoral artery pulse and deep inguinal ring. ASIS, anterior superior iliac spine.

4. To measure the **popliteal pulse**, the patient's knee is flexed to 30% and the weight of the limb is taken in the clinician's hands with the thumbs placed on the tibial tubersosities and the fingertips of both hands on the midline of the back of the knee, slightly below the popliteal fossa. Gently pressing the artery against the head of the tibia enables the pulsating artery to be felt. The popliteal pulse may be difficult to feel in normal individuals; if it is obvious there is a popliteal aneurysm. Little time should be wasted on this in an OSCE before moving on to the pedal pulses: if these are present then the popliteal must also be there. If the pedal pulses are absent then you need to show that you have tried to find a popliteal pulse.

5. The **posterior tibial pulse** can be felt 1.5 cm posterior and 1.5 cm inferior to the medial malleolus. Stand at the end of the bed and feel both together.

6. The **dorsalis pedis pulse** is felt lateral to the ligament of the extensor hallucis longus.

Auscultation for bruits over the abdominal aorta and femoral vessels can be left until the end. In an OSCE, you should also offer to auscultate the carotid and popliteal arteries.

Move

Buerger's angle and **Buerger's test** (the sunset sign; Fig. 3.24.2) is used to gauge the presence of critical limb ischaemia. A positive test is when the limb changes colour; a normal limb will not change colour throughout the test.

1. With the patient lying flat, the examiner elevates the patient's leg until the blood drains. Low arterial pressure will not be able to overcome gravity and **pallor** and **venous guttering** will occur.

2. The angle at which the blood has drained is called Buerger's angle; the lower the angle the worse the disease state (measure between the sternum and the heel).

3. If the patient sits up quickly, with their legs hanging over the side of the bed, the blood will quickly refill the feet with a marbled deep red appearance; this is called **reactive hyperaemia**. This is called Buerger's sunset sign because of the deep red colour and the fact the leg is cool to touch.

Arteriogram

The appearance of an arteriogram (Fig. 3.24.3) is predicatable from feeling the pulses; additionally, examining the arteriogram first will allow prediction of which pulses will be absent.

Concluding the examination

It should be possible now to state at which level the arterial blockage is occurring. An examination should proceed to examine the other pulses, the cardiovascular system, the ankle brachial pressure index and to obtain a duplex scan.

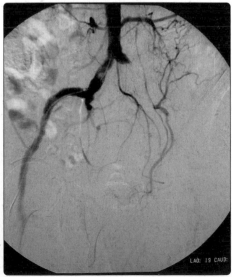

Fig. 3.24.3 Arteriogram showing occlusion of the left common iliac artery. Absent pulses in an examination would be the femoral, popliteal, and foot pulses on the left side.

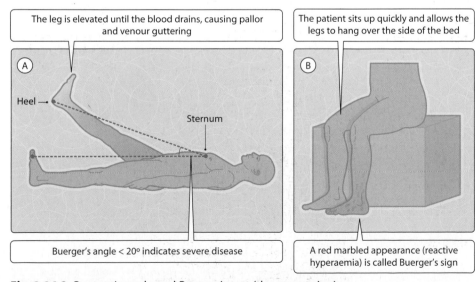

The leg is elevated until the blood drains, causing pallor and venour guttering

Heel →

Sternum

Buerger's angle < 20º indicates severe disease

The patient sits up quickly and allows the legs to hang over the side of the bed

A red marbled appearance (reactive hyperaemia) is called Buerger's sign

Fig. 3.24.2 Buerger's angle and Buerger's test (the sunset sign).

25. Aneurysms

Questions
- What are the different types of aneurysm?
- How is a patient with a ruptured abdominal aortic aneurysm initially managed?
- What are the complications of elective abdominal aortic aneurysm repair?

Aneurysms are permanent, localized dilatations in an arterial wall. They commonly occur in the abdominal aorta and popliteal arteries and are most common in males over 65 years (Fig. 3.25.1).

Aetiology

The most common cause is **atherosclerosis**. Other causes are connective tissue disorders (Marfan's syndrome, Ehler–Danlos syndrome), congenital (Berry aneurysms in the circle of Willis), or infective (e.g. syphilis; now rare).

◼ ABDOMINAL AORTIC ANEURYSM

Clinical features

Abdominal aortic aneurysms may present either as an asymptomatic pulsatile abdominal mass diagnosed incidentally or as an emergency with pain, distal embolization or rupture. Over 90% are **infrarenal**, which means surgical repair is easier;

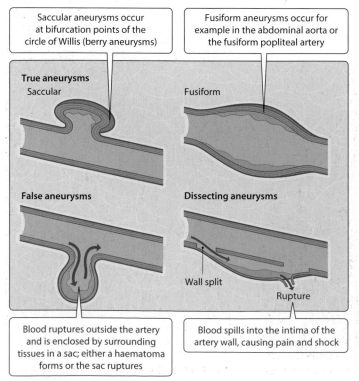

those above or involving the renal arteries are much more difficult to repair and have higher mortality.

Acute presentation:

- ruptured abdominal aortic aneurysm: pain is the most common symptom, which may be abdominal (with guarding) or sudden-onset back pain
- patients may collapse and be hypotensive with a tachycardia
- an acutely ischaemic limb: the aneurysm may 'spit out' emboli that block distal leg arteries (Ch. 23).

Non-acute presentation occurs in asymptomatic patients (e.g. during ultrasound scan or plain radiograph (showing calcification in the aortic wall) performed for another reason) or as a complaint of a mildly bloated abdomen, back pain or pulsation.

Investigations

Examination to detect an abdominal aortic aneurysm is described in Ch. 6. **Ultrasound** shows its diameter and should be repeated at regular intervals to monitor growth if it is below the threshold for repair (< 5.5cm). The use of ultrasound in screening for abdominal aortic aneurysm is currently being assessed. CT is performed preoperatively to check for renal artery involvement and assess suitability for endovascular repair (Fig. 3.25.2). In an emergency presentation, the only investigations that are performed preoperatively are FBC, clotting studies, cross-matching for 6–8 units of blood and electrocardiograph. If the patient is stable with back pain, there may be time for CT.

Management

Elective surgery is undertaken in the fit patient to prevent rupture for aneurysms > 5.5 cm in diameter, for those which are growing faster than 1 cm/year or if symptomatic (pain or emboli). Mortality associated with elective surgery is approximately 5%.

Emergency management of a ruptured abdominal aortic aneurysm

Initial management is ABC with oxygen, intravenous access (two large-bore cannulae in two large arm veins) and careful fluid management.

Fluid management. A haematoma may have formed around the aorta, and increasing the patient's blood pressure may dislodge it, causing the patient to bleed to death. Therefore, the patient's systolic blood pressure should be maintained carefully at or below 100 mmHg.

Fig. 3.25.1 Classification of aneurysms.

Surgery. The patient should be taken to theatre immediately where a conventional aneurysm repair is used (Fig. 3.25.3): 50% of those with a rupture reach hospital, and 50% of these patients survive emergency repair (overall mortality is 75–85%).

1. the patient is given intravenous heparin for anticoagulation
2. The aorta is cross-clamped above the aneurysm; the limbs are supplied by collateral (alternative) arteries
3. The aneurysm is cut open and the thrombus removed
4. A dacron graft is sewn inside the aorta, and the clamp removed to check for leaks
5. The rest of the aorta wall is sewn around the dacron graft.

In selected patients, an endovascular option exists, where the stent is placed within the aneurysm via the femoral artery. The complications are described on p. 8.

■ OTHER ANEURYSMS

If one aneurysm is found, the rest of the peripheral vascular system should be carefully examined to identify others.

Popliteal aneurysms. These are the second most common and often bilateral. They may cause distal emboli, or may thrombose, presenting as an acutely ischaemic limb. If asymptomatic but > 3 cm in diameter, some advocate repair with a bypass graft.

Thoracic aortic aneurysms. These may be of the aortic arch or the ascending or descending thoracic aorta. They may present as chest pain, back pain, aorto-oesophageal fistula (with lethal haematemesis), obstruction of the superior vena cava or recurrent laryngeal nerve and tracheal compression. Assessment is with chest radiograph, CT and transoesophageal echocardiography. Under cardiac bypass, the aneurysm is partially excised and a synthetic graft inserted. These aneurysms may dissect (blood splits the intima of the artery wall), causing severe chest and upper back pain, and severe shock. Mortality is high and emergency surgery is required. Traumatic damage to the thoracic aorta by high-energy trauma is immediately life-threatening, requiring urgent surgery.

Femoral aneurysm. One cause of a groin lump (Ch. 33).

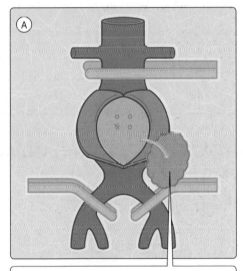

The aneurysm is opened, the thrombus removed and the lumbar arteries are oversewn

The clamps are loosened to check for leaks *before* final closure of the aorta

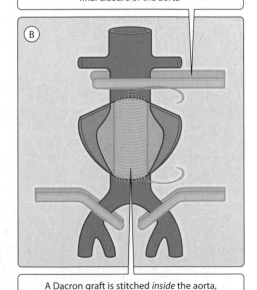

A Dacron graft is stitched *inside* the aorta, proximal anastomosis first

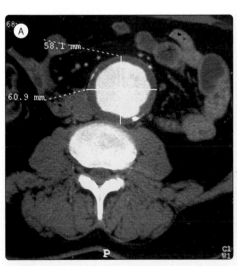 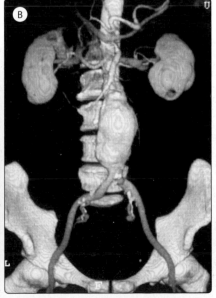

Fig. 3.25.2 An infrarenal abdominal aortic aneurysm, shown on conventional CT scan (A), and on three-dimensional CT reconstruction (B).

Fig. 3.25.3 The repair procedure for an abdominal aortic aneurysm.

26. The carotid artery and upper limb vascular diseases

Questions
■ How may carotid artery disease present?
■ What are the indications for surgery in carotid artery disease?
■ What is Raynaud's phenomenon?

Carotid artery disease

Disease of the carotid arteries is a common cause of stroke. It is caused by atherosclerosis of the carotid artery, most commonly at its bifurcation (Fig. 3.26.1).

Pathology

Atherosclerosis occurs most commonly at the carotid artery bifurcation. A subsequent embolism from the plaque (atheroma) leads to carotid territory ischaemia. Global ischaemia caused by hypoperfusion may occur if there is severe bilateral carotid stenosis and disease of the vertebral arteries.

Clinical features

Main features are shown in Fig. 3.26.1B, C.

Investigations

Initial investigations are blood pressure, glucose, cholesterol, cross-match for blood. This is followed by duplex scan to show degree of stenosis, angiography (confirms duplex findings and defines arterial anatomy) and CT/MRI (identifies cerebral infarcts).

Management

Conservative and medical management. This approach is suitable for asymptomatic patients with less than 70% stenosis: stop smoking, take aspirin and statin and control hypertension.

Surgical management. **Carotid endarterectomy** is used for stenosis > 70% and for symptomatic disease with any degree of stenosis. The carotid artery is opened and thrombus and diseased intima removed (often using a temporary shunt to bypass the operative field and maintain cerebral perfusion). A patch graft (e.g. from a forearm vein) is placed. Stroke and mortality rate should be < 5%. The risk of stroke with surgery and best medical therapy is considerably less than with best medical therapy alone.

Raynaud's phenomenon

Raynaud's phenomenon is cold-induced spasm of the arterioles, most commonly of the hands but also the feet. The primary condition, **Raynaud's disease**, is a benign condition and almost

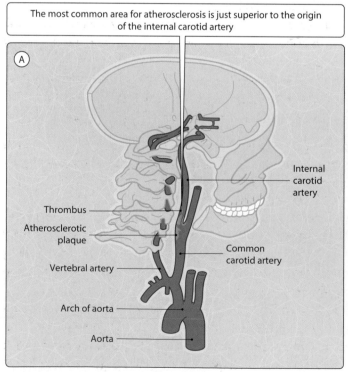

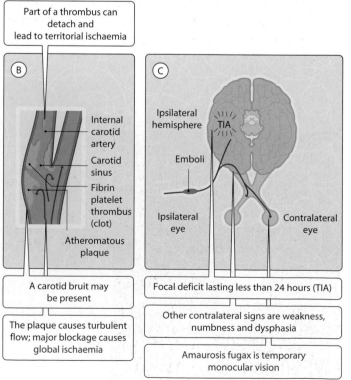

Fig. 3.26.1 Carotid artery disease. (A) Stenosis of the carotid artery from atheroma and an associated thrombus; (B) stenosis can lead to clots breaking off from the thrombus; (C) symptoms. TIA, transient ischaemic attack.

always affects females. The secondary condition **Raynaud's syndrome**, is associated with an underlying disease process; symptoms are often more severe and tissue damage may occur.

Pathology

Vasospasm causes typical colour changes of the digits. Raynaud's disease affects up to 5% of young females, and is precipitated by cold and relieved by warmth. It is usually bilateral and does not lead to any tissue damage. Causes include connective tissue diseases (scleroderma/CREST (<u>c</u>alcinosis, <u>R</u>aynaud's phenomenon, (o)<u>e</u>sophageal dysmotility, <u>s</u>clerodactyly, <u>t</u>elangectasias), polyarteritis nodosa), cervical rib, rheumatoid arthritis and atherosclerosis.

Clinical features

The colour changes in Raynaud's phenomenon are:

- white: as blood supply is interrupted to the digits
- blue: as cyanosis occurs because of the reduced blood flow.
- red: vasospasm relaxes and blood reenters the digits; this reactive hyperaemia causes a red colouration.

Management

Conservative management. The effects of cold are reduced by using gloves and hand-held heat packs. Stopping smoking is essential.

Medical management. Nifedipine (a calcium channel antagonist) prevents vasospasm and may be used as maintenance therapy in those severely affected. Iloprost infusion (synthetic prostacyclin analogue) can improve circulation, relieve pain and quicken ulcer healing in severe Raynaud's syndrome.

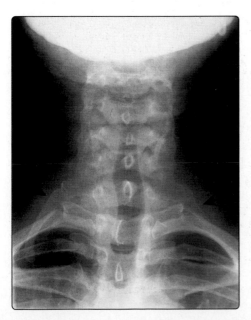

Fig. 3.26.2 Bilateral cervical ribs. These ribs compress the subclavian artery between themselves and the first rib and are also causing deviation of the trachea.

Surgical management. Surgical intervention is uncommon for Raynaud's disease. For Raynaud's syndrome, the underlying pathology is treated and digital amputation may be required. **Thoracoscopic cervical sympathectomy** (cutting the sympathetic nerve supply to the fingers to prevent the vasospasm) may improve symptoms but is not long lasting and is rarely used.

Thoracic outlet syndrome

Thoracic outlet syndrome is caused by compression of the subclavian artery, vein or brachial plexus as they pass through the narrow gap between the thoracic outlet and the first rib. The most common cause is a cervical rib, although other causes include a healed fractured first rib or muscle occlusion/adhesions (salenus anterior). It may present as a combination of neurological and vascular symptoms (as below).

A **cervical rib** is an extra rib that is present above the first rib (Fig. 3.26.2) and so it can compress and damage the subclavian artery, giving rise to cervical rib syndrome. There is stenosis of the subclavian artery at the site of occlusion, with a poststenotic dilatation that behaves like an aneurysm, with luminal thrombus that may break off to form emboli in the upper limb. Clinical features are:

- vascular signs: exercise pain leading to rest pain; the pulse increases when the arm is raised, and the radial pulse on the affected side may disappear on abduction and external rotation of the shoulder, which increases the angle between the neck and shoulder
- neurological signs: pain, tingling in a dermatome of the brachial plexus, weakness in the muscle group supplied by the brachial plexus
- multiple emboli: emboli to the distal circulation of the upper limb may cause acute ischaemia
- a rib in the supraclavicular fossa may be palpable.

Treatment is initially conservative with exercise regimens, but if these fail surgery to excise the cervical and first rib is indicated.

Buerger's disease

Buerger's disease (thromboangitis obliterans) is an aggressive inflammatory disease of the small and medium-sized arteries and veins of the hands and feet. It almost always affects young men who are heavy smokers. Its symptoms are similar to peripheral vascular disease, usually affecting the hands and fingers. Both veins and arteries become inflamed, and rapid claudication, critical ischaemia and/or ischaemic ulcers occur. Smoking must be completely stopped; analgesia and prevention of foot damage are important. Surgery is largely ineffective.

27. The acute limb

Questions
■ What are the key signs of an acute ischaemic limb?
■ How may a deep vein thrombosis present?
■ How is cellulitis treated?

An acutely painful limb is a common presentation to many specialties, especially to general practice and casualty.

The acute ischaemic limb

Sudden blockage of an artery by an embolus or thrombus causes acute ischaemia, with rapid tissue death (**necrosis**). This is a surgical emergency. A **thrombus** is a clot that forms locally (in situ), usually on a plaque of atheroma, and occludes a vessel; an **embolus** is a clot that has broken from a proximal source (e.g. an aneurysm) and occludes a distal vessel.

Aetiology

The disease may be *acute* in a previously asymptomatic individual, or *acute-on-chronic* where the patient has evidence of previous peripheral vascular disease (PVD). Sources of blockage (Fig. 2.27.1) are:

■ embolus: most commonly from the left atrium in atrial fibrillation or the left ventricle in postinfarct thrombus or aneurysm (90% of all emboli), but also from an aortic aneurysm, proximal arterial disease or in intravenous drug abusers
■ thrombosis: of a peripheral aneurysm, atheromatous plaque or a previous surgical graft; may also occur in a hypotensive patient or a patient with thrombophilia
■ dissection: aortic dissection may present with limb-threatening ischaemia.

Clinical features

This is a surgical emergency and characterized by the '6Ps' (Fig. 3.27.1).

Emboli may also travel to other sites, possibly causing stroke (**cerebral artery**), amaurosis fugax (**retinal artery**), pulmonary embolism (lungs), mesenteric ischaemia (**mesenteric artery**) or loin pain (**renal artery**).

Management

The definitive treatment is to revascularize the limb, normally with urgent surgery. If time permits, an arteriogram is useful before surgery.

Initial **medical management** treatment is with analgesia (opiate with an anti-emetic), aspirin and anticoagulation (5000 U intravenous heparin initially, warfarin in the long term). Thrombolysis with streptokinase or tissue plasminogen activator (t-PA) may revascularize a threatened limb if used early (12–24 h).

Surgical management
Embolectomy. Revascularization is possible if the affected artery is exposed and the embolus is removed using a Fogarty balloon catheter.
Bypass surgery. This may be required in those with acute-on-chronic ischaemia.
Amputation. This is needed if ischaemia has been prolonged and the limb is considered to be non-viable (Fig. 3.27.2). The lower limb requires amputation more often than an upper limb. Other general indications for limb amputation are trauma (e.g. after an accident), gangrene (in severe PVD (with relentless critical limb ischaemia or gangrene), often with coexisting diabetes; p. 9), when necrosis sets in or for bone tumours (e.g. osteosarcoma) where clear margins and limb salvage cannot be achieved.

Complications of surgery
Reperfusion injury. If the limb has been ischaemic for some time (> 24 h), there may be significant areas of necrosis

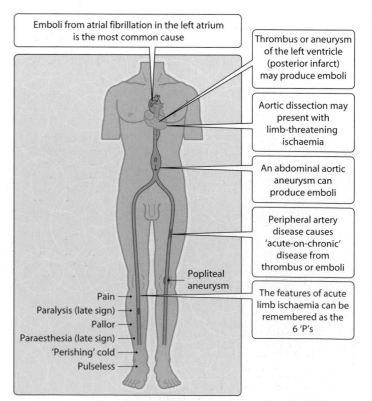

Fig. 3.27.1 Sources and clinical features of an acute ischaemic limb.

(rhabdomyonecrosis). Reperfusion may lead to sudden release of 'toxins' into the systemic circulation, which cause massive cardiovascular collapse, renal failure, acute respiratory distress syndrome (ARDS) and subsequent death. If large areas of necrosis are identified, amputation may be a life-saving alternative.

Compartment syndrome. Following reperfusion, compartment syndrome may develop (Ch. 52).

Prognosis

Limb salvage techniques are suitable for 80% of patients, the remainder will require amputation or palliative care. The overall mortality is high, at 20–30%.

Deep vein thrombosis

Deep venous thrombosis (DVT) affects the deep veins in the lower leg and the thigh. **Virchow's triad of clotting** predispose to thrombus formation:

- **venous stasis**: injury or inflammation, air travel
- **endothelial damage**: surgery, malignancy, trauma
- **raised clotting factors**: malignancy, congenital disease, drugs, thrombogenic state.

The **risk factors** are obesity, age, smoking, female sex, family history, previous DVT and cooccurring conditions (pregnancy or pelvic tumour (causing venous stasis), malignancy,

pelvic/lower limb orthopaedic surgery or thromboembolic disease (e.g. hypercoagulability)).

Clinical features. DVT often presents with sudden-onset of pain, calf tenderness, swelling, redness and tight skin. The superficial veins may be engorged, and there may be a low-grade pyrexia. There is variable oedema in and below the calf and Homan's sign my be positive. Some patients are asymptomatic and collapse from a pulmonary embolism.

Investigations. Clotting should be assessed and a duplex scan should be performed to identify the thrombosis. A patient with shortness of breath that suggests a pulmonary embolism should be checked for a DVT in the calf.

Management. Low-molecular-weight heparin (LMWII) is initially used; this is subsequently converted to warfarin therapy. Warfarin is continued for 3–6 months after a first DVT but is needed lifelong after a second. Measures to prevent DVT are outlined on p. 3.

Cellulitis

Cellulitis is an inflammatory reaction usually to a bacterial infection of the skin and underlying soft tissues, most often caused by *Streptococcus pyogenes* or *Staphylococcus aureus*. It occurs more often in those with diabetes (increased susceptibility to infection), existing PVD or venous disease, or it may arise spontaneously. Cellulitis may be caused by insect or animal bites or local trauma that has been secondarily infected.

It commonly presents with the four signs of swelling: heat, redness, swelling and pain. In more advanced disease (particularly in the immunosuppressed or elderly), systemic infection with fever and malaise may occur. A diffusely red and swollen area is visible. When affecting the legs, it is usually unilateral. A source of infection may be visible: insect/animal bite, laceration.

For simple cellulitis, outpatient treatment with oral antibiotics and follow-up is sufficient (e.g. 10 days of oral flucloxacillin). More extensive cellulitis with systemic symptoms requires admission for intravenous antibiotics. Any signs of necrosis, circumferential cellulitis or crepitus (indicating anaerobic microorganisms) require surgical evaluation for urgent debridement.

Ruptured popliteal aneurysm

A ruptured popliteal aneurysm may present as claudication and distal embolic effects, or less commonly as an acute rupture (see Ch. 25).

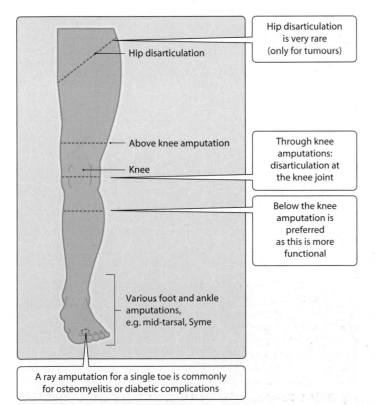

Hip disarticulation is very rare (only for tumours)

Hip disarticulation

Above knee amputation

Through knee amputations: disarticulation at the knee joint

Knee

Below the knee amputation is preferred as this is more functional

Various foot and ankle amputations, e.g. mid-tarsal, Syme

A ray amputation for a single toe is commonly for osteomyelitis or diabetic complications

Fig. 3.27.2 Amputation.

28. Ulcers and the diabetic foot

Questions
- What are the different types of ulcer?
- What are the differences between venous and arterial ulcers?
- What is a Charcot's joint and why does it occur?

Ulcers

An ulcer is a full-thickness loss of an epithelial surface. Leg ulcers are particularly common problems in the elderly, in whom there are many different types (Table 3.28.1): venous (70% of leg ulcers), arterial, mixed arteriovenous, neuropathic, malignant, traumatic infective (rare) and pressure sores.

Examination for ulcers

Ulcers are common on the wards and in OSCE stations. It is difficult to differentiate ulcers visually and the patient's history must be considered (age, disease history, particularly diabetes, peripheral vascular disease, neurological disorders, drugs, malignancy, venous disease). Examination of an ulcer looks at site, size, shape, surface, edge, surrounding skin, depth, base and discharge. The heel and between the toes and associated varicose veins are examined. The area is **felt** for temperature, pain and sensation around the ulcer, capillary refill, foot pulses and local lymph (malignancy). Buerger's test (Ch. 24) is applied if an arterial ulcer is suspected.

Venous ulcers

Venous ulcers are caused by chronic venous insufficiency and hypertension in the lower limb, which is associated with superficial venous disease (60%) and/or deep venous insufficiency (40%): which may be caused by previous DVT (Ch. 27).

The ulcer is debrided (usually chemically) and four-layer compression bandaging applied, which squeezes the blood out of the leg, thus preventing chronic venous hypertension. If significant arterial disease coexists, compression bandaging is contraindicated and so it is essential to check the **ankle brachial blood pressure index**.

Arterial ulcers

Arterial (ischaemic) ulcers occur when the arterial blood supply is compromised (Fig. 3.28.1 and Ch. 22). Critical limb ischaemia is often present, and these ulcers occur in association with diabetes, Buerger's disease, and some of the vasculitides.

Management aims to reestablish the arterial supply, most commonly with bypass surgery or angioplasty. Arterial disease is treated first and then any venous disease.

Neuropathic ulcers

A loss of sensation means that the patient cannot tell when skin is being damaged, and so healing is delayed (Fig. 3.28.2). Causes include peripheral neuropathy (diabetes (most common cause), leprosy, alcohol, nerve injuries, multiple sclerosis) or spinal disease (spina bifida, syringiomyelia).

Table 3.28.1 DIFFERENTIATING ULCERS

	Venous	Arterial (ischaemic)	Neuropathic
Site	Occur in 'gaiter area', especially on the medial side	Forefoot and toes (including pressure areas)	Pressure points (heel, head of 1st and 5th metatarsal, tips of toes, lateral edge of the foot)
Size	Small or (very) large	Often small, 'punched out'	Often small
Shape	Irregular; sloping, pale purple/blue	Regular; 'punched out'	Regular
Depth	Shallow	Deep; ligaments and bone may be visible	Deep; tendons and bones may be visible
Base	Granulation tissue; white tissue on a pink base	No granulation tissue; flat and pale	Variable
Skin temperature	Normal	Cold	Normal
Surrounding Skin quality	Poor; signs of chronic venous insufficiency	Pale; poor arterial supply	Healthy
Skin Sensation	Normal	Normal	Diminished or absent
Pulses	Present	Absent	Present (may be absent with coexisting arterial disease)
Painful	Painless	Painful	Painless

Careful wound control with measures to avoid trauma is important and tight diabetic management if appropriate. Total contact plaster cast (with a hole cut for the ulcer) prevents further damage and aids healing.

Malignant ulcers

Malignant ulcers are often associated with a raised rolled edge; most are caused by the three main types of skin cancer (Ch. 68).

Other types of ulcer

Traumatic ulcers. These often occur on the shin and follow minor trauma, often in the elderly where the wound does not heal well, particularly if there is coexisting venous or arterial insufficiency or malnutrition. This group includes sacral pressure sores and bedsores.

Infection. Inflammatory reactions in tuberculosis.

Pyoderma gangrenosum. This involves multiple necrotic ulcers, which turn black as tissue dies and may be very deep and widespread. They are associated with ulcerative colitis, Crohn's disease and rheumatoid arthritis.

The diabetic foot

The feet in diabetic patients often suffers from mixed pathology (Fig. 3.28.3). One-third of ulcers in diabetic patients are arterial, one-third are neuropathic and one-third are mixed arterial and neuropathic disease. The foot is often warm, and the pulses may be present (if not, this may be a critically ischaemic limb). Trauma to the feet of these patients may go unnoticed, allowing neuropathic ulcers and gangrene to develop.

Charcot's joint

A Charcot's joint has lost sensation (a neuropathic joint) in a chronic, painless, disorganized, dysfunctional joint. In long-standing neuropathy, the ankle and foot undergo multiple unnoticed fractures giving rise to a joint with poor mobility. It occurs in diabetics, syringomyelia, leprosy, late syphilis and other denervating diseases.

Charcot's joints occur as OSCE stations:

- look for an abnormal joint, and signs of PVD and infection (cellulitis, abscesses, osteomyelitis)
- feel for abnormal bony positions, temperature cold (PVD), diminished or absent sensation (glove and stocking distribution), absent vibration and joint position sense; check the foot pulses
- move the joint (limited and painless although some sensation may remain).

Surgery is uncommonly used, although options include osteotomies, arthroplasty and Ray amputations (for osteomyelitis of a single toe).

Fig. 3.28.1 Necrotic arterial ulcer which has a 'punched out' edge and is black. The skin is pale and flaking; there is dry gangrene.

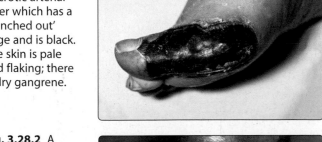

Fig. 3.28.2 A neuropathic ulcer on the heel of a diabetic. The ulcer is small, deep and covered in poor-quality tissue. An initial break in the skin was not noticed (peripheral neuropathy); it failed to heal and became infected.

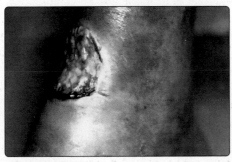

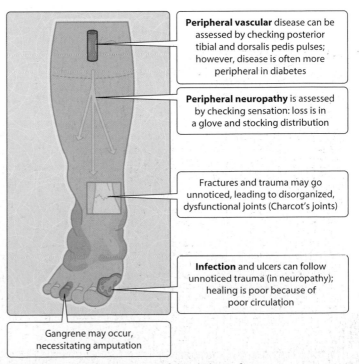

Peripheral vascular disease can be assessed by checking posterior tibial and dorsalis pedis pulses; however, disease is often more peripheral in diabetes

Peripheral neuropathy is assessed by checking sensation: loss is in a glove and stocking distribution

Fractures and trauma may go unnoticed, leading to disorganized, dysfunctional joints (Charcot's joints)

Infection and ulcers can follow unnoticed trauma (in neuropathy); healing is poor because of poor circulation

Gangrene may occur, necessitating amputation

Fig. 3.28.3 Pathophysiology of the diabetic foot.

29. Benign prostatic hyperplasia

Questions
■ How might benign prostatic hyperplasia present?
■ What are the management options for these patients?
■ What is transurethral resection of the prostate (TURP) and what are its complications?

Benign prostatic hyperplasia (BPH; Fig. 3.29.1) affects 50% of men over 50 years of age. The enlarged prostate pushes against the urethra and the bladder, obstructing or blocking urine flow (Fig. 3.29.2). It is a diagnosis made histologically.

Clinical features

Lower urinary tract symptoms are often present, plus:

■ filling/storage symptoms: <u>f</u>requency, <u>u</u>rgency, <u>n</u>octuria (the FUN symptoms), secondary to overactivity of the detrusor
■ bladder outflow obstruction symptoms: <u>h</u>esitancy, <u>i</u>ntermittency, <u>t</u>erminal dribbling, <u>s</u>tream reduction (remember by HITS), caused by obstruction of the bladder neck.

Patients with BPH may present with **acute urinary retention** (see below). A urinary catheter should be promptly passed to provide immediate relief. **Overflow incontinence** presents more gradually, often as a progressing nocturia; it is caused by a painless chronically distended and atonic bladder. Continued bladder neck obstruction and chronic retention may lead to upper tract obstruction and chronic **renal impairment**.

Investigations

Symptom questionnaires are widely used (e.g. International Prostate Scoring System (IPSS)). Other investigations are:

■ digital rectal examination to determine size and consistency
■ prostate specific antigen (PSA; Ch. 30)
■ urinalysis: infection and renal function
■ flow rates: flow velocity and post-void residue scan to assess bladder emptying.

More specific tests are transrectal ultrasound to determine the size and consistency of the prostate and urodynamics to assess more complex lower urinary tract symptoms.

Management

Around 50% of those affected deteriorate, 30% remain stable and 20% improve, although it is impossible to determine which

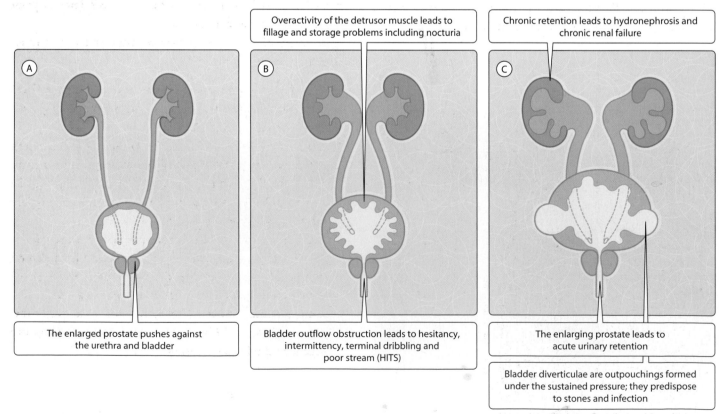

Overactivity of the detrusor muscle leads to fillage and storage problems including nocturia

Chronic retention leads to hydronephrosis and chronic renal failure

The enlarged prostate pushes against the urethra and bladder

Bladder outflow obstruction leads to hesitancy, intermittency, terminal dribbling and poor stream (HITS)

The enlarging prostate leads to acute urinary retention

Bladder diverticulae are outpouchings formed under the sustained pressure; they predispose to stones and infection

Fig. 3.29.1 Symptoms and sequalae of benign prostatic hyperplasia. (A) Asymptomatic enlargement. (B) Prostatic enlargement and diverticular formation, causing lower urinary tract symptoms. (C) chronic renal impairment.

patients will follow a particular course. **Conservative management** is suitable for some men with tolerable symptoms who may be satisfied with active surveillance, where follow-up is 6 monthly.

Medical management is suitable for moderate symptoms:

- alpha-blockers (e.g. tamsulosin, alfusozin) treat the dynamic component (smooth muscle contraction)
- 5α-reductase inhibitors (e.g. finasteride, datasteride) treat the static component; they decrease formation of the active dihydrotestosterone, delaying further hyperplasia
- herbal treatments: limited evidence exists for the use of saw palmetto, rye grass and pumpkin seed extracts.

Surgical management

Transurethral resection of the prostate (TURP) is the gold standard treatment. Tissue is removed from the prostate where it obstructs the urethra using a diathermy cutting loop (passed via the urethra). It is suitable for moderate and severe symptoms; mortality is < 1%. Early complications include: haemorrhage (most common), septicaemia (secondary to chronic urinary tract infection) and **transurethral resection (TUR) syndrome**. This is massive cardiovascular collapse with hyponatraemia and metabolic acidosis caused by entry into the circulatory system (through diffusion) of the irrigation fluid; it is treated with furosemide and fluid restriction. Late complications of TURP include retrograde ejaculation (in > 80%), impotence, urethral stricture and incontinence (5%).

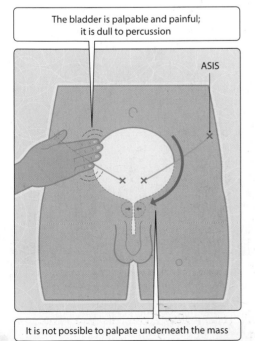

The bladder is palpable and painful; it is dull to percussion

ASIS

It is not possible to palpate underneath the mass

Fig. 3.29.2 Benign prostatic hyperplasia obstructing the urethra, causing acute urinary retention.

■ ACUTE URINARY RETENTION

Acute urinary retention is the sudden inability to pass urine and is a urological emergency. It is common in older men, where it may be the acute presentation of BPH, but it may also follow any operation (particularly pelvic surgery) or anaesthetic (especially spinal anaesthesia). Rarely (but very important to recognize), neurological conditions such as spinal cord compression or cord trauma may be the cause. The patient has the urge to pass urine but cannot and subsequently develops lower abdominal pain that becomes severe as the bladder continues to distend. The bladder is palpable and is dull to percussion, and it may be enlarged up to the umbilicus.

Management

Immediate management

The patient requires urgent urinary catheterization in order to empty the bladder and thus prevent damage to the upper urinary tract (i.e. acute renal failure). Urethral catheterization is attempted first but if this repeatedly fails, suprapubic catheterization is indicated. If the patient has chronic retention (a distended, painless, overflowing bladder), the bladder requires controlled emptying or renal failure may be precipitated. Digital rectal examination after bladder decompression indicates whether the prostate enlargement is benign or malignant. PSA will be artificially high as the prostate will be irritated and so it is measured after a 4 week interval from catheterization or rectal examination.

The cause of the acute urinary retention must be treated before the catheter is removed.

- *BPH.* TURP is performed electively once symptoms have subsided. If the man is unfit for surgery, long-term catheterization is possible.
- *Postsurgical retention.* No urine output, or decreasing output, occurs but the patient has the urge to pass urine and/or a palpable bladder is found. A catheter should be passed and fluid output monitored; the normal voiding mechanism should return within a few days.
- *Neurological retention.* In the presence of bilateral sciatica or known cancer, there may be buttock anaethesia and bowel symptoms, usually constipation with overflow. Perianal dermatomes should be assessed for sensation, anal sphincter tone (lax) and other features of **spinal cord compression** (Ch. 74). This is a surgical emergency and requires urgent surgical decompression.

30. Prostate cancer

Questions
- How may prostate cancer present?
- Under what conditions would prostate specific antigen (PSA) be raised?
- What are the alternatives to surgery for prostate cancer?

Prostate cancer is the most frequently diagnosed cancer in men, and the leading cause of cancer-specific deaths in men. It may be asymptomatic, and postmortem studies show that 80% of men over 80 years die *with* prostate cancer, but not necessarily *of* it. The 5-year survival is 80% with localized disease but 20–30% if metastases are present.

Aetiology

Generally prostate cancer is dependent on androgens (testosterone) for growth. The incidence is higher in African-Americans than in Europeans, and least frequent in Asians. Genetic factors play a role in 10% of cases, particularly in the young (initial mutation in chromosome 8).

Pathology

Prostate cancers are adenocarcinomas and typically grow around the periphery of the gland. They are staged based on the histology of the cancer (Fig. 3.30.1).

Clinical features

The main symptoms are:

- prostate specific antigen (PSA) screening/testing
- bone pain caused by metastatic deposits: the first presentation of prostate cancer in 30% of men; the diagnosis of prostate cancer should be considered in an elderly man presenting with recent-onset lower back pain (also look for weight loss, lethargy and anaemia)
- lower urinary tract symptoms: if the prostate grows large enough, it may cause bladder outflow obstruction symptoms (as in Ch. 29). Thus for patients with benign prostatic hyperplasia (BPH), prostate cancer screening with PSA can be considered.

A tumour may be an incidental finding while performing transurethral resection of the prostate to treat suspected benign prostatic hyperplasia (10%).

Investigations

Digital rectal examination. The patient lies on one side for the examination (Fig. 3.30.2). An enlarged, hard and craggy prostate suggests cancer.

PSA. This protein is produced by the prostate to convert semen into liquid. Men with prostate cancer tend to have higher plasma levels of PSA but it is an imperfect marker for prostate cancer (Table 3.30.1). PSA is also raised by urinary tract infections, BPH, ejaculation, acute urinary retention, prostatic massage and increasing age. Asymptomatic men who request PSA screening require careful counselling. The PSA level is highest in those with metastatic disease (> 50 ng/ml); levels > 10 need investigating. There are current trials assessing PSA as a screening method.

Renal function. U&E and creatinine.

Transrectal ultrasound. Ultrasound is used to estimate prostate volume and to guide needle biopsy (10 or more biopsies are taken via the perineum for staging).

Bone isotope scan. Bone pain should be assessed for the presence of metastatic disease.

Staging

The Gleason score differentiates stage based upon histological examination, the lowest count indicating well-differentiated and the highest count least-differentiated tissue. The score is a combination of two assessments, the most predominant type of cancer cell and the next most frequent type of cell (therefore,

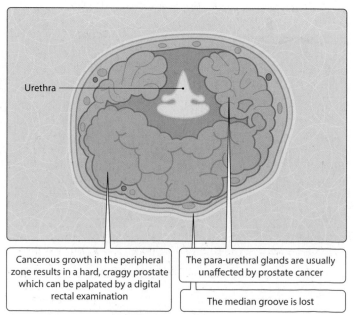

Urethra

Cancerous growth in the peripheral zone results in a hard, craggy prostate which can be palpated by a digital rectal examination

The para-urethral glands are usually unaffected by prostate cancer

The median groove is lost

Fig. 3.30.1 The prostate in cross-section.

Table 3.30.1 USE OF PROSTATE-SPECIFIC ANTIGEN (PSA)

PSA (ng/ml)	Interpretation
0.5–4	Normal (but 30% of men with prostate cancer have a normal values)
4–10	20–30% chance of cancer
10	> 60% chance of cancer
Rise of 20% per year	Refer for immediate biopsy

1 + 1 is the minimum score). Local invasion occurs to adjacent tissues and organs (bladder, urethra, seminal vesicles), and rarely to the rectum. Haematogenous spread is more common and mainly to bone, liver and lung. Lymphatic spread is via the iliac and para-aortic nodes.

Management

Radical management

Radical options are suitable for younger patients with a life expectancy greater than 10 years, or for small tumours confined to the prostate:

- **radical radiotherapy**: external beam radiation therapy or brachytherapy (an implanted radioactive seeds delivers radiation directly to the gland)

- **radical retropubic prostatectomy**: removes the entire prostate gland and surrounding tissue (including seminal vesicles and obturator nodes) via a retropubic approach; long-term complications are infertility (100%), impotence (30%) and incontinence (5%), but nerve-sparing surgery may prevent impotence
- **laparoscopic prostatectomy**: is a increasingly performed.

Non-curative management

Active surveillance is appropriate for men whose life expectancy is relatively short (e.g. < 10 years for over 70 years of age) or for a tumour that is slow growing and well differentiated. Monitoring is with 6-monthly clinical review (PSA then digital rectal examination). Many clinical trials show the benefit of active monitoring and conservative management of symptoms.

Hormone therapy

Therapy to reduce testosterone action should decrease tumour progression. It may be used as the primary intervention or in combination with other treatments:

- bilateral orchidectomy eliminates androgen production
- hormone-manipulating drugs (medical castration)
  — luteinizing hormone releasing hormone (LHRH) agonists (e.g. goserelin) decrease testosterone release; initial stimulation of testosterone may produce a 'tumour flare' (increased risk of spinal cord compression, urinary retention, bone pain)
  — anti-androgen treatment (e.g. bicalutamide) alone or with LHRH agonists to reduce tumour flare.

Side-effects of hormone treatments include loss of libido, impotence, gynaecomastia, cardiac failure and liver damage.

Palliative measures for advanced disease

Hormone treatments (e.g. goserelin) reduce symptoms. Metastatic bone disease can be treated with short courses of external beam radiation therapy and radioisotopes or bisphosphonates. Severe backache should be taken as a warning of possible spinal cord compression. Chemotherapy can be considered for men with hormone-refractory prostate cancer (one in five tumours). Transurethral resection of the prostate can be used to relieve urinary obstruction.

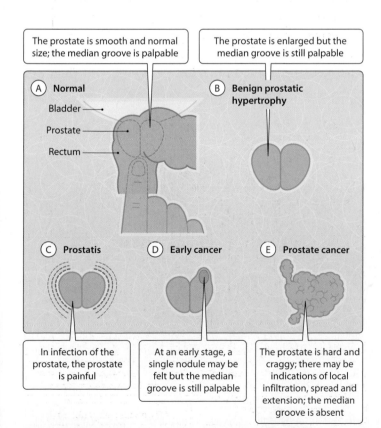

The prostate is smooth and normal size; the median groove is palpable

The prostate is enlarged but the median groove is still palpable

(A) **Normal**
Bladder
Prostate
Rectum

(B) **Benign prostatic hypertrophy**

(C) **Prostatis**

(D) **Early cancer**

(E) **Prostate cancer**

In infection of the prostate, the prostate is painful

At an early stage, a single nodule may be felt but the median groove is still palpable

The prostate is hard and craggy; there may be indications of local infiltration, spread and extension; the median groove is absent

Fig. 3.30.2 Digital rectal examination of the prostate.

31. Testicular and penile tumours

Questions
- What features of a testicular lump suggest malignancy?
- What are the tumour markers for testicular tumours?
- What are the risk factors for penile cancer?

Testicular cancer

Although rare, testicular cancer is the most common cancer of men aged 20–40 years. The incidence is increasing, but the overall 5-year survival is excellent (> 95%). Any lump within the testis should be treated as a tumour until proved otherwise.

Aetiology

There is a 10 times increased risk of cancer in an undescended testis; repositioning the testis at an early age does not alter the risk of cancer but the testis is now palpable. There is a clear genetic link: the relative risk in brothers is 8–10 and in father and son is 4. Virtually all cases show amplification of the chromosome 12q.

Clinical features

The presentation can vary (Fig. 3.31.1):

- painless, firm lump: there may also be a feeling of heaviness in the scrotum and a dull ache in the groin or abdomen; most present with a painless lump
- painful swollen testes: 10% present as an acutely swollen testis
- history of trauma: identifies a problem to the patient, who then presents with a lump
- back pain: caused by para-aortic lymph node metastases
- gynaecomastia: rare, caused by increased circulating hormones
- breathlessness from massive secondary deposits in the lungs
- bone pain from bony metastases.

Pathology

Almost all (95%) testicular cancers are germ cell tumours, which spread first to the para-aortic lymph nodes and then to the lungs. They are classified as seminomas (40%) or non-seminoma germ cell tumours (NSGCT; 60%): including teratomas (32%; more common in the young), combined seminoma and teratoma, and other rare tumours (e.g. yolk cell carcinomas).

Investigations

Investigations provide diagnosis and staging (Table 3.31.1):

- ultrasound scan: of both testes at rapid access clinics
- tumour markers: used to aid diagnosis and monitor progression (75% have elevation)

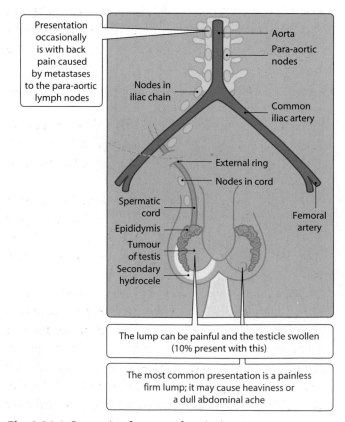

Fig. 3.31.1 Presenting features of testicular tumours.

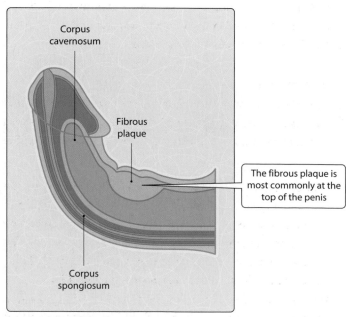

Fig. 3.31.2 Peyronie's disease. The plaque most often occurs at the top of the penis.

— α-fetoprotein: useful for teratomas as not elevated with seminomas; is present in 45–65% of NSGCT
— β-human chorionic gonadotrophin: present in 30–60% NSGCT and in 10% of seminomas
— lactate dehydrogenase: less specific and less useful as a marker of tumour progression

- CT scan: of the chest, abdomen and pelvis for staging.

Management

Surgical management. Treatment is in specialist centres with multidisciplinary teams. Radical orchidectomy (removal of the testis and spermatic cord) is the initial treatment performed in all cases. Option of biopsy in the contralateral testis should be discussed at presentation.

Adjuvant treatments. Seminomas are very radiosensitive:

- stage I/II disease: adjuvant radiotherapy to the para-aortic nodes
- stage III: adjuvant radiotherapy with chemotherapy using the BEP regimen (bleomycin, etoposide, cisplatin)

Teratomas (NSGCT). These are only monitored if they are stage I. Stage II/III disease is treated with adjuvant chemotherapy: two courses of BEP if blood or lymph invasion is found.

Complications

'Dry ejaculation' and psychological problems affect one-third of men. Sperm storage (**cryopreservation**) should be offered to all patients who may wish to father children.

Prognosis

Overall 5-year survival is high: 95% with metastatic disease and approaching 100% without metastases. A subgroup of NSGCT does poorly. Up to 5% of men develop cancers in the remaining testis within 25 years of initial diagnosis.

Penile cancer

Cancer of the penis is rare and affects men aged 60–80 years. It almost always affects uncircumcised men and is associated with poor hygiene and infection with human papilloma virus (genital warts).

Clinical features. Presentation is with suspicious penile lesions or growths: most often squamous cell carcinoma of the glans or foreskin that do not appear to be caused by infection. There may be rash, bumps, plaques or flat growths on the penis/foreskin or foul-smelling discharge underneath the foreskin. Diagnosis is through biopsy.

Management. Partial amputation is performed for localized lesions, but more widespread lesions require radical penectomy. If lymph nodes are involved, prognosis is poor.

Table 3.31.1 STAGING BY THE UK ROYAL MARSDEN SYSTEM

Stage	Clinical features
I	Confined to testes
II	Infradiaphragmatic lymph nodes involved
III	Supradiaphragmatic lymph nodes involved
IV	Distant metastases (lung, liver)

Otherwise, these cancers tend to be noticed earlier so survival is fairly high (5-year survival, 60–75%).

Eponymous urological conditions

Peyronie's disease. In this benign non-tumourous penile disorder, hard fibrous plaques in the tunica of the corpus cavernosa cause angulation toward the affected side, which results in painful erections (Fig. 3.31.2). The cause is not known, but it affects 4% of men over 40 years and may be caused by previous trauma (almost always occurs after penile fracture); there is an association with Dupuytren's contracture in 5%. There is often an initially painful phase after which there is a prolonged painless period during which calcification and rarely bone formation may occur. Treatment is conservative if the patient wishes, and the condition may remit in some patients after 3–5 years. Medications offer limited help, and **Nesbitt's operation** can be performed to correct the deformity.

Balanitis xerotica obliterans. This autoimmune condition is characterized by ivory–white patches on the glans, typically around the meatus. Treatment is with steroid creams or circumcision.

Balanitis. Inflammation of the glans is usually associated with a tight foreskin (phimosis).

Fournier's gangrene. A bacterial infection of the scrotum can result in necrotizing fasciitis, which can be fatal if it spreads systemically. Urgent surgical debridement and intravenous antibiotics are necessary.

Hydatid of Morgagni. This is an embryological remnant in the upper pole of the testes. Torsion of this epididymal appendage is of no consequence but presents in a similar fashion to a full torsion and surgical exploration is indicated if there is any doubt.

Paraphimosis. An inability to replace the foreskin when it has been retracted behind the glans is caused by a narrowed or inflamed foreskin (e.g. failure to replace the foreskin following urethral catheterization); it can lead to gangrene.

Phimosis. A tight foreskin cannot be drawn back over the underlying glans, predisposing to inflammation (balanitis). It is either congenital or caused by infection; definitive treatment is with circumcision.

32. Testicular lumps

Questions
- What is a hydrocele and how can it be treated?
- On what side does a varicocele normally occur, and what does it feel like?
- If ultrasound was unavailable, how would you manage a teenager who presents with a suddenly painful testis?

Any lump within the testes is treated as a tumour until proved otherwise. All lumps should be scanned with ultrasound at rapid access clinics if any suspicion of malignancy exists. A suddenly painful testis in a young male may be a torsion, and urgent surgery is indicated; do not wait for confirmation.

Hydrocele

A hydrocele is an accumulation of fluid within the *tunica vaginalis* (Figs. 3.32.1 and 3.32.2A). Most hydroceles are primary (idiopathic) caused by local increased production of serous fluid, although some may be secondary to a tumour or infection. They are not separate from the testis; they are brilliantly transilluminable and normally it is possible to feel above the lump (unless the hydrocele is within the spermatic cord).

Management

Aspiration reveals a straw-coloured fluid. As hydrocele often recurs, aspiration is suitable for those unfit for surgery but the treatment of choice is surgery. The tunica vaginalis is opened to release the fluid, and then the sac is sewn back onto itself (*placation* of the sac) or excised, so that fluid cannot reaccumulate. The most common complication is haematoma formation, which occasionally may become more painful than the original hydrocele.

Varicocele

A varicocele is dilatation of the veins of the **pampiniform plexus** within the spermatic cord (a 'varicose vein' of the testes) (Fig. 3.32.2B). The patient may become subfertile as a result. Almost all varicoceles are left sided (95%) as there is increased venous pressure in the left testicular vein as it drains at a right angle into the left renal vein, causing turbulent flow; the right testicular vein drains at a lesser angle directly into the inferior vena cava and so does not suffer this problem. Very rarely, the venous drainage of the left testicular vein into the left renal vein may be disrupted by a left renal tumour, giving rise to a secondary varicocele.

The varicocele feels like a bag of worms, and disappears on lying down. It may rarely give rise to haematospermia (blood in the ejaculate).

Management

Conservative: reassurance may suffice for the patient. Surgery is used for heavy or aching varicoceles or for men who are subfertile as a result of the varicocele. The affected testicular veins are divided and embolized. Radiological embolization is also used.

Epididymal cysts and spermatoceles

Epididymal cysts (Fig. 3.32.2C) occur more often in men over 40 years. One or multiple swellings are felt in the scrotum behind the testis; these lumps are transilluminable. Spermatoceles are similar but contain sperm and so are not as transilluminable. A cyst that causes discomfort or is very large can be removed by surgery (enucleation). However, since surgery poses a potential risk to fertility in young men, small and asymptomatic cysts may be left untreated with the patient reassured.

Hernia

A hernia in the scrotum is an indirect inguinal hernia (Fig. 3.32.2D); it has a cough impulse, is not transilluminable and it is not possible to feel above it (Ch. 33).

Tumour

A tumour often presents with a painless lump that is often not separate from the testis (Fig. 3.32.2E), in a patient between 20 and 40 years of age (Ch. 31).

Testicular torsion

Testicular torsion (Fig. 3.32.2F) is most common in those under 20 years of age (although it may occur in older men). The testis

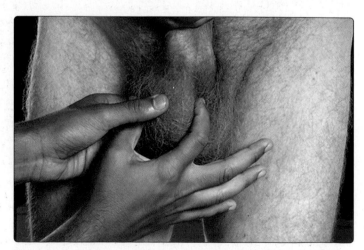

Fig. 3.32.1 Palpating the testes. A small hydrocele is present.

rotates around its vascular base, leading to acute pain. It is characterized by sudden-onset severe testicular pain, abdominal pain and often vomiting. The testis may retract, leading to the classic 'bell clanger' position.

If Doppler ultrasound scan is immediately available, it can be used to confirm a torsion. However, in the presence of a positive clinical diagnosis, management is by urgent surgical exploration (*do not wait for investigation*). Both testes should be sutured to the tunica vaginalis to prevent further torsion (**orchidopexy**).

The **differential diagnosis** of painful testicular lump is torsion, epididymitis, strangulated hernia and testicular tuberculosis (may also be painless).

Epididymitis and orchitis

Infection of the epididymis leads to scrotal discomfort and pain during micturation (Fig. 3.32.2G). It is more common in those over 20 years, in whom the most common cause is chlamydial infection (sexually transmitted); in older men it is more likely to be caused by *Escherichia coli*. Treatment in young men with uncomplicated disease is with a 2-week course of doxycycline.

Orchitis is infection of the testis and is mostly caused by viral infection, particularly paramyxovirus (mumps). If the swelling does not settle, the testis should be examined further for the possibility of tumour. If epididymitis spreads to the testes, it is termed **epididymo-orchitis**.

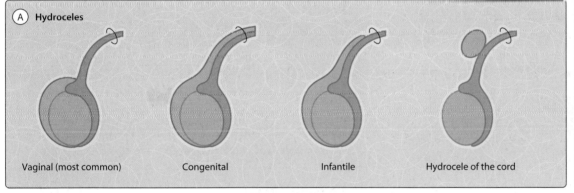

A Hydroceles

Vaginal (most common) Congenital Infantile Hydrocele of the cord

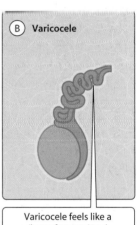

B Varicocele

Varicocele feels like a 'bag of worms' and disappears when the patient lies down

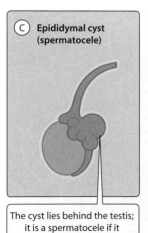

C Epididymal cyst (spermatocele)

The cyst lies behind the testis; it is a spermatocele if it contains sperm

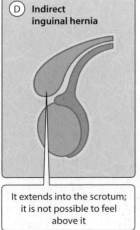

D Indirect inguinal hernia

It extends into the scrotum; it is not possible to feel above it

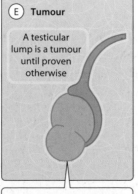

E Tumour

A testicular lump is a tumour until proven otherwise

Tumours are painless lumps not separated from the testis; they are often hard, irregular and may cause a dull ache

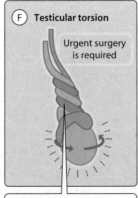

F Testicular torsion

Urgent surgery is required

Torsion presents with sudden-onset severe pain, abdominal pain and vomiting

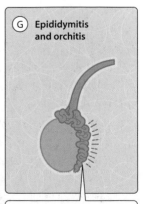

G Epididymitis and orchitis

Infection leads to gradual onset of a dull ache or pain

Fig. 3.32.2 Testicular lumps. (A) hydrocele; (B) varicocele; (C) epididymal cyst; (D) indirect inguinal hernia; (E) tumour; (F) torsion; (G) epididymitis and orchitis.

33. Examination of the groin and scrotum

Questions
- How do you test for reducibility of an inguinal hernia?
- If a hernia extends into the scrotum, is it direct or indirect?
- What is a tense, fluctuant, brilliantly transilluminable testicular lump likely to be?

The groin

Introduction

The patient should be asked about any pain and then asked to stand up and unclothe from nipples to knees. The locations of groin hernias are shown in Fig. 3.5.1. Causes of groin lumps are:

- inguinal and femoral hernias
- lymph node: look for generalized lymphadenopathy
- lipoma: subcutaneous, mobile, variable size, may be fluctuant
- femoral aneurysm: expansile pulsation, may be bilateral
- lymphocele: following femoral artery surgery in the groin, the local lymphatics may become disrupted, and a local collection of lymphatic fluid forms a lump; it can be simply aspirated
- ectopic testis: the testis is absent from the scrotum; feeling along the line of the inguinal ligament should detect an undescended testes
- saphena varix: bluish tinge, has a cough impulse, disappears on lying; varicose veins may be present
- psoas abscess: in the psoas muscle (Crohn's disease or tuberculosis): deep and fluctuant, causing fixed flexion of the hip.

Inspection

Both sides of the groin are inspected for lumps and scars. Differentiate between inguinal and femoral hernias and inspect the scrotum for obvious swellings. The patient is asked to cough. First inspect the lump to see if it bulges; then look on the other side for any bulges.

Palpation

The cough impulse is repeated while placing a hand over the lump to feel its movement. This is repeated on the other side to check for a less-obvious bilateral hernia.

Reducibility. A reducible hernia can be returned into the abdomen; there is an increased risk of strangulation in an irreducible hernia. The patient should be asked if they have tried pushing it back in before. Ask them to try to do so now. If they fail, the clinician should attempt to reduce it

from behind using a flat palm, being careful not to cause any pain. If the hernia is reducible, it should come back out again if the patient coughs.

Direct or indirect inguinal hernias (Fig. 3.33.1).   The patient is asked to reduce the lump again. Cover the *deep inguinal ring* with two fingers. If the lump comes out when the patient coughs again, the hernia is direct. If it stays in place, it is an indirect inguinal hernia (coming through the deep ring) but it should reappear when the patient coughs if the deep ring is uncovered. Indirect hernias may descend into the testis.

At this point it should be clear if the lump is inguinal (direct or indirect) or femoral, reducible or irreducible.

Transillumination is a useful examination for groin and testicular lumps: hernias are non-transilluminable.

Percussion and **auscultation** over a large inguinal hernia will indicate whether it contains loops of bowel (resonant with bowel sounds; do not percuss the testis).

Concluding the examination

In an OSCE, a student would follow this by suggesting that the scrotum and abdomen should be examined for other hernias. Hernias are surgically corrected because they are at constant risk of strangulation. The *surgical* difference between an indirect and direct inguinal hernia is that the former arises laterally to the inferior epiastric artery (i.e. arises through the deep ring).

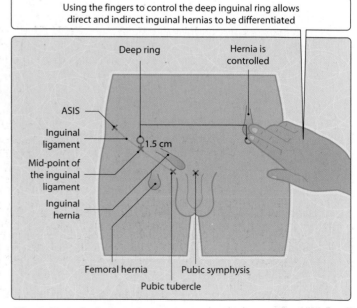

Using the fingers to control the deep inguinal ring allows direct and indirect inguinal hernias to be differentiated

Deep ring   Hernia is controlled

ASIS

Inguinal ligament   1.5 cm

Mid-point of the inguinal ligament

Inguinal hernia

Femoral hernia   Pubic symphysis

Pubic tubercle

Fig. 3.33.1 Groin lumps.

The scrotum

An OSCE of a scrotal lump may be on a real patient, a simulated patient or a plastic model.

Inspection

The scrotum is inspected for obvious lumps, swelling or old scars. The patient is asked to move his penis aside to allow inspection of the scrotum for any sinuses, subcutaneous nodules or ulcers.

Palpation

Each testis is palpated, starting on the unaffected side (although the condition may be bilateral, e.g. hydrocele). If the testis is absent, look for scars of previous surgery and then palpate along the line of the inguinal ligament to identify an undescended testis. A diagnosis is tested with a cough impulse (positive for a hernia) and transillumination (positive for a hydrocele and epididymal cyst) for both testes.

The algorithm in Figure 3.33.2 will help in diagnosis. Painful lumps could be a torsion or epididymitis, where the epididymis and spermatic cord are swollen and painful (If the testis is involved it is epididymo-orchitis). Indirect hernias may also move into the testis (Fig. 3.33.3). Some hydroceles are instantly recognizable but they can be more subtle (see Fig. 3.32.1).

Concluding the examination

If the diagnosis is an indirect inguinal hernia, a further examination of the abdomen for hernias should be suggested. If there is any confusion over what the lump is, an ultrasound scan would exclude an underlying tumour.

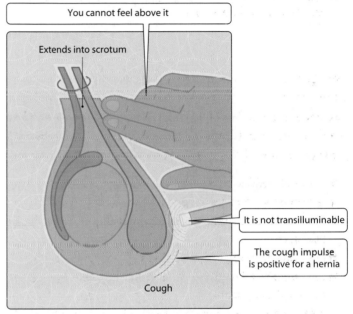

Fig. 3.33.3 Assessing an indirect inguinal hernia extending into the scrotum.

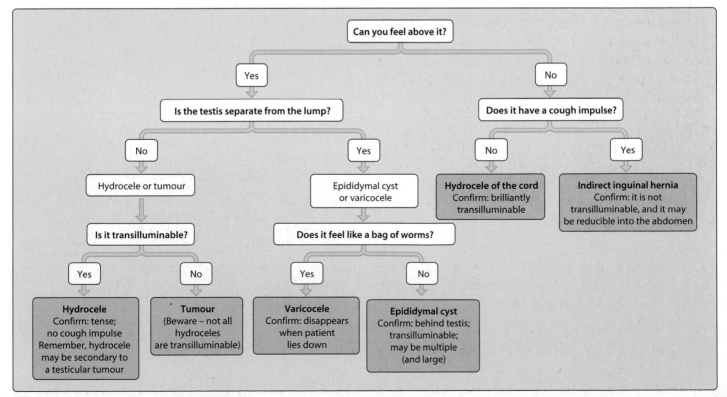

Fig. 3.33.2 Differentiating testicular lumps.

34. Haematuria and urological tumours

Questions
- What are the causes of haematuria and how should it be investigated?
- What are the causes of bladder tumours?
- What is intravesical therapy?

The urological tumours involve the bladder, ureters and kidney. The most common presenting symptom of these tumours is painless haematuria (blood in the urine); one in five of those with macroscopic haematuria have a urinary tract malignancy.

Haematuria

Haematuria is either macroscopic (frank) or microscopic (detectable on dipstick). All patients with macroscopic haematuria and those over 40 years with microscopic haematuria should be referred to rapid access clinics. The causes of haematuria are shown in (Fig. 3.34.1):

The following investigations are performed:

- mid-stream urine: microscopy and culture for urinary tract infection causing haematuria
- ultrasound and intravenous urogram: to identify anatomy and filling defects of the upper tract
- flexible cystoscopy with biopsy: cancer can be detected

using a cystoscope to view inside the bladder; multiple biopsies are taken.

Bladder tumours

Transitional cell epithelium lines the bladder and ureters; a carcinoma arising from this lining is a **urothelial tumour**. The bladder is the most commonly affected site (95%).

Aetiology

Bladder tumours are associated with:

- male:female ratio of 2:1; most common in men aged 60–80 years
- cigarette smoking: most common proven association
- aromatic amines: increased risk with rubber industries (tyre and rubber manufacturers); dyes, paints and plastics; diesel fumes; tumours may arise up to 20 years later
- schistosomiasis (bilharzia): in some countries (e.g. Egypt), bladder tumours are associated with this waterborne parasite, giving rise to squamous cell carcinomas.

Clinical features

Presentation of bladder tumours can be with:

- painless macroscopic haematuria (in 90%)
- recurrent urinary tract infections and chronic renal failure (secondary to chronic ureteric obstruction)
- pelvic and back pain: indicating metastatic spread.

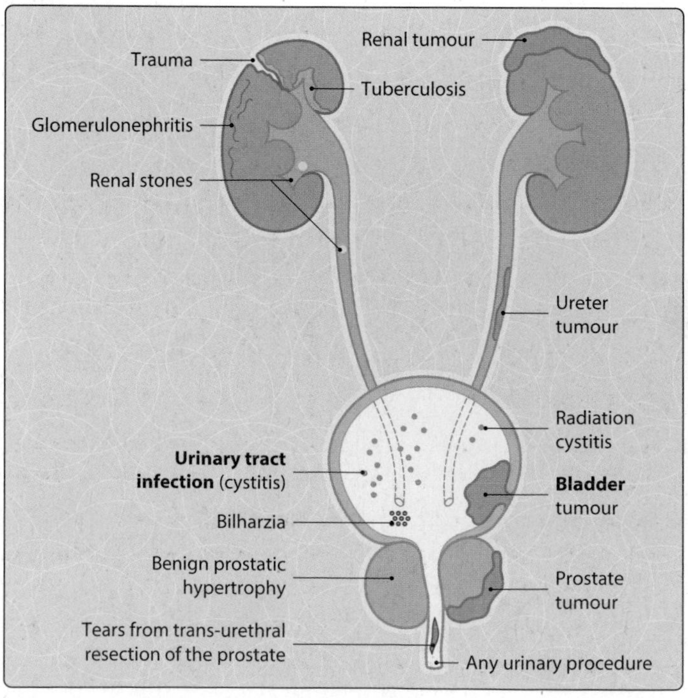

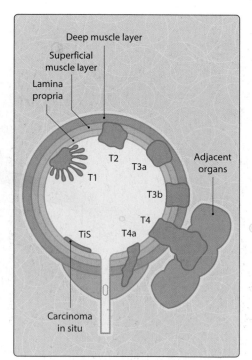

Fig. 3.34.2 Staging of bladder tumours.

Fig. 3.34.1 The causes of haematuria (common causes in bold).

Pathology

Approximately 75% are superficial (they do not invade the muscle wall; Fig. 3.34.2) and most are transitional cell carcinomas (Fig. 3.34.3). Carcinoma in situ is flat and has not yet invaded the bladder epithelium, although is is very aggressive and needs to be managed aggressively, sometimes with cystectomy.

Management

Surgical management depends on the stage and grade of the tumour (Fig. 3.34.2).

Superficial bladder tumours: T1

Transurethral resection of a bladder tumour (TURBT) involves endoscopic resection to leave a clear margin of tissue. Follow-up is 6 weeks later and then with regular cystoscopy. The bladder is irrigated with a chemotherapy solution (for 8–10 weeks), which decreases recurrence:

- **bacille-Calmette-Guérin** (BCG) activates the immune system; side-effects are influenza-like symptoms, cystitis and fever.
- **mitomycin C** reduces the risk of local recurrence by 50%, although local inflammation causes frequency, urgency, haematuria or pain; it can eradicate low-grade (T1) tumours.

Muscle-invasive tumours: T2, T3, T4

Radical surgery. Cystectomy is removal of the bladder. Urine is removed from the body with either an ileal conduit or bladder reconstruction. In an ileal conduit, a short section of ileum is resected, and the ureters are attached to it. The ileum is brought to the skin and the urine drains into a stoma bag (a urinary diversion). In bladder reconstruction, a neo-bladder is created using a piece of bowel.

Radical radiotherapy. Deep radiotherapy is appropriate for patients who are not fit for surgery or who wish to avoid cystectomy.

Transitional cell carcinoma of the ureter is treated with radical resection (nephroureterectomy) and carcinoma in situ with BCG.

Metastatic disease

Palliation is with surgery for relief of obstruction, radiotherapy, chemotherapy and management of metastatic bone disease.

Prognosis

Survival is 75% at 5 years for superficial tumours and 20% at 5 years for muscle-invasive tumours.

Renal cancer

Renal cancer is often found incidentally while investigating other problems (e.g. ultrasound or radiography of the abdomen). Most are adenocarcinomas and 10% are transitional cell carcinomas.

Aetiology

There is an association with cigarette smoking, polycystic kidney disease and genetics. **Von Hippel–Lindau syndrome** is a rare inherited disorder (chromosome 3) in which patients have a higher risk of developing kidney and other types of cancer. **Wilm's tumour** is a nephroblastoma of the kidney in infants and children, often presenting as an abdominal mass; a positive family history increases risk.

Clinical features

The symptoms of renal cancer are macroscopic haematuria, the most common symptom, loin pain and abdominal mass. However, this triad is not often found. There may also be pyrexia of unknown origin, hypertension, weight loss and metastatic symptoms.

Management

Treatment is primarily surgical, where partial nephrectomy is used for small tumours and radical nephrectomy for larger tumours with part of the inferior vena cava if there is extension beyond the renal vein. Radiotherapy and chemotherapy are ineffective. Immunotherapy is a promising new approach that has been shown to increase survival. Survival is 50% at 5 years if disease is confined to the organ at presentation.

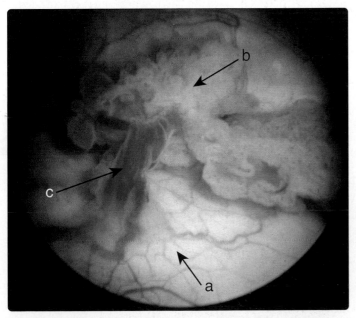

Fig. 3.34.3 Cytoscopic appearance of a superficial transitional cell carcinoma of the bladder: normal bladder epithelium is visible (a); tumour (b); bleeding (c).

35. Urinary stone disease

Questions
- What are the different types of urinary stone?
- How is the acute phase managed?
- Do stones always need treating and why?

Urinary stone disease (**urolithiasis**) is a common disorder where stones form in the kidney or bladder but may present anywhere in the urinary tract. While stones often cause pain at some point, many can remain asymptomatic. They affect 1–5% of the population, with Caucasian men being particularly affected.

Aetiology
Urinary stone disease is usually idiopathic, with low fluid intake promoting stone formation, but it can be associated with metabolic disorders (hyperparathyroidism, prolonged immobilization, irritable bowel disease, gout, cystinuria) and dietary factors (high oxalate: tea, nuts, chocolates, strawberries).

Pathology
There are several types of stone:

- calcium oxalate (80%): mostly idiopathic (also secondary to metabolic disorders, e.g. hyperparathyroidism)
- calcium phosphate (10%): mostly idiopathic

- triple phosphate (staghorn) stones (5%): calcium, magnesium and ammonium phosphates; these are often large and fill the renal pelvis, resulting in hydronephrosis (mostly secondary to infection)
- uric acid (< 5%): occur in gout and are radiolucent
- cystine: rare (1%); in metabolic disorders or indinavir therapy (for AIDS).

Clinical features
The features are:

- ureteric colic: loin to groin pain, which may radiate into the testes or labia, is the acute presentation, where ureteric smooth muscle contracts against the blocked stone causing colic; this pain is intense and agonising, and the patient is unable to find relief in any position
- microscopic haematuria: occurs in > 90% of patients
- gravelly urine: small stones passed painlessly in the urine
- urinary tract infections: recurrent cystitis or pyelonephritis
- chronic renal failure: from progressive renal damage.

Investigations
Urinary stones are investigated by:

- urinalysis: identifies urinary tract infection and haematuria

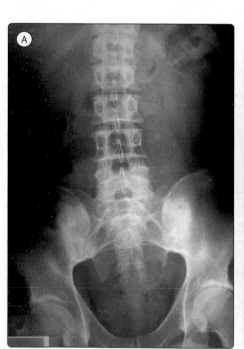
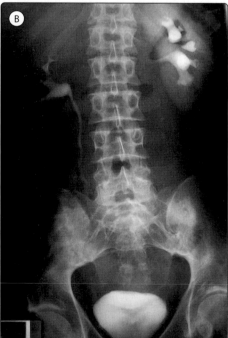
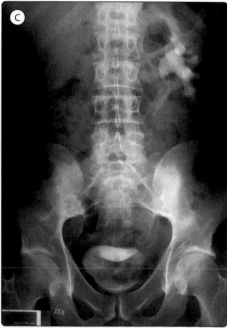

Fig. 3.35.1 Plain film radiographs of the kidneys, ureters and bladder (KUB). (A) A stone in the left ureter. (B) Film at 40 min: the right kidney is draining normally and filling the bladder. The left kidney is filling with dye, which shows hydronephrosis (dilatation of the upper tracts), but has not yet drained. (C) Postmicturation film: the right system has completely finished draining, which is normal. The left side is slowly draining and is hydronephrotic. The stone is obstructing drainage of the left kidney.

- blood tests: FBC, U&E (renal function); calcium, phosphate and uric acid (metabolic disturbances)
- radiography: a plain radiograph (Fig. 3.35.1) is taken as 90% of stones are radioopaque; CT shows a stone and any hydronephrosis (modern test in the acute phase)
- intravenous urogram: outlines the urinary tract and shows function and any obstruction or hydronephrosis
- renal ultrasound and renogram: ^{99m}Tc-mercapto-acetyltriglycine (MAG3) to assess renal excretion).

Management

The initial **acute management** of the patient comprises analgesia with oral/rectal diclofenac or morphine, fluids and broad-spectrum antibiotics (e.g. cefotaxime). An obstruction, particularly if infection is present, is an urological emergency and must be relieved to prevent permanent renal damage. This is done by **percutaneous nephrostomy**: a small tube is passed into the upper renal pelvis (under ultrasound guidance with the patient sedated), and the urine is collected in an external bag (Fig. 3.35.2). Once the acute stage is passed, active measures are commenced, treatment depending on the size and site of stones. Almost all stones < 5 mm will pass conservatively within 6 weeks and so require only supportive management. Larger stones in 10–20% of affected patients require removal.

Extracorporeal shockwave lithotripsy (ESWL; Fig. 3.35.3). This is a non-invasive procedure used in more than 80% of patients with stones. Shockwaves are focused, using ultrasound guidance, onto the stone, which is fragmented and passed during micturition; as this may cause pain, analgesia is required. Pregnant women and patients taking warfarin cannot undergo this treatment.

Ureteroscopy. A flexible ureteroscope is passed via the urethra to retrieve the stones using collecting baskets, or to fragment them with intracorporal lithotripsy or lasers.

Percutaneous nephrolithomy (PCNL). A tract is formed via a small loin incision directly from the loin into the renal pelvis (under general anaesthesia), and a nephroscope is passed under radiograph control. The stone is retrieved with a basket or fragmented. This technique is suitable for large stones or staghorn stones in the renal pelvis.

Open surgery. This is rarely needed and only indicated when the above procedures have failed, or for those with other disease (e.g. obesity, spina bifida, scoliosis). Laparoscopy is performed for some stone extraction procedures.

Prognosis

Stones will recur in 50% of patients, and patients should be advised of measures to prevent recurrence: high fluid intake to produce > 2 litres of urine per day, avoid foods with high oxalate content and manage hypercalcaemia with thiazide diuretics.

Gout (uric acid) is managed with allopurinol and infections should be treated.

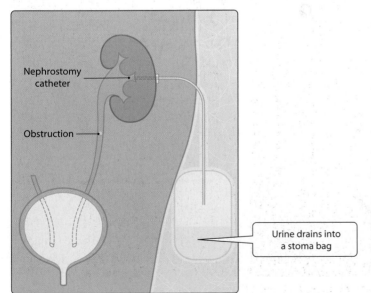

Fig. 3.35.2 Percutaneous nephrostomy to relieve obstruction of the kidney.

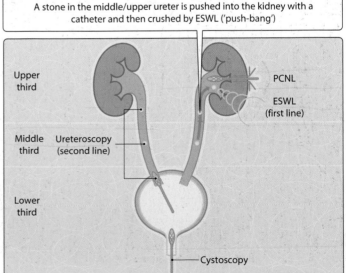

Fig. 3.35.3 Active measures to remove stones. Stones < 2 cm are mostly suitable for extracorporeal shock-wave lithotripsy (ESWL). PCNL, percutaneous nephrolithomy.

36. Urinary tract infection

Questions
- Where might infection of the urinary tract occur?
- Why are women much more commonly affected than men?
- What is the treatment for simple cystitis in females?

Urinary tract infection (UTI) is defined as the presence of bacteria in the urine (**bacteriuria**) > 100 000 organisms/ml in the presence of symptoms. It is a very common problem and 50–70% of women can expect at least one infection in their lifetime. Infection normally starts in the lower urinary tract (urethra and bladder) and if untreated may progress to the upper tracts (ureter and kidneys) and become life-threatening. Common sites of infection are kidney (pyelonephritis), bladder (cystitis) and urethra (urethritis); in men prostatitis, orchiditis and epididymitis also occur.

Pathology

Most causative microorganisms are migratory bowel gut bacteria from the perineum, with *Escherischia coli* being the most common (in 80%). Other organisms include *Proteus mirabilis*, *Staphylococcus epidermis* and *Streptococcus faecalis*. Culture of infected urine characteristically produces a monoclonal growth; multiclonal growth may indicate a contaminated sample.

Women are much more commonly affected than men; they have a shorter urethra than men (Fig. 3.36.1) and this, and its position, makes contamination with bowel organisms more likely. Consequently, females should only be investigated if they have recurrent lower infections (> 3/year) while a single infection in a male should be investigated further. Other causes are:

- urinary catheter: this may introduce organisms into the bladder; the risk increases if a long-term catheter is necessary
- immunosuppression, e.g. diabetes
- chlamydial infection: a sexually transmitted UTI
- bladder outflow obstruction, e.g. kidney stones or benign prostatic hyperplasia
- structural abnormalities: including **posterior urethral valves**, causing bladder outflow obstruction, or **vesicoureteric reflux**.

Lower tract infections

Acute cystitis

Acute cystitis is an infection of the bladder. It is normally an uncomplicated infection where organisms spread from the perineum and ascend the urethra. Females outnumber males 20:1, and women can expect at least one infection in their lifetime.

Clinical features include:

- frequency, urgency and dysuria (stinging and burning): these are the key signs
- haematuria: may be present
- abdominal pain: may be the first presentation, especially in children where it may be the only sign
- lack of fever: patients with cystitis tend not to become pyrexial (unlike those with pyelonephritis) and have few systemic symptoms.

Urethral syndrome occurs when cystitis symptoms are present but no organisms can be cultured.

Investigations include clean catch mid-stream urine sample; this must be taken *before* starting broad-spectrum antibiotics in order to identify organisms and sensitivities. Children and men should be investigated further. The likelihood of anatomical abnormalities is high.

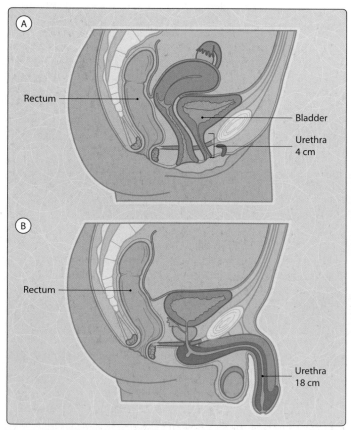

Fig. 3.36.1 The female urethra is 4 cm long (A); the male urethra is 18 cm long (B).

Management of acute cystisis include increased oral fluid intake and antibiotics. A 3-day course of antibiotics (trimethoprin) is adequate for simple UTI in women but males require longer courses of antibiotics (at least 2 weeks) and further investigation; there is evidence that a single dose of trimethoprin is effective in women.

Preventative measures include encouraging micturation immediately after intercourse and teaching females to wipe from 'front to back'. Recurrent infections in any gender may require trimethoprin prophylaxis once anatomical and functional abnormalities are excluded.

Sterile pyuria

A sterile pyuria (infective symptoms where no organisms are cultured) may be caused by tuberculosis (incidence increasing as HIV increases), malignancy (e.g. bladder cancer), appendicitis, any inflammatory lesion adjacent to the bladder (diverticulitis or Crohn's disease) or inadequately treated infection.

Epididymitis

Epididymitis is infection of the epididymis; orchitis is infection of the testes (Ch. 32).

Prostatitis

Bacterial prostatitis is either acute or chronic. Acute infection presents with irritative voiding symptoms, fever or acute urinary retention; chronic infection may present with recurrent low-grade UTI and it may be difficult to clear the organism. Abacterial prostatitis is a different diagnosis and is part of the chronic pelvic pain syndrome, which requires special investigations and exclusion of other diagnoses.

Upper tract infections

Acute pyelonephritis

Acute pyelonephritis is an acute infection of the kidney and can damage kidney function; it may be fatal if left untreated (Fig. 3.36.2). It commonly affects young women idiopathically at puberty, although it may affect older adults with stones or obstruction. The route of infection may be:

- ascending infection: from the lower urinary tract
- haematogenous: from a blood-borne infection (uncommon).
  Clinical features. Unilateral loin pain, fever, rigors and irritative voiding symptoms (frequency, urgency, dysuria).
  Management. Initial ultrasound to exclude hydronephrosis and kidney abnormalities. Prompt intravenous antibiotics (e.g. ciprofloxacin) and fluids are given until the acute episode settles, followed by oral antibiotics for 2 weeks. Obstruction in the presence of infection (e.g. infected kidney stones) is an emergency and should be promptly

relieved (percutaneous nephrostomy) to prevent permanent damage.

Chronic pyelonephritis

Chronic pyelonephritis results from repeated infections causing renal scarring and progressive renal impairment; it is commonly associated with vesicoureteric reflux. It may cause low-grade symptoms or may be silent, only noticed when hypertension or chronic renal failure develops. Recurrent infection can be caused by inadequate treatment of an acute infection, underlying anatomical abnormality or urinary stones (often in the renal pelvis).

The **investigations** required are:

- cystogram: identifies vesicoureteric reflux micturating disease (especially in children)
- mid-stream urine: identifies organisms and sensitivity
- renal ultrasound: identifies abnormal anatomy
- renogram with labelled MAG3: identifies renal scarring and assesses renal function.

The current infection should be treated with antibiotics. Surgical correction of anatomical deformities may be necessary (Teflon injections for reflux, or relocation or ureters if severe). Long-term prophylaxis of UTI may be necessary.

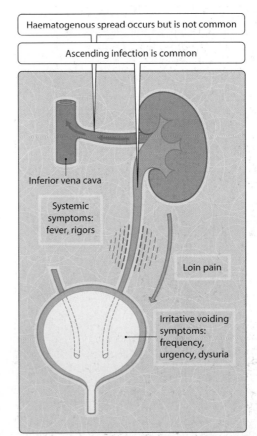

Fig. 3. 36.2 Spread and features of acute pyelonephritis.

Haematogenous spread occurs but is not common

Ascending infection is common

Inferior vena cava

Systemic symptoms: fever, rigors

Loin pain

Irritative voiding symptoms: frequency, urgency, dysuria

37. Urinary incontinence

Questions
- What are the different types of incontinence?
- What are the treatment options for someone with genuine stress incontinence?
- What is the immediate treatment of acute urinary retention?

Incontinence is defined as the involuntary loss of urine and is a symptom, not a diagnosis.

The bladder wall is formed from the detrusor muscle, which is smooth muscle, and is *compliant,* stretching to allow urine to fill the bladder. There are several forms of incontinence (Fig. 3.37.1), although it may be multifactorial in the elderly:

- common causes
  — stress
  — urgency
  — mixed (stress and urge)
  — chronic retention/overflow
- rare
  — fistulae
  — ectopic ureter.

Social embarrassment is often a major patient concern and patients feel ashamed to seek help.

Stress incontinence

Stress incontinence is the involuntary loss of urine when the pressure inside the bladder is greater than the urethral closing pressure. A sudden increase in intra-abdominal pressure (e.g. a cough or sneeze) raises the bladder pressure and causes a small amount of urine to be lost. It is common in middle-aged multiparous women and is caused by pelvic floor weakness, which is most commonly secondary to childbirth.

Investigations
Investigations include:

- examination: incontinence occurs when the patient coughs; there may be a cystocele
- bladder diary: records frequency and volumes
- mid-stream urine: identifies urinary tract infection
- cystometry/urodynamics: shows flow of urine when patient coughs.

Management
Conservative management. Pelvic floor strengthening exercises are required for at least 6 months, plus weight loss and fluid advice.

Medical management. Topical oestrogen creams are used to treat atrophic vaginitis plus selective serotonin and nor-adrenaline (norepinephrine) uptake inhibitors and duloxetine.

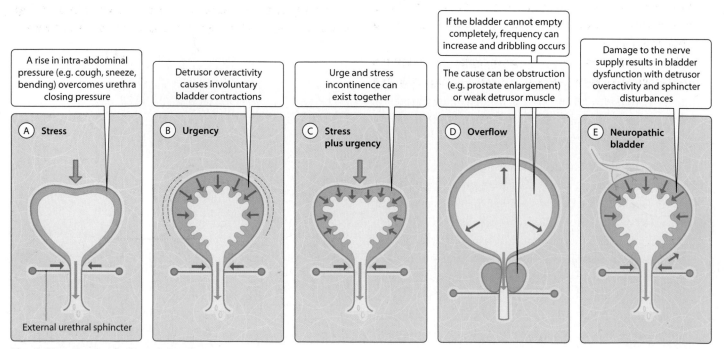

Fig. 3.37.1 Types of urinary incontinence.

Surgical management.

- artificial urinary sphincters and urethral-bulking agents (e.g. collagen)
- vaginal slings: a low-morbidity transvaginal procedure carried out under local anaesthesia and as a day case; the urethra is suspended in a sling formed from cadaver or porcine implants, human tissues (e.g. fascia lata) or, more commonly, synthetic tape (e.g. prolene transvaginal-tape and SPARC)
- Burch colposuspension: although this is the gold standard treatment to elevate the bladder neck and prevent it from opening, it is a major operation with associated morbidity.

Urge incontinence

Urge incontinence is involuntary bladder contractions during the filling phase. The underlying abnormality is an overactive detrusor muscle. There is a sudden urge to pass urine, which often results in incontinence. The overactive detrusor muscle is most often idiopathic. During urge incontinence, the normal control of detrusor contraction is lost. Rarely it is caused by an underlying neurological abnormality.

Urge incontinence is most common in middle-aged women, where small amounts of urine are passed frequently. Urodynamics are performed to confirm the diagnosis, showing regular contractions of the detrusor while the bladder is filling. Note that urge and stress incontinence may exist together.

Management

Conservative management. Bladder retraining attempts to 'educate' the bladder to hold more urine, thus reducing frequency and urgency. The patient is also advised to avoid excessive tea and coffee.

Medical management. This is the mainstay of treatment. Anticholinergic drugs prevent detrusor overactivity but cause side-effects (e.g. blurred vision, dry mouth, constipation). Oxybutynin, tolterodine and solifenacin (antimuscarinic action) may help. More recently botulinum toxin A has been used very successfully; it is injected into the bladder via cystoscopy.

Surgical management. Surgery is rarely performed and only as a last resort. Bladder enlargement utilizes a section of ileum (**clam ileocystoplasty**).

Overflow incontinence

When the urinary bladder cannot empty fully, there is 'overflow' of urine, leading to frequency of small amounts of urine and constant dribbling; this often occurs during the day and the night. The passage of urine is often of low volume and weak, and there is a high residual volume in the bladder. The cause is usually chronic, either a hypotonic bladder or bladder outflow obstruction (e.g. benign prostatic hyperplasia).

Cystometry confirms the diagnosis, showing an overfull bladder with weak contraction and weak detrusor activity. Treatment is by relieving the obstruction (e.g. transurethral resection of prostate for benign prostatic hyperplasia) or with intermittent self-catheterization.

The neuropathic bladder

Damage to the nervous supply of the bladder causes neurological loss of control, resulting in bladder dysfunction with detrusor overactivity and sphincter disturbance. Causes include dementia, Parkinson's disease, multiple sclerosis, diabetic neuropathy, spinal cord injury and lesions, spina bifida and malignancy. Treatment depends on the cause. There is a risk of incontinence and recurrent urinary tract infection; high vesical pressure leads to upper tract damage and renal failure.

38. Breast cancer

Questions
- Who is screened for breast cancer?
- How is a presurgical diagnosis of breast cancer formed?
- How is lymph node status determined?

Breast cancer is the commonest cancer affecting women: 1 in 10 women develop the disease in the UK. All women aged 50 to 70 years in the UK are currently invited for mammography. Less than 1% of breast cancers occur in males, where prognosis is worse because they present later.

Aetiology

Risk factors include:

- age: higher over 50 years; rare under 35 years
- family history: first-degree relatives
- genetics: 5% of cancers are caused by breast cancer genes (*BRCA1* and *BRCA2*); they give an 80–90% risk of developing cancer
- oestrogen exposure: early menarche (< 12 years), late menopause (> 55), oral contraceptives, hormone replacement therapy, obesity.

Clinical features

Breast cancer can present with specific features (Fig. 3.38.1), during screening (mammography; Fig. 3.38.2), which has reduced mortality by 30%, or as metastatic disease (back pain (vertebrae), breathlessness (lungs), jaundice/abdominal distension (liver)).

Pathology

Ductal carcinoma is the most common type. The rarer variants (lobular, tubular, cribriform, mucinous, medullary) have distinctive histological appearances and a better prognosis.

Oestrogen receptor (ER) expression.   A tumour expressing ERs is dependent on oestrogen and susceptible to hormone therapies. The ER status is determined histologically; ER-positive tumours (more common) have a better prognosis.

Ductal carcinoma in situ.   This is a non-invasive cancer where malignant cells have not penetrated the epithelial basement membrane and so have not yet extended out of the breast duct system. It may be detectable by mammography and biopsy of microcalcification before invasion occurs and is usually asymptomatic.

Paget's disease of the nipple.   This is a skin manifestation (patch of eczema around the nipple) of an underlying breast malignancy (1% of cancers). Ductal carcinoma in situ is often associated early on, but it will develop into invasive cancer if untreated. An underlying lump may be palpable (not always), and mammography and nipple biopsy should be performed.

Inflammatory disease of the breast.   Lymphatic invasion by a highly malignant carcinoma can lead to a rapid-onset red, hot and swollen breast. These tumours are often non-resectable and prognosis is poor.

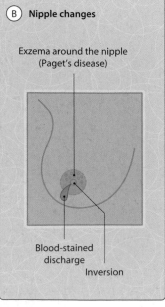

Fig. 3.38.1 Presentation of breast cancer.

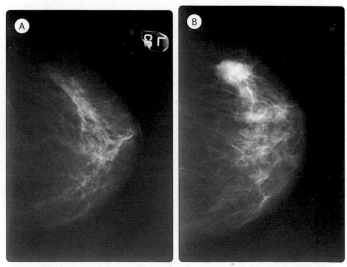

Fig. 3.38.2 Mammography: (A) normal (craniocaudal view); (B) a spiculated mass.

Investigations

Presurgical diagnosis is formed by triple assessment:

- Clinical examination: skin tethering, nipple changes, asymmetry of the breast, a painless, hard, irregular lump
- imaging: screened mammography uses craniocaudal and oblique views; ultrasound differentiates cysts from solid lesions and is useful in women under 35 years as their breast tissue is more dense
- biopsy: a fine needle aspiration, core (tru-cut) biopsy or open biopsy; fine needle aspiration will distinguish benign from malignant cells and core biopsy indicates whether the cancer is invasive.

Management

The patient is managed by a multidisciplinary team. A 'curative' approach is used when there is either no lymph node involvement or only the axillary nodes are involved. A palliative approach is used for symptom relief when distant metastases are present.

Curative approach

There are two surgical options that have equivalent survival:

- breast-conserving surgery: the lump is removed with a wide margin of excision followed by radiotherapy; it is suitable for smaller tumours (< 5 cm) and for patients who wish for minimal surgery
- mastectomy (removal of the whole breast): suitable for large (> 5 cm), central or multifocal tumours.

Breast reconstruction is either immediate or delayed, with muscle flaps such as the rectus abdominis myocutaneous (TRAM) flap.

Palliative treatment in metastatic disease

Hormonal therapies, radiotherapy and chemotherapy all play a role in reducing pain and progression. A 'toilet' mastectomy removes fungating lesions, and pathological fractures of long bones may be fixed.

Assessment of lymph node status

Axillary lymph node clearance. The axillary nodes are cleared in invasive cancer, which controls local disease and allow for staging (thus directing further treatment). **Lymphoedema** of the affected arm is a potential complication.

Sentinel lymph node biopsy. The first node in a lymphatic chain is the *sentinel node*. A radioactive blue dye injected into the axilla causes the sentinel node to turn blue first, which is identifiable at surgery by the blue dye and radioactivity. This is biopsied for metastasis; if negative, the rest of the lymphatic

Table 3.38.1 THE NOTTINGHAM PROGNOSTIC INDEX (NPI)

NPI score	Prognosis	5 year survival (%)
< 3	Excellent	> 90
3–3.4	Good	70
3.4–5.4	Intermediate	50
> 5.4	Poor	20

The NPI score is (0.2 × size in cm) + grade (1–3) + lymph node status (1–3).
Grade of differentiation: 1, good; 2, moderate; 3, poor.
Lymph node involvement: 1, none; 2, 1–3 nodes; 3, ≥ 4 nodes.

trunk is probably free of metastases; if positive, all nodes are removed from the axilla. The false-negative rate for sentinel lymph node biopsy is about 5% in the best series.

Adjuvant therapies

Adjuvant therapies reduce recurrence and increase survival.

Hormonal treatments:

- tamoxifen is an anti-oestrogen (it in fact has a weak agonist action) that decreases cancer recurrence; it is currently given for 5 years
- aromatase inhibitors (e.g. anastrazole) block oestrogen synthesis; this is possibly more effective than tamoxifen
- trastuzumab (Herceptin): a monoclonal antibody that blocks HER2 receptors on the surface of HER2-positive tumour cells; it slows cell growth and is given with chemotherapy
- ovarian ablation: luteinizing hormone releasing-hormone (LHRH) agonists and oophrectomy (removal of ovaries) eliminate oestrogen production.

Radiotherapy. Chest wall and breast radiotherapy is given after wide local excision, and sometimes following mastectomy.

Chemotherapy. Anthracycline-based chemotherapy is used to treat women with any poor prognostic factors.

Special conditions

Ductal carcinoma in situ. Either wide local excision with radiotherapy or mastectomy can be used, depending on extent of disease.

Carriage of BRCA. Either annual surveillance with mammography or prophylactic bilateral mastectomy (reduces risk by 90%) can be used.

Paget's disease. Patients with an underlying invasive breast cancer undergo mastectomy and lymph node clearance.

Prognosis

The Nottingham Prognostic Index (Table 3.38.1) is a system that combines assessment of size, grade and lymph node status.

39. Benign breast disease and breast examination

Questions
■ What is the most common of cause of a breast lump in a 25-year-old woman?
■ What is fibrocystic change?
■ How do you examine a breast?

The majority of women who present with a breast problem have a benign disease. They can present with a lump, breast enlargement, pain, nipple changes or discharge (Fig. 3.39.1). Any suspicious lump should be investigated with triple assessment (Ch. 38) to exclude malignancy. The causes of single lumps are:

■ breast cancer: *firm, fixed, irregular*
■ fibroadenoma
■ breast cyst: *fluctuant, mobile.*

The causes of multiples lumps are:

■ fibroadenomas
■ fibrocystic change (cyclical symptoms)
■ breast cysts.

Benign breast conditions

Fibroadenoma.   This benign tumour is the most common breast lump in women under 30 years. It is a hard, mobile and painless lump. If a definite diagnosis of fibroadenomas is confirmed, the lump need not be excised.

Fibrocystic change.   This is a common presentation and is now considered to be simply a variant of normal (it is not premalignant). It is caused by cyclical proliferation and involution of breast tissue, and so symptoms change with the menstrual cycle. It occurs in women between 25 and 45 years, and may present with:

■ cyclical breast pain
■ multiple or single lumps: triple assessment is performed if a solitary lump is present
■ cysts: treat with aspiration.

Pain relief, oral contraceptives and evening primrose oil may also be used in its treatment.

Breast cysts.   Cysts are a very common abnormality, and are predominately seen in women aged 40–60 years, when 50% develop one or more cysts. They are fluctuant and are diagnosed with ultrasound scanning. They are treated with needle aspiration during triple assessment if palpable.

Breast pain (mastalgia).   Pain is associated with benign disease and may be unilateral or bilateral. Cyclic mastalgia relates to the menstrual cycle and pathology is excluded by examination and imaging. Treatment is conservative (firm bras, paracetamol, evening primrose oil), and hormone therapies may help with chronic pain.

Nipple discharge.   This is a common symptom and is only rarely caused by an underlying carcinoma (Table 3.39.1). **Duct ectasia** is the most common cause of nipple discharge. It is breast duct dilatation accompanied by periductal inflammation. Nipple retraction, periareolar inflammation

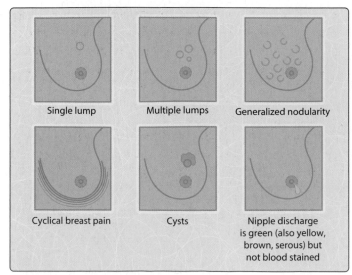

Fig. 3.39.1 Features of fibrocystic change.

Table 3.39.1 CAUSES OF NIPPLE DISCHARGE

Colour of discharge	Cause	Management
Green	Duct ectasia	Excision of affected ducts
Green/yellow/brown	Fibrocystic change	Excision of affected ducts
Blood (red)	Carcinoma Duct papilloma (a benign tumour with hyperplasia of the epithelial lining)	As for cancer Excise ducts (microdochectomy)
White/clear	Lactation; galactorrhoea	Test plasma prolactin if bilateral (it could be a prolactinoma)
Serous	Physiological Fibrocystic change Duct ectasia	Conservative Conservative Excision
Purulent	Breast abscess	Antibiotics

(red and tender nipples) and green discharge occur, and a lump may be found (which undergoes triple assessment). Antibiotics may be tried, but definitive treatment is surgical excision of all the major ducts.

Breast infection. Breast infections are usually caused by a common bacteria found on normal skin (*Staphylococcus aureus*). The bacteria enter through a break or crack in the skin, usually the nipple. Breast infections usually occur in women who are breast-feeding. Breast infections that are not related to breast-feeding must be differentiated from a rare form of cancer, inflammatory breast cancer, which is a highly malignant carcinoma. Infections include:

- **mastitis**: mostly occurs during lactation and is caused by *S. aureus*; breast feeding can be continued
- **cellulitis**: the initial stages of an infection, which can be arrested with antibiotics (flucloxacillin); if not promptly treated, an abscess may develop
- **abscess**: infection followed by pus accumulation, leading to mass formation; the abscess should be aspirated and followed by antibiotic therapy; breast feeding is continued from the other breast.

Fat necrosis. Trauma damages fat cells and causes an immune reaction, followed by fibrosis and painless lump formation. The lump should be aspirated to exclude malignancy, and then can be excised.

Gynaecomastia. This is hypertrophy of breast tissue in males (occasionally painful). It can occur at puberty (as a result of normal growth). In older men it is caused by chronic liver disease, drugs (digoxin, spironolactone, cimetidine) or tumours (pituitary, testicular, lung).

Examination of the breast

Introduction
The patient should initially be sitting at 45° and exposed from the waist up with her bra removed.

Inspection
Look for asymmetry, nipple changes (retraction, discharge), skin dimpling, local depression and oedema (Fig. 3.39.2). Then inspect:

- with her arms resting down by her sides
- with her arms above her head
- with the patient pressing her arms into her hips (tensing the pectoral muscles).

Palpation
Ask if the breasts are painful, and if the patient has noticed a lump; if so ask the patient to indicate where it is. Both breasts are palpated, starting with the normal breast and using the flat of the fingers.

Assessing the breast for lumps. The normal breast is palpated in each quadrant, and then towards the centre around the nipple, until finally over the nipple. Palpate the nipple carefully, and note the characteristics and source of any discharge. Palpate the axillary tail between a finger and thumb as it extends into the axilla. The affected breast is then palpated in all areas away from the lump. Finally the lump is assessed for site, size, shape, surface, overlying skin, tethered, fluctuant/fixation/mobility.

Assessing the axillary lymph nodes (Fig. 3.39.2B). The clinician uses one arm to take the entire weight of the patient's arm. The axilla is then palpated fully (apex, medial, anterior, posterior, lateral) for any lymph nodes. This is repeated on both sides. The cervical, supra- and infraclavicular lymph nodes are also examined.

Concluding the examination
Further examination that should be suggested is for evidence of metastases, by palpating the liver for enlargement, examining the vertebrae for pain and auscultating the lungs.

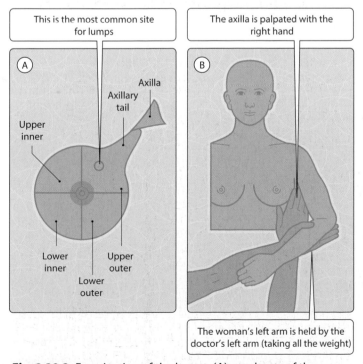

Fig. 3.39.2 Examination of the breast. (A) quadrants of the breast; (B) palpating the axilla.

40. Thyroid disorders

Questions
- What are the causes of thyroid lumps?
- What are the complications of thyroid surgery?
- What are the features of thyroid dysfunction?

Patients with thyroid disease typically present with symptoms of hyperthyroidism, hypothyroidism or a thyroid enlargement (Table 3.40.1). Patients with a goitre may be hyperthyroid, euthyroid (neutral) or hypothyroid (Fig. 3.40.1). Goitres can give rise to mechanical problems: palsy of the recurrent laryngeal nerve (**hoarseness**), tracheal compression (**stridor**) and oesophageal compression (**dysphagia**) (Fig. 3.40.2).

Management
Medical management.   **Hyperthyroidism** is managed using:
- propanolol (a beta blocker) to control symptoms
- carbimazole or propylthiouracil: both interfere with the synthesis of thyroid hormones; bone marrow suppression (**agranulocytosis**) is a rare but potentially lethal side-effect, so patients must be counselled to report sore throats, mouth ulcers, fever and malaise promptly
- radioactive iodine: causes localized destruction of thyroid tissue after uptake; this leads to a decrease in the release of thyroid hormones and is used when repeated medical treatment fails (it is contraindicated in pregnancy);

patients must be warned that hypothyroidism is very common in the long term.

Surgical management.   Thyroidectomy is indicated for:
- diagnosis: thyroid follicular adenomas and follicular carcinomas are not distinguishable on fine needle aspirants
- thyroid cancer
- hyperthyroidism: uncontrolled by medication
- cosmetic reasons (goitre debulking)
- tracheal and superior mediastinal decompression.

Complications of thyroid surgery.   The early complications of thyroid surgery are:
- laryngeal swelling: oedema or haemorrhage compress the trachea, causing stridor (an inspiratory rasping noise caused by upper airway obstruction)
- thyroid crisis (storm): may lead to sudden lethal hyperthyroidism
- hypocalcaemic tetany: caused by accidental removal of the parathyroid glands
- recurrent laryngeal nerve damage: unilateral damage causes hoarseness of voice; bilateral damage (rare) may present as laryngeal obstruction
- superior laryngeal nerve damage: change in quality of voice.

Hypothyroidism is a long-term complication and requires lifelong thyroxine replacement.

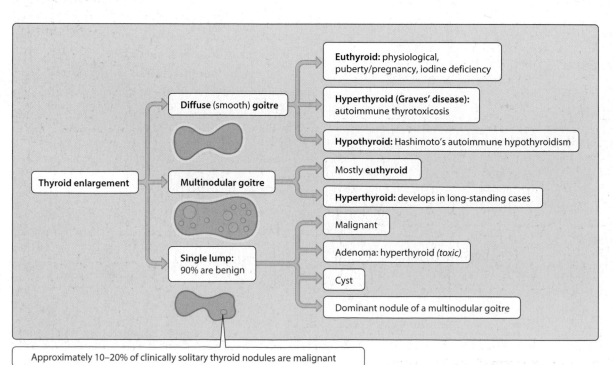

Fig. 3.40.1 Assessment of goitre. Fine needle aspiration and cytology has 90% accuracy in diagnosis.

Thyroid enlargement

Diffuse (smooth) goitre
- **Euthyroid:** physiological, puberty/pregnancy, iodine deficiency
- **Hyperthyroid (Graves' disease):** autoimmune thyrotoxicosis
- **Hypothyroid:** Hashimoto's autoimmune hypothyroidism

Multinodular goitre
- Mostly **euthyroid**
- **Hyperthyroid:** develops in long-standing cases

Single lump: 90% are benign
- Malignant
- Adenoma: hyperthyroid *(toxic)*
- Cyst
- Dominant nodule of a multinodular goitre

Approximately 10–20% of clinically solitary thyroid nodules are malignant

Thyroid cancer

Suspicious symptoms are single neck lump, lymphadenopathy, neck pain, dysphagia, dysphonia, bone pain and haemoptysis.

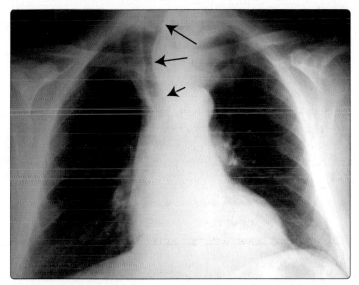

Fig. 3.40.2 Retrosternal goitre. The trachea is deviated to the right by a large retrosternal mass (M), which is an enlarged left lobe of the thyroid gland with retrosternal extension.

Pathology

There are various types of thyroid cancer:

- papillary: most common type, presents between 20 and 30 years, best prognosis
- follicular: presents at 30–40 years, metastasizes early
- medullary: uncommon, associated with multiple endocrine neoplasia 2 (Ch. 41)
- anaplastic: rare, age 60–80 years, very aggressive, poor prognosis
- lymphoma: non-Hodgkin's, women > 50 years, good prognosis unless widespread.

Management

Treatment is primarily surgical after patient is rendered euthyroid. Papillary, follicular and medullary cancers are treated by total thyroidectomy with lymph node clearance followed by radioactive iodine. Anaplastic cancer is palliated with chemotherapy and radiotherapy to relieve tracheal symptoms.

Differentiated thyroid tumours are sensitive to thyroid-stimulating hormone (TSH), so patients should be given thyroxine to suppress its secretion from the anterior pituitary gland, which is monitored by following TSH levels postoperatively.

Table 3.40.1 FEATURES OF THYROID DYSFUNCTION

Feature	Hyperthyroid	Hypothyroid
General	Thin, anxious, wasted facial muscles	Overweight, lethargic, slow speech, hoarseness
Hands	Sweating Fine tremor, seen if the hands are outstretched Thyroid acropachy: thyroid finger clubbing associated with Graves' disease Onycholysis: nail is lifted out of its bed (also in psoriasis) Palmar erythema	Cold and dry; the fingertips may be blue Non-pitting oedema of congestive heart failure
Pulse	Tachycardia, atrial fibrillation	Bradycardia
Eyes	Exophthalmos: protruding eyes as a result of retro-orbital oedema; sclera is visible all the way around the iris Lid retraction: raised upper eyelid where sclera is not visible all the way around the iris Proptosis: the eye protrudes forward so far it is visible beyond the supraorbital ridge when viewed from above Chemosis: periorbital oedema with redness Lid lag when performing eye movements: on vertical gaze (possible double vision) Opthalmaplegia occurs as eye movements are weak (especially upward gaze)	Enophthalmos: loss of the outer third of the eyebrow
Reflexes	Brisk reflexes at the knee	Slow relaxing reflexes
Ankles	Pre-tibial myxoedema: thickening of the tissues in front of tibias (rare)	Signs of non-pitting oedema of congestive heart failure

Thyroid hormones
  Free T_3 or T_4 ↑
  Total T_3 or T_4 ↑
  TSH ↓
		↓
		↓
		↑

T_3, triiodothyronine; T_4, thyroxine; TSH, thyroid-stimulating hormone.

41. Lymph nodes and endocrine disorders

Questions
- What are the causes of hypercalcaemia?
- What tumours affect the adrenal gland?
- What are the causes of an enlarged lymph node in the head and neck?

Lymph nodes

The body has approximately 500 lymph nodes, around 200 of these are in the head and neck (Fig. 3.41.1). Causes of enlarged head and neck lymph nodes are important to remember as an OSCE might well include a node in the neck (remember LIST: lymphoma/leukaemia, infection, sarcoidosis, tumour); they include infections (e.g. tonsillitis, tuberculosis), malignancy (skin cancers, lymphoma, metastases) and sarcoidosis.

Lymph nodes of the head are examined by palpation from behind the patient, using gentle rotation movements of the fingertips (Ch. 42). If enlarged lymph nodes are found, then an examination should look for general lymphadenopathy (e.g. by palpation of the axilla and groin).

Cervical metastases from a distant tumour

Tumours metastasize to the cervical nodes from the lips, tongue, oral cavity, larynx, pharynx and nasopharynx. Tumours in these areas are linked to smoking and chewing carcinogens.

Parathyroid glands

There are four parathyroid glands, which lie behind the thyroid gland. They secrete parathyroid hormone, a substance that helps to maintain the correct balance of calcium and phosphorous in the body. In **hyperparathyroidism**, blood calcium rises and it is this hypercalcaemia that usually signals that something may be wrong with the parathyroid glands.

Hyperparathyroidism can be:

- **primary**: the parathyroid gland excretes excess parathyroid hormone, resulting in high calcium levels; adenomas cause 90% and treatment is with surgical excision of the adenoma
- **secondary**: hypocalcaemia (e.g. from renal failure, vitamin D deficiency) causes the parathyroid gland to increase production of parathyroid hormone
- **tertiary**: once the long-standing cause of calcium loss in secondary hyperparathyroidism has been stopped and calcium returns to normal, the parathyroids continue to secrete excess parathyroid hormone.

Hypercalcaemia can be caused by:

- malignancy: multiple myeloma, bone metastases
- primary hyperparathyroidism
- excess dietary vitamin D
- Addison's disease
- thiazide diuretics
- Paget's disease.

In patients who are symptomatic, these are remembered as 'bones, stones, moans and groans':

- bones: bone pain and pathological fractures from bone cysts
- stones: increased production of calcium urinary stones, renal failure, polyuria
- moans: psychiatric disturbance (depression, lethargy, confusion)
- groans: abdominal pain.

The radiological features of hyperparathyroidism are:

- subperiosteal bone resorption
- pepperpot skull
- brown tumours: osteoclast resorption is stimulated, causing holes in the bone that are filled with fibrous tissue; these can link together, leaving a large defect called a brown tumour.

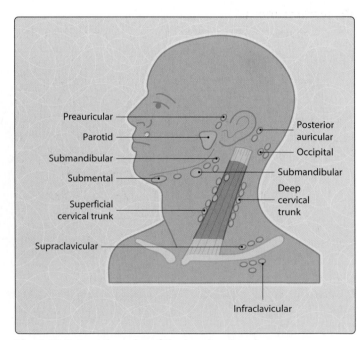

Fig. 3.41.1 Lymph nodes of the head and neck.

Adrenal disorders

Neuroblastoma. This malignant tumour of neural crest tissue most commonly arises in the adrenal medulla. It mostly presents in children < 2 years, with an abdominal mass or failure to thrive. Treatment is with surgical resection and chemo/radiotherapy. Prognosis is poor at 30–35%.

Phaeochromocytoma. This neoplasm of the chromaffin cells of the adrenal medulla produces high levels of catecholoamines (noradrenaline and adrenaline) and typically presents in early adulthood or middle age, with either sustained or intermittent symptoms of headache, sweating, palpitation, vomiting, anxiety, weakness (where 'attacks' last minutes to hours). Hypertension is the most common feature. Diagnosis is with 24-h urine collection, which will show raised catecholamines. Surgical resection is performed.

Multiple endocrine neoplasia type 2 (MEN-2). This is a syndrome of phaeochromocytoma, medullary thyroid tumour and hyperparathyroidism existing together.

Conn's syndrome. Conn's syndrome or primary hyper-aldosteronism is most often caused by a unilateral adrenocortical adenoma. It causes hypokalaemia and is a secondary cause of hypertension. Unilateral adrenalectomy (usually laparoscopically) is the treatment of choice. (If bilateral hyperplasia is the cause (one-third), treatment is medical.)

Pituitary tumours

Pituitary tumours are uncommon tumours that oversecrete hormones. Symptoms are:

- overproduction of hormones: the specific symptoms will depend on the type of hormone that is being overproduced
- visual deficits: caused by local pressure, a large tumour grows in a superior direction and compresses the optic chiasm (causing bitemporal hemianopia)
- hypopituitarism: a non-functioning adenoma can compress the pituitary gland, depressing normal hormone production
- non-specific symptoms of headaches or a sensation of pressure or fullness behind the eyes.

Pituitary tumours are almost always benign adenomas. They are assessed by MRI to determine size and anatomical information and by full endocrinological evaluation to determine whether hormone levels have been affected. Symptoms and classification depend on the hormones produced.

Adrenocorticotrophic hormone (ACTH)-secreting tumour. Excess glucocorticoid (cortisol) secretion from the adrenal cortex is stimulated by excess secretion of ACTH from a pituitary tumour. **Cushing's disease** is an ACTH-secreting pituitary tumour. **Cushing's syndrome** is when the symptoms are caused by hormone excess from another source, an adrenal adenoma/carcinoma, ectopic ACTH secretion (e.g. small cell lung cancer) or prolonged steroid use (iatrogenic; the most common cause of Cushing's syndrome). Cushingoid features include a moon face, central weight gain with peripheral weight loss, purple striations, poor wound healing, hypertension, diabetes, osteoporosis, a buffalo hump, oedema and psychiatric disturbance. A dexamethasone suppression test confirms the diagnosis.

Growth hormone. Overproduction of growth hormone causes acromegaly (gigantism in a child); treatment is with pituitary surgery.

Prolactin-secreting tumour (prolactinoma). Excess prolactin will cause infertility or galactorrhoea.

Management

Medical treatment is available for pituitary adenoma that overproduce prolactin (bromocriptine) and growth hormone (octreotide). For Cushing's disease, the treatment of choice is surgery using a **trans-sphenoidal** approach (via the nose) to resect as much of the tumour as is safe. It is followed by radiotherapy.

42. Neck lumps

Questions
- What is a midline lump that moves on tongue protusion likely to be?
- What is a non-midline lump with a fistula likely to be?

Neck lumps are examined with a specific scheme (Ch. 43), to differentiate thyroid lumps from other neck lumps. Lumps can be differentiated into midline and non-midline lumps (Fig. 3.42.1) and whether they are in the anterior or posterior triangle of the neck (see Fig. 3.43.1).

■ MIDLINE LUMPS

Thyroid goitre. A goitre is an overgrowth of the thyroid gland, which may be a diffuse or multinodular, or a single thyroid lump (Ch. 40).

Thyroglossal duct cyst (and sinus). This is a remnant of the embryological thryroglossal duct. It is higher than the normal position of a goitre, and 40% present in the first decade. The lump moves up on swallowing and on tongue protrusion, because the lump is still attached to the **thyroglossal tract** and **hyoid bone**, part of which must be removed as well as the track at surgery. Fine needle aspiration for cytology and ultrasound can be performed if there is any doubt about the diagnosis (e.g. cancer). If the cyst ruptures, a thyroglossal sinus may form.

Dermoid cyst. Dermoid cysts arise where an embryonic dermatome has fused. Consequently, they often occur in the midline of the trunk and also in the head (typically around the eyebrow and behind the ear) and neck. They are normally 1–2 cm in diameter, may be firm or soft and are smooth. Treatment is with surgical excision. Not all dermoid cysts are midline.

Pharyngeal pouch. This arises at the junction of the pharynx and oesophagus and is a rare cause of dysphagia. Diagnosis is with barium swallow and treatment is by surgical excision or endoscopic stapling.

■ NON-MIDLINE LUMPS

Lymph nodes are covered in Ch. 41.

Salivary gland lumps

There are three pairs of salivary glands: the **parotid**, **submandibular** and **sublingual glands**. Swellings of these glands may also be apparent on the face as well as neck.

Clinical features. The lump should be assessed in relation to the anatomical landmarks and the position of one of the three salivary glands. Initially the lump is inspected from in front and then palpated from behind the patient. The special tests are:
- bimanual palpation of the lump: observe in the oral cavity, looking for swellings, discharge, salivary ducts,

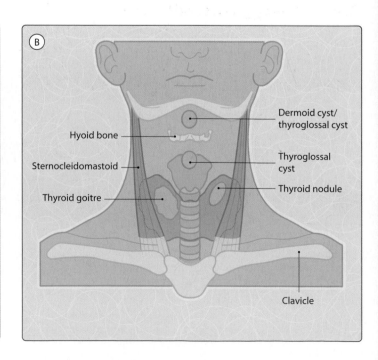

Fig. 3.42.1 Neck lumps: (A) non-midline and (B) midline lumps.

pigmentation and inflammation; palpate with one gloved finger in the mouth, one finger underneath the mandible

- assessment of the facial nerve: ask the patient to perform these tests (while demonstrating yourself): raise eyebrows high, screw eyes shut, blow out cheeks, show teeth (gritted).

Causes of salivary gland swelling:

- infection: bacterial, viral (mumps)
- benign and malignant tumours: 80% of all salivary gland tumours are in the parotid gland; 80% are benign and 80% are pleomorphic adenomas
  - pleomorphic adenoma: benign tumours (most common of all salivary gland tumours); as the tumour often grows outside of the capsule, treatment is by surgical excision including the area around the capsule (otherwise there is risk of recurrence); the main complication is damage to the facial nerve, and its branches should be carefully identified
  - adenoid cystic carcinomas: the most common malignant tumour, highly invasive, metastasizes early and perineurally
  - Warthin's tumour: an adenolymphoma (benign cystic tumour); it is soft and well differentiated, and treatment is with surgical excision
- stones: most commonly in the submandibular gland; they present with intermittent pain and swelling on eating, or with pain if infected
- rare autoimmune causes: Sjögren's syndrome (also with dry eyes and mouth), sarcoidosis.

Branchial cysts, sinuses and fistulae

Modern thinking is that a **branchial cyst** represents a degenerative lymph node (older theories are that it is a remnant of the second branchial cleft). Patients are often in their 20s. Presentation is with a painless swelling (or a red tender swelling if infected) underneath the anterior border of the sternocleidomastoid muscle at the level of the hyoid, and the lump is transilluminable. If the branchial cyst fails to close off embryologically, a **branchial sinus** forms that discharges anywhere along the anterior border of the sternocleidomastoid. Treatment for both is by surgical excision. A **branchial fistula** arises from a persistent second pharyngeal pouch and opens onto the inferior third of the anterior border of the sternocleidomastoid.

Other causes of non-midline lumps

Lymphatic malformations. These are also known as **cystic hygromas** and are found in children in the posterior triangle. They are multiple congenital cysts filled with lymphatic fluid, which remain within the jugular lymphatic sac. They may be very large and are soft, fluctuant and brilliantly transilluminable. Treatment is with surgical excision, although this may prove difficult.

Carotid body tumour. Also known as a chemodectoma, these are very rare. They are often pulsatile, move from side to side (*not* up and down) and empty when compressed. Approximately 5% are malignant, and they may be bilateral. Treatment is by excision (vascular surgeon) with care not to damage cranial nerves IX and XII.

Sternocleidomastoid tumour. An ischaemic, fibrous mass can develop within the sternocleidomastoid muscle. Following a traumatic delivery, damaged muscle fibres contract and heal to form a fibrous mass. It causes fixed rotation of the head towards the affected side (**torticollis**) and is very hard upon palpation and within the muscle. It should be removed by surgical excision to prevent asymmetry of the face and visual complications.

Cervical rib. This extra rib (typically attaching to C7) may present as a neck lump. Other symptoms include neurovascular problems of the affected limb (Ch. 26).

43. Examination of the neck

Questions
- How can you identify a thyroid lump?
- What are the boundaries of the neck triangles?
- How do you assess the thyroid status?

The scheme shown in Fig. 3.43.1 contains the steps needed to differentiate neck lumps. These can be considered as midline or non-midline (Ch. 42) and whether they are in the anterior or posterior triangle of the neck (Fig. 3.43.2). The **anterior triangle** is bordered by the midline of the neck (anterior border), the anterior border of sternocleidomastoid (posterior border) and the inferior border of the mandible (superior border). The **posterior triangle** is bordered by the posterior border of sternocleidomastoid (anterior border), the anterior border of the trapezius (posterior border) and the superior border of the clavicle (inferior border).

The most effective investigations for an unknown lump are CT, MRI and fine needle aspirate cytology.

An OSCE might involve thyroid goitre, surgically corrected goitre, lymph nodes, thyroglossal cyst or other neck lump, usually a salivary gland swelling. The patient should be asked to expose the neck fully or remove their top.

Inspection
Inspection needs to consider the lump, swallowing and tongue protrusion:

- lumps: look for obvious swellings or lumps; note the size, shape, site and overlying skin
- site: is the lump in the midline; is it in the anterior or posterior triangle (see Fig. 3.41.2); is it in the anatomical position of the thyroid gland?
- scars: a horizontal scar is the most common sign of previous thyroid surgery (the patient is now euthyroid or hypothyroid)

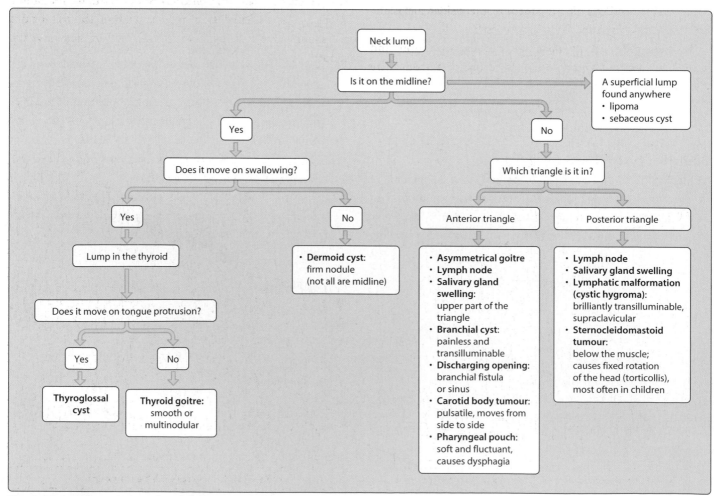

Fig. 3.43.1 Differentiation of neck lumps.

- distended neck veins: as a result of thoracic outlet obstruction.

A potential thyroid swelling is assessed by:

- swallowing: ask the patient to take a sip of water, hold it in their mouth and then swallow; if the lump moves, it is in the thyroid gland
- tongue protrusion: Ask the patient to 'stick their tongue out'; if the lump moves upwards, it is attached to the hyoid cartilage (possibly a thyroglossal cyst); if it does not move (but does with swallowing), the lump is within the thyroid.

Palpation

The clinician (or student in an OSCE) stands behind the patient to feel the neck (Fig. 3.43.3). Both hands are used gently to palpate the lump and assess its surface. Is it diffuse, multinodular or a single lump?

The water swallowing and tongue protrusion tests are repeated while palpating the neck.

The lymph nodes are examined to identify lymphadenopathy (Ch. 42). If local lymphadenopathy is found, generalized lymphadenopathy should be assessed. At this point in an OSCE, list the causes and examine for them (e.g. consider metastatic cancer, possibly from the thyroid or breast).

From in front of the patient, tracheal deviation and transillumination of a lump are assessed (cystic hygromas are brilliantly transilluminable). Tracheal deviation is identified by palpating gently the suprasternal notch. Deviation is caused by a large mass (e.g. goitre). Cystic hygromas are brilliantly transilluminable.

Percussion

Retrosternal extension of a mass is assessed by percussing downwards from the goitre, over the clavicle to the second rib. Such extension could cause obstruction of the superior vena cava.

Auscultation

A bruit over a goitre indicates Graves' disease.

Concluding the examination

At the end of an OSCE station, a student would state that the patient's thyroid status should be assessed (Table 3.40.1). Investigation of a thyroid lump would include bloods, ultrasound, fine needle aspiration (for a solid single lump to identify malignancy and to remove fluid from a cyst), diagnostic lobectomy (to detect adenomas and carcinomas if follicular cells identified), thoracic inlet radiography (tracheal deviation and retrosternal extension) and MRI/CT (for preoperative anatomical detail). It is essential that an examination should include (or should state that it should include) the eye, ear, nose and mouth.

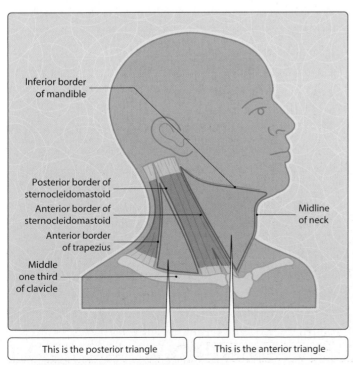

| This is the posterior triangle | This is the anterior triangle |

Fig. 3.43.2 Triangles of the neck.

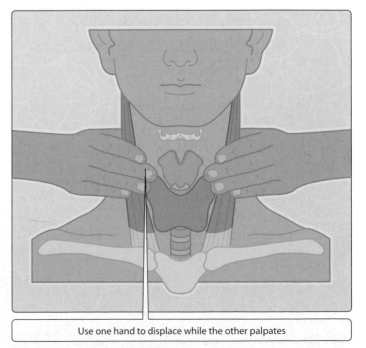

| Use one hand to displace while the other palpates |

Fig. 3.43.3 Palpating the neck.

44. Managing trauma

Questions
- What is the primary survey?
- What is the secondary survey, and when is it commenced?
- How can you control an airway?

Management of major traumas arriving in hospitals is standardized so that the team's priorities in the initial care of the patient are set and nothing is missed.

The primary survey

The initial management is with ABC:

A: airway (with cervical spine control)

B: breathing with ventilatory support

C: circulation with haemorrhage control.

Also consider:

D: dysfunction (neurological status)

E: exposure.

The primary survey is repeated until the patient is stable. Only then are radiographs and the secondary survey initiated.

Airway

The first step in evaluating and treating any trauma patient is to assess airway patency and, if compromised, restore it. If the patient can speak, this suggests a patent airway.

Stridor is indicative of upper airway obstruction. Obstruction such as the position of the tongue, a foreign body or vomit is assessed. The tongue is controlled with adjuvants (see below) and foreign objects are removed with suction or Magill forceps. All patients should be given 100% oxygen at 15 l/min.

Management of the airway

- simple measures
  — chin lift, jaw thrust manoeuvres
  — Guedel airway
  — nasopharyngeal tube
- definite airway (Fig. 3.44.1)
  — endotracheal intubation: orotracheal, nasotracheal
  — surgical airway: cricothyroidotomy; this is a last resort and is only effective for 30–45 min.

Indications for a definitive airway are:

- the presence of apnoea
- inability to maintain a patent airway by less-invasive means
- to protect the lower airway from aspiration of blood or vomitus
- impending or potential airway compromise (e.g. following inhalational injury, facial fractures)
- presence of a closed head injury requiring assisted ventilation
- inability to maintain adequate oxygenation by face mask oxygen supplementation
- any patient with a Glasgow Coma Score (GCS) of 8 or less; see Ch. 72) will have loss of airway protective reflexes (e.g. gag reflex).

Cervical spine control

Full cervical spine immobilization is required with a hard collar and lateral supports with straps across the forehead and chin (a collar alone will *not* do). The cervical spine is checked carefully for fractures by radiograph and clinical examination during the secondary survey; if either is positive, a fracture is assumed.

Breathing

Breathing is assessed by:

- respiratory rate: count and record, look for tachypnoea
- chest expansion: decreased on side of tension pneumothorax
- tracheal position: shifted to side of tension pneumothorax (a late sign)
- percussion: hyperresonant in an area of collapse or pneumothorax
- auscultation: no breath sounds in area of collapse.

Life-threatening respiratory conditions are remembered as ATOM FC:

- **a**irway obstruction
- **t**ension pneumothorax
- **o**pen pneumothorax
- **m**assive haemothorax
- **f**lail chest: a segment of ribs is detached and moves in an opposite direction to the rest of the chest
- **c**ardiac tamponade: bleeding into the non-distensible pericardial sac, thus compressing the heart; Beck's triad is shock, distended neck veins and muffled heart sound; if pericardiocentesis is positive, urgent thoracotomy is needed.

Circulation

Circulation is assessed by looking at skin colour, peripheral temperature, capillary refill, consciousness level, pulse, blood pressure, presence of hypovolaemic shock (falling blood pressure, rising heart rate) and evidence of acidosis.

Initial management is by

- controlling haemorrhage

- intravenous access with two large cannulae (14G) in two large peripheral veins
- taking bloods for FBC, U&E, glucose, cross-matching (pregnancy test if appropriate)
- a fluid challenge for a rapid response: 250 ml in 10 min
- fluid resuscitation with warmed crystalloids (Hartmann's solution, 4:1 blood replacement), colloids or O-negative blood (before cross-matched blood arrives)
- if an intravenous line cannot be sited, a **saphenous cutdown** may be required (dissect down to the great saphenous vein behind the medial malleolus); in the hypovolaemic child, an intraosseous infusion may be needed
- monitor closely for a response.

Haemorrhage control is by

- direct compression of external bleeding
- splint long-bone fractures and stabilize pelvic fractures
- stop intra-abdominal bleeding: may require a laparotomy
- stop intra-thoracic bleeding: may require a sternotomy.

Dysfunction: assessment of neurological status

In the immediate primary survey, neurological status can be assessed rapidly by the AVPU test:

- alert
- verbal: response to verbal stimuli
- painful: response to pain
- unresponsive.

The GCS is recorded and reassessed. A finger-prick blood sample is taken for glucose measurement (BM stix).

Exposure

Remove all clothing and check for major bleeding sources or obvious wounds and warm hypothermic patients with air blankets and warmed intravenous fluids.

Trauma series radiographs

Radiography must assess the lateral cervical spine, followed by anteroposterior (A-P) and odonoid peg view; all three must be clear to remove the collar. A-P views of chest and pelvis are then taken.

Secondary survey

Every part of the patient is examined meticulously from head to toe, including a log-roll to examine the spine and orifices (rectal and vaginal examination). This only begins when the primary survey is complete, resuscitation is progressing well and the patient is stable. Patients are given analgesia, anti-tetanus, antibiotics as required.

As required, tubes will be sited: two for intravenous access, a urinary catheter, a nasogastric tube, chest drain, central venous line and arterial line.

Limb injuries are immobilized and reduced. Open fractures are photographed and samples taken for culture before covering them with iodine-soaked dressings (p. 15 and Ch. 45).

An AMPLE history is taken: allergies, medication, past medical history, last meal, events of injury.

 EMERGENCY TREATMENT OF A PATIENT HAVING DIFFICULTY BREATHING

A motorcyclist involved in an accident becomes increasingly short of breath over 15 min. Chest examination reveals a deviated trachea to the right side, with decreased chest expansion, absent breath sounds and hyperresonant percussion on the left side.

Clinical diagnosis is a **tension pneumothorax**, which requires immediate treatment (it is life threatening; Ch. 76). Initial treatment is to decompress the 'tension' with **needle thoracocentesis**.

1. A wide-bore venflon (orange or brown) is passed 'above the rib below' (so avoiding the intercostal neurovascular bundle) into the second intercostal space on the side of the pneumothorax
2. When the needle enters the expanded intrapleural space, air escapes (often with an audible hiss) and the patient's breathing should ease.

This temporary measure is followed by a chest drain insertion of into the 5th intercostal space at the mid-axillary line.

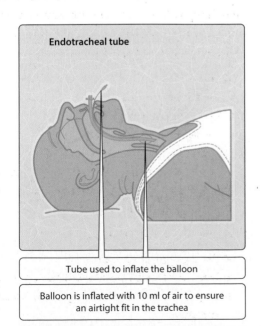

Endotracheal tube

Tube used to inflate the balloon

Balloon is inflated with 10 ml of air to ensure an airtight fit in the trachea

Fig. 3.44.1 Airway management with an endotracheal tube.

45. Describing fractures

Questions
- What is a fracture?
- How do you describe fractures?
- Why are open fractures important?

A fracture is defined as a soft tissue injury with a disruption in the continuity of a bone. *The soft tissue injury is just as important as the break in the bone.* The common fractures of various areas of the body are shown in Fig. 3.45.1. These are covered in more detail in later chapters:

- shoulder: Ch. 47
- forearm: Ch. 48

- lower limb: Ch. 49
- neck of femur: Ch. 50
- axial: Ch. 51
- skull: Ch. 72
- rib: Ch. 77.

Fractures are described in terms of:

- open and closed fractures
- the bone involved
- position on the bone
- pattern
- deformity
- associations.

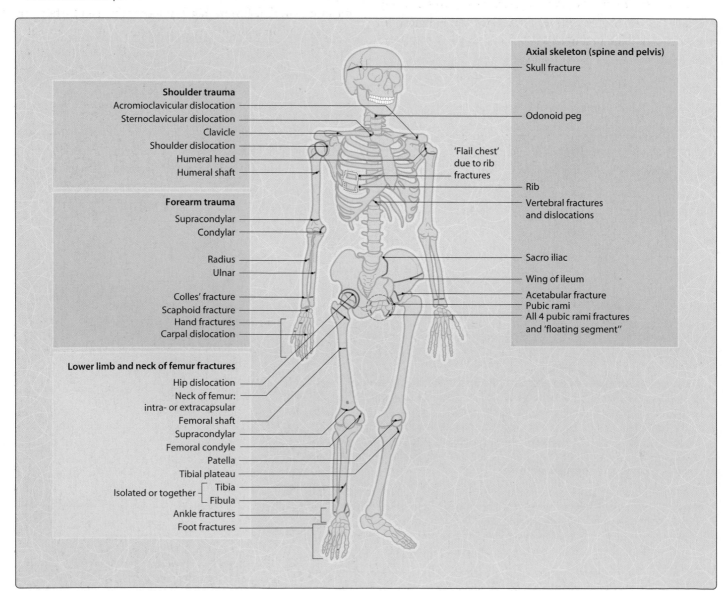

Fig. 3.45.1 The common fractures.

Open and closed fractures. This is determined by clinical examination the time of the injury. Open fractures are exposed. There is a wound in continuity with the bone and there is a risk of infection. The bone ends are typically more displaced and have a much higher risk of infection and, therefore, require operative treatment. The potential for associated soft tissue damage must be assessed: neurovascular damage, muscle bulk damage, compartment syndrome.

The bone involved. The damaged bone must be identified and named. One or more bones can be fractured if they occur closely together (e.g. radius and/or ulna).

The position of the fracture. Typically split into the proximal, middle or distal third of the bone.

The pattern of the fracture. Figure 3.45.2 show the different types seen: transverse, spiral (oblique), comminuted (more than two fragments), wedge (e.g. osteoporotic wedge fracture of the vertebrae), avulsion, pathological, or greenstick (common in children).

Deformity (Fig. 3.45.3). This is defined in several ways:
- displacement: the percentage loss of end-to-end contact of the distal and proximal bone ends (pole); displacement can be minimal or significant
- shortening: if shortening has occurred and to what extent (in centimetres)
- angulation: of the distal to the proximal pole (degrees)
- rotation: rotation upon clinical examination and rotation on a radiograph (degrees).

Associations. This describes other associated features: involvement of the joint (intra- or extra-articular); associated dislocation (a fracture–dislocation); if in a long bone, is the epiphysis, diaphysis or metaphysis affected. Soft tissue associations must also be described (ruptures of muscle, blood vessels or nerves).

A good description of a fracture is as follows. 'This is a closed fracture of the left femoral shaft. It affects the middle third and is a spiral fracture. The distal pole is displaced by 50%, is rotated by 30°, is shortened by 1 cm and clinically the limb is externally rotated. There is no intra-articular involvement, no associated dislocation and no soft tissue complications.'

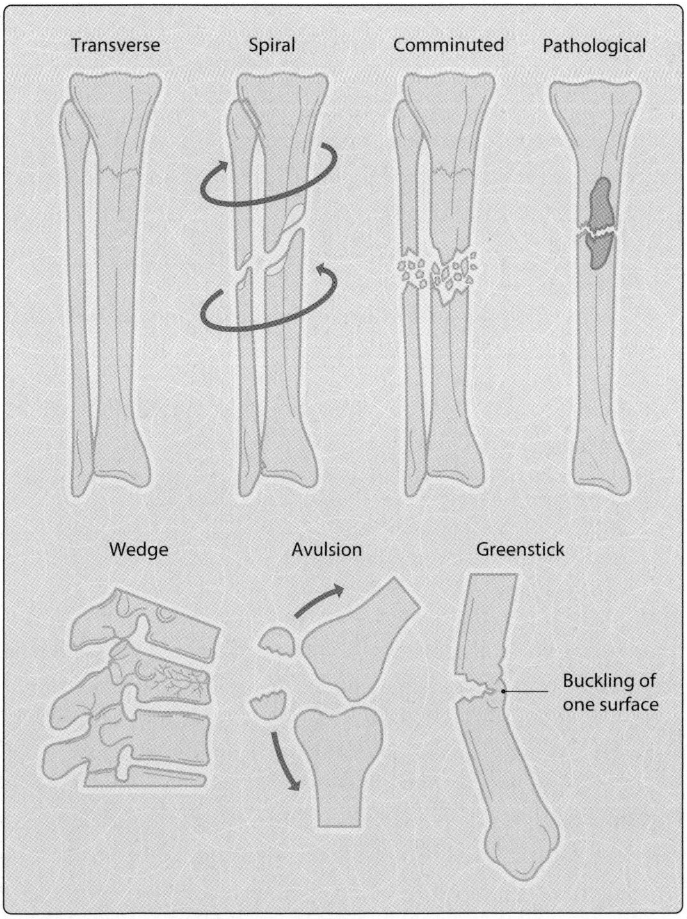

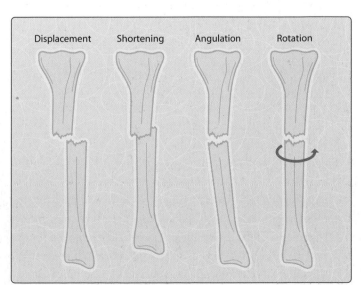

Fig. 3.45.2 The different shapes of a fracture.

Fig. 3.45.3 Deformity of a fracture.

46. Managing fractures

Questions
- How is an open fracture managed?
- What are the methods of reduction?
- How can a fracture be immobilized?

A fracture is defined as soft tissue injury with a disruption in the continuity of a bone. This is an important definition, as the soft tissue injury is just as important as the fracture; open fractures, neurovascular damage or compartment syndrome all require special management.

The rate at which fractures heal depends upon a number of factors: the patient (increasing age and adverse health factors slow healing), the fracture (closed fractures heal faster than diaphyseal) and the treatment (good blood supply and immobilization). On average, fractures of lower limbs take 6 weeks in children and 12 weeks in adults, and those of upper limbs take 3 and 6 weeks, respectively.

Imaging
Plain radiographs following the rule of 2s:
- 2 views, A-P and lateral: to assess displacement; some areas require specific views
- 2 joints: joint above and below to identify joint extension
- 2 times: one film prereduction and one film postreduction, to assess the effectiveness of reduction
- 2 sides: to compare normal and abnormal.

MRI is used to assess spinal injury and CT is used to assess visceral injury in pelvic and lower rib fractures.

Interpretation of an orthopaedic radiograph
The ABCS system is used.

Adequacy and alignment.   The radiograph should include the joint above and below to identify fully the features of the injury including the alignment of the bones with each other (e.g. when looking at the aligment of one cervical vertebrae with the vertebrae below).

Bone margin and density.   The bone margins are followed to note any disruptions indicating fractures. The fracture pattern and deformity (Ch. 45) should be noted and the radiographs examined closely for other fractures and in other bones. The general density and architecture should be noted and any suspicious lesions, which might suggest the possibility of pathological fractures.

Cartilage and joints.   Any widening/disruption of joint spaces and surfaces may indicate intra-articular involvement or dislocation, which may alter management.

Soft tissues.   Air in the tissues may indicate an open wound, fracture, visceral injury or synergistic infection; gross swelling of the soft tissues may produce local complications.

Management

Initial management
The initial management of all patients with a traumatic injury should be the emergency assessment ABC.

The soft tissue injury is just as important as the fracture and **compartment syndrome** must be recognized early.

Open fractures require treatment to prevent infection. The wound is swabbed, photographed and covered with antibiotic dressings and a temporary splint. Tetanus prophylaxis is given and intravenous antibiotics commenced. The wound must be immediately debrided and irrigated meticulously in theatre, where the fracture is stabilized. The wound is packed and left open; it is reinspected and debrided 24–72 h later. If it is clean, the wound can be closed. Repeat debridement may be needed.

Neurovascular compromise must be considered by examining the distal limb; rapid reduction of the fracture may be needed to save the limb from ischaemia.

Management of the fracture
Fractures are treated with the RIR principle: reduction, immobilization and rehabilitation.

Reduction

If a fracture is significantly displaced, shortened or angulated, it needs to be reduced:

- closed reduction is by traction or manipulation under anaesthesia
- open reduction with internal fixation (ORIF): the fracture is manually reduced and then internally fixed; typically this is used when displacement is too severe for closed reduction (see below).

There are some fractures that do not need to be reduced even if displaced, as the functional outcome is not improved: mid-clavicle (uncomplicated), ribs, scapular blade and pubic ramus (not all).

Immobilization

In order for the fracture to heal, the two ends of bone must be immobilized (fixation) in place. Fractures can be fixed either externally or internally (where the fracture is also reduced).

Non-operative immobilization is achieved with:

- splints: relieves pain and prevents further damage
- sling or collar and cuff (e.g. for mid-clavicular fractures)
- casts: plaster of Paris, backslab
- traction: gravity, skin traction, skeletal traction (e.g. Gallows traction for paediatric femoral shaft fractures); this is uncommon in general fracture management
- cast bracing: a plaster cast on the thigh and calf, joined by a brace.

Operative immobilization is achieved by external (Fig. 3.46.1) or internal (Fig. 3.46.2) fixation.

External fixation. This approach is good for complex or open fractures. Screws are drilled into the bones and held in place externally. Ring fixators (Illizarov fixators) are suitable for complicated fractures (e.g. comminuted tibial fractures), where the bones are held firmly in place from multiple directions.

Internal fixation. This follows open reduction in ORIF and uses:

- plates and screws: suitable for articular and comminuted long-bone fractures (e.g. ankle fractures)
- intramedullary nails: for fractures of long bones (femur, tibia, humerus) as it allows early mobilization
- Kirschner (K) wires: commonly used for foot, wrist and hand fractures; wires are inserted percutaneously and can be placed under tension.

Rehabilitation

Physiotherapy plays a crucial role to allow the other joints to remain mobile, and to regain muscle tone, ensure good joint alignment and maximize joint function once the fracture has healed. A fracture is united when:

- clinically there is an absence of pain, tenderness or swelling
- radiologically there is new bone visible on radiograph (may lag behind clinical union).

Fracture healing

There are three sequential but overlapping stages of bone healing.

1. *Inflammatory phase.* This occurs in the first 24–72 h. Bleeding immediately after the fracture causes swelling and cytokine release; this stimulates the rest of the repair mechanism.
2. *Reparative phase.* Repair of the fractured bone depends on the stability of the fracture:
   - **healing by callus in unstable fractures:** occurs between 4 and 8 weeks; necrotic bone is resorbed and weak woven bone is laid down, which is the precursor for highly organized and very strong lamellar bone
   - **healing by primary bone healing in stable fractures:** *contact healing* can occur when the two ends are in direct contact and 'cutting cones' cross the fracture.
3. *Remodelling phase.* This starts 8–12 weeks after the fracture, at the end of the repair phase, and continues for years. Strong lamellar bone replaces woven bone (osteoclasts remove existing bone; osteoblasts lay down new bone).

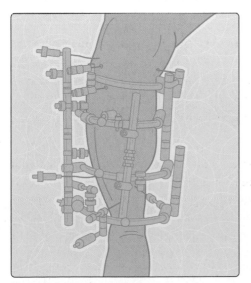

Fig. 3.46.1 External fixation.

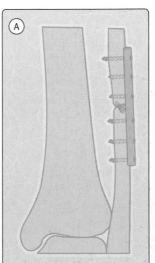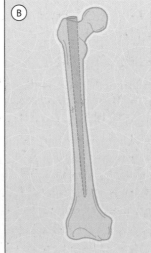

Fig. 3.46.2 Internal fixation. (A) Plate and screws; (B) intramedullary nail.

47. Shoulder trauma

Questions
- How do you manage a clavicle fracture?
- In what direction do most shoulders dislocate?
- How would you manage a displaced humeral shaft fracture?

Trauma around the shoulder is very common. The glenohumeral joint is a shallow ball and socket joint, where stability is sacrificed to allow a wide range of movement.

Many of the fractures and dislocations in this region are the result of falls, commonly a fall on an outstretched hand ('FOOSH').

Fractures of the clavicle
Fractures of the clavicle are common and often occur in a FOOSH (Fig. 3.47.1). Most occur in the middle third because ligaments firmly attach the medial and lateral ends. Neurovascular compromise of the distal limb is rare but may damage the **subclavian artery** and **brachial plexus** (check distal sensation and pulses).

Treatment is conservative with a broad arm sling for 3 weeks and analgesia. A 'bump' forms in the healed bone. Surgical reduction with ORIF is only needed if the fracture is open or there is neurovascular compromise, as it causes greater disability than conservative treatment.

Fractures of the humerus
Humeral fractures are common in those with osteoporosis, mainly occurring at the proximal humerus and the shaft of the humerus. Patients present with pain, tenderness, swelling and deformity, and an inability to move the shoulder.

Proximal humerus. Fractures of the neck of the humerus are usually caused by indirect trauma (e.g. a fall onto the shoulder in the elderly). Fractures through the *surgical neck* of the humerus are common, and since they are extra-capsular, the blood supply is not disturbed and avascular necrosis is rare. Fractures through the *anatomical neck* are less common but have a high risk of avascular necrosis. Axillary nerve injury may occur with these fractures, hence deltoid sensation should be assessed. Most fractures are undisplaced and stable and are treated conservatively with a collar and cuff, which provides traction by gravity. Shoulder stiffness is a common complication, and so early physiotherapy in the elderly is important.

Humeral shaft. The humeral shaft can fracture following a direct blow during a FOOSH. The fracture is usually oblique and displaced. Treatment is initially conservative with a collar and cuff for 3 weeks, which reduces the fracture in 95%. Occasionally ORIF with plates or an intramedullary nail is required, particularly if the fracture is pathological. Radial nerve damage occurs in 5–10% and is most common with spiral fractures; the patient cannot extend the fingers and wrist, although recovery usually occurs with time.

Shoulder dislocation
A **dislocation** is complete loss of contact between the articular surfaces of a joint whereas a **subluxation** is partial loss of contact. The shoulder is the most commonly dislocated joint (Fig. 3.47.2). There is pain, loss of function and loss of shoulder contour. Dislocations can either be anterior (by far the more common) or posterior.

Anterior dislocation of the shoulder is the most common shoulder dislocation and is a common injury. The humeral head dislocates anteriorly and then medially to lie underneath the coracoid process. The main complication is damage to the **axillary nerve**, which causes a loss of sensation over the deltoid muscle (regimental patch). The patient holds the arm in abduction, and shoulder movement is impossible. **Posterior dislocations** are much less common and are easily missed.

Investigation. Two radiograph views are essential (A-P and lateral view) to confirm the direction of dislocation and identify a fracture; careful examination for fracture of the humeral head is important, as otherwise a fracture–dislocation may be missed and incorrectly reduced as a simple dislocation, with potentially disastrous results.

Management:
1. analgesia
2. assess neurovascular status of the distal limb (pulse and sensation): compromise requires urgent reduction
3. radiograph
4. early reduction: closed or open
5. reassess neurovascular status
6. confirm reduction with a radiograph.

The humeral head is reduced with the patient sedated. There are several methods (Fig. 3.47.3):

- **modified Kocker's method**: the elbow is flexed and adducted into the patient's side, and the shoulder is then externally rotated, stopping every few degrees to allow spasm to subside; at full external rotation, the humeral head is easily replaced with some traction, and then the arm is internally rotated. The arm is held in a sling for 3 weeks, followed by physiotherapy

- **traction/countertraction**: a useful method where one clinician provides traction down the axis of the affected arm, while another provides counter-traction on the chest wall; as traction is gently applied, the humeral head slips back into place
- **Hippocratic method**: traditionally used when only one physician was available but is now considered unsafe; the arm is pulled forcefully against traction (the clinician's shoeless foot in the patient's armpit) and the foot pushes the humeral head into place.

Recurrent shoulder dislocation

Repeated anterior dislocation is common in young patients: 90% in those under 20 years but only 10% in those over 40. Recurrence is linked to a soft tissue defect (Bankart lesion: damage to the anterior portion glenoid labrum of the capsule) or a bony deformity of the humeral head (Hill–Sachs' lesion). The **apprehension test** is positive (Ch. 63).

Treatment for shoulder instability depends on the cause. Surgery is required for physical damage (torn loose), which is remembered as TUBS: traumatic, unidirectional instability, Bankart lesion, surgery. Surgery is only used if conservative measures fail for congenital dislocations (born loose), remembered as AMBRI: atraumatic, multidirectional instability, bilateral (asymptomatic shoulder is also loose), rehabilitation treatment, inferior capsular shift (surgery is required if conservative measures fail). Surgical repair of the weakened capsule can be performed, depending on patient factors and preference.

Acromioclavicular joint subluxation/dislocation

This often occurs in rugby players, causing pain and a step in the shoulder. Treatment is a sling with strapping over the joint. Occasionally open reduction with repair of the ligament is performed.

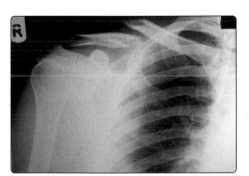

Fig. 3.47.1 A fractured clavicle following a fall onto the shoulder.

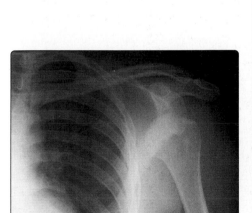

Fig. 3.47.2 Anterior dislocation of the shoulder. A lateral view is also needed to confirm the direction.

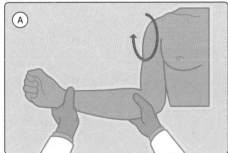

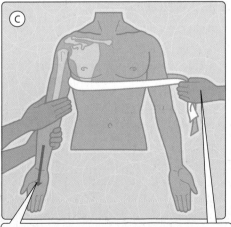

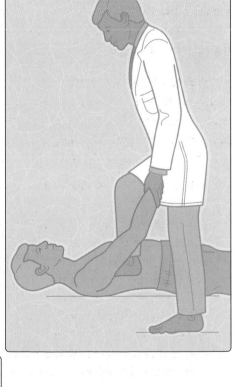

Traction is applied down the axis of the affected arm, allowing the humeral head to slip back into place

One person provides counter-traction

Fig. 3.47.3 Methods of reducing a dislocated shoulder. (A) Modified Kocker's method; (B) Hippocratic method; (C) traction/countertraction.

48. Forearm trauma

Questions
- What is a Galaezzi fracture?
- What is a Colles' fracture and how is it managed?
- How is a scaphoid fracture managed?

Fractures

If there is one obvious fracture of the forearm, the arm should be examined to see if there is another fracture or a dislocation; radiographs of the distal and proximal joint must be taken.

Fractures around the elbow

Supracondylar fractures. Supracondylar fractures occur chiefly during childhood but may occur in adults (Ch. 51).

Olecranon. The olecranon is easily fractured as the result of a FOOSH or a direct blow. The fracture is commonly displaced and requires ORIF with K-wire fixation.

Radial head. The radial head easily fractures. Undisplaced fractures can be treated with a support bandage and early immobilization. Displaced fractures may need ORIF.

Condylar fractures. **Medial epicondylar fractures** are often missed, especially in young children. They are often intra-articular and, consequently, need careful examination followed by ORIF with K-wires. **Lateral condylar fractures** most commonly occur in preschool children; if significantly displaced, ORIF is required. Condylar fractures can cause growth arrest, mal-union, stiffness and *ulnar nerve palsy*.

Mid-shaft fractures

Fractures involving both the radius and ulnar are common and are often open; complications are frequent (mal-union, compartment syndrome, cross-union). A **Galeazzi fracture–dislocation** is a radial fracture with dislocation of the distal radioulnar joint (Fig. 3.48.1). Mal-union is common, so ORIF is indicated. The **Monteggia fracture–dislocation** is the mirror image of this and is frequently missed in children. These two fractures should not be confused with a simple Colles' fracture, and they illustrate the need for a full set of radiographs. They are often unstable, and so ORIF is the treatment of choice with plates and/or intramedullary nail.

Distal radius fractures

Fractures of the distal radius (and/or ulna) are commonly seen in A&E. Wrist fractures are mostly caused by a FOOSH.

Colles' fracture. A Colles' fracture occurs within 2.5 cm of the distal end of the radius, with dorsal angulation (Fig. 3.48.2). It is common in females over 50 years (osteoporosis) following a FOOSH. A classic dinner fork deformity is visible. **Management** is by reduction of the fracture under regional anaesthesia (a Bier's block) or local anaesthesia (haematoma block) to reverse the deformities; radiograph confirms satisfactory reduction. The area is held in a plaster backslab from the elbow to the metatarsophalangeal joints for 6 weeks. Intra-articular involvement, failed reduction or mal-union require surgical intervention. **Complications** include carpal tunnel syndrome, mal-union, stiffness and rupture of the extensor pollicis longus.

Smith's fracture. A Smith's fracture is a reverse Colles' fracture with anterior angulation and tilt, but it is uncommon. Treatment is with manipulation under anaesthesia and a plaster cast above the elbow for 6 weeks.

Barton's fracture. This is an intra-articular fracture of the wrist, causing the hand and part of the distal radius to displace proximally. Many require ORIF.

Chauffeur's fracture. Chauffeur's fracture is a fracture of the radial styloid.

Carpal fractures and dislocations

The most commonly fractured carpal bone is the **scaphoid**. It is usually damaged in a FOOSH in young adults. A tender

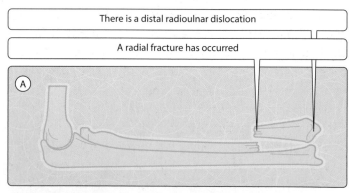

> There is a distal radioulnar dislocation

> A radial fracture has occurred

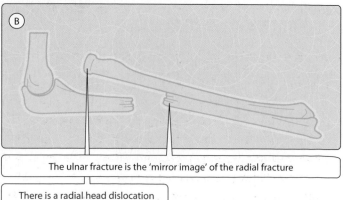

> The ulnar fracture is the 'mirror image' of the radial fracture

> There is a radial head dislocation

Fig. 3.48.1 Mid-shaft fractures. (A) The Galeazzi fracture–dislocation; (B) a Monteggia fracture is a 'mirror image'.

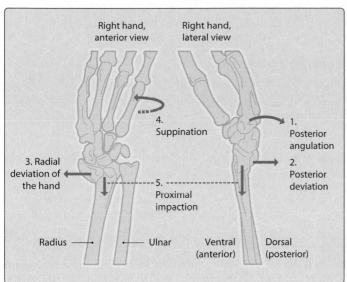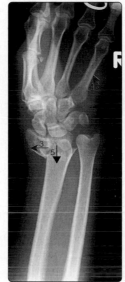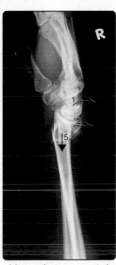

Fig. 3.48.2 The Colles' fracture. Radiographs to show the right hand (anterior view on left and lateral view on right). There are five deformities: 1, posterior angulation; 2, posterior deviation; 3, radial deviation of the hand; 4, suppination; 5, proximal impaction.

anatomical snuff box may be the only sign. The scaphoid is most likely to fracture across its narrow waist. As the blood supply to the scaphoid is retrograde (it enters via the distal end), a complete fracture may disrupt the blood supply to the proximal pole causing avascular necrosis. Subsequent non-union is common and causes premature wrist osteoarthritis, which may require ORIF and bone grafting.

Four radiographic views are necessary, although the fracture may still not be visible and a fracture is assumed if there is tenderness over the anatomical snuffbox. A scaphoid plaster is applied (from the elbow to knuckles). The radiograph is repeated at 2 weeks to try to identify the fracture, although a bone scan may be needed. If this shows a fracture, the plaster cast remains for a further 8 weeks. If the fracture has not united at 12 weeks, internal fixation is needed (Fig. 3.48.3).

Anterior dislocation of the **lunate** is the commonest carpal dislocation. Check for associated scaphoid fracture and acute median nerve compression. Reduction is either closed or open.

Hand
Complicated hand injuries require a specialist hand surgeon.

Bennett's fracture. This fracture of the first metacarpal, extending into the carpometacarpal joint, is caused by a blow to the point of the thumb. It is unstable and should be reduced; if this fails, a percutaneous pin can be inserted.

Metacarpal and phalangeal injuries. These are often caused by direct blows (e.g. punching; check for a 'fight bite'). Most are managed with closed reduction where necessary, followed with immobilization by splinting to the neighbouring finger (a plastic back-slab can be added for extra stability). Unstable fractures and multiple metacarpal involvement indicate percutaneous K-wires.

Flexor tendon injury. The flexor tendons of the hand lie within a tight fibrous sheath. If there is a tendon injury (with or without an associated fracture), this indicates surgical exploration and repair by a specialist hand surgeon.

Hand infections. Infections of the hand are potentially very serious and must be admitted for intravenous antibiotics and/or washout, under the care of a specialist hand surgeon:

■ **fight bite**: a puncture by a tooth so oral organisms contaminate the wound; if ignored, it later presents with severe pain, swelling and discharge; treatment is with antibiotics and surgical toilet

■ **nail fold infections** (paronychia): both nail fold and pulp space infections respond well to elevation and antibiotics, with occasional need for irrigation and drainage.

Fig. 3.48.3 A scaphoid fracture.

49. Lower limb fractures

Questions
- What is the mechanism of femoral shaft fractures?
- What is the most common direction of hip dislocation?
- How are tibial shaft fractures managed?

Fractures of the lower limb are common. Fractures of the neck of femur are extremely common and because of its importance and prevalence, it has a dedicated chapter (50).

Femoral shaft fracture

Femoral shaft fractures most commonly occur in young people as a result of high-energy impacts (e.g. road traffic accidents (RTA; Fig. 3.49.1)), but they may also occur in those with oesteoporosis. The risk of **complications** is high: shock (a femoral fracture results in blood loss of 1–2 litres, and the femoral artery may be damaged), fat embolus, thrombo-embolism and infection. **Treatment** is commonly surgical with an intramedullary nail, where screws can be passed through the bone and nail to prevent rotation (a locking nail). Traction, cast bracing and external fixation are also sometimes used.

Hip dislocation

The majority of hip dislocations are posterior and follow impact directed along the femoral shaft, commonly during a RTA when the knee strikes the dashboard and the femoral head is forced backwards. Associated femoral and acetabular fractures should be sought. The leg is shortened, adducted, internally rotated and in slight hip flexion. The femoral head may be palpable in the buttock, and the **sciatic nerve** may become damaged. The femoral head is reduced under general anaesthesia as soon as possible, and held in traction for 3 weeks; an associated acetabular fracture requires ORIF.

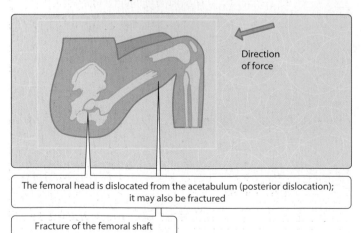

Direction of force

The femoral head is dislocated from the acetabulum (posterior dislocation); it may also be fractured

Fracture of the femoral shaft

Fig. 3.49.1 Road traffic accidents often lead to traumatic hip dislocation and an associated femoral shaft fracture.

Around the knee

Intra-articular joint involvement is common in knee trauma, and any disruption in the joint line must be accurately reduced to prevent post-traumatic osteoarthritis. The fractures around the knee can be divided into supracondylar, femoral condyle, patellar and tibial plateau fractures. The last range from simple to very complicated (Fig. 3.49.2), involving both the tibia and femur; there are often depressed, crushed and cleaved off segments, which must be accurately elevated and fixed into position to ensure a good joint line.

Management

Supracondylar fractures are commonly managed with ORIF, allowing early mobilization and discharge.

Femoral condyle fractures are fixed with closed reduction, using either skeletal traction or screw fixation to follow.

Tibial plateau fractures are difficult to manage and prolonged rehabilitation may be needed. Large fragments may need ORIF (the loose segment is drilled back and pinned into place, possibly with a bone graft to fill any defect).

Non-displaced patellar fractures with an intact knee extensor mechanism can be treated in a plaster cast. If extensor mechanism is damaged, ORIF with K-wires and repair of the extensor mechanism are required. If the patella is severely comminuted, it may need to be removed — **patellectomy**.

Knee dislocations

Knee dislocations usually only occur after major trauma. Particular attention must be paid to the state of the **popliteal vessels and nerves**. The capsule can be repaired, and the joint immobilized for 6 weeks; ligamentous reconstruction is frequently needed.

Patella dislocations

Almost all patella dislocations are lateral; they can be either:

- traumatic: reduction is under anaesthesia, followed by repair of ruptured ligaments and immobilization
- recurrent: usually affect adolescent girls and are related to tibial deformities and valgus knees; the dislocation is spontaneous or from minor trauma, and it usually responds to physiotherapy.

Tibial shaft fractures

Tibial shaft fractures are common and often follow RTAs or sporting injuries; they are often open. Fractures are spiral, oblique or transverse; there is a danger of compartment syndrome, with both open and closed injuries and minimally displaced fractures. (No limb should have regional anaesthesia as it may mask this.) Unstable fractures are treated with internal fixation using an intramedullary nail. Stable fractures can be treated with closed reduction using a plaster cast. External fixation can be used to treat open and/or comminuted fractures.

Ankle fractures, dislocations and sprains

Ankle fractures can be complicated and may involve bones, ligaments and dislocations; they are best classified using the simple Weber system (Fig. 3.49.3) based on the relationship of the fibula fracture to the **syndesmosis** (the ligamentous attachment between the tibia and fibula). The greater the disruption to the syndesmosis, the more unstable the fracture and the increasing need for ORIF.

Type A. The fibular fracture is below the syndesmosis. They are avulsion fractures found below the mortise (joint line) and are stable, thus requiring only closed reduction.

Type B. The fibular fracture is at the level of the syndesmosis. They are spiral fibular fractures that start at the level of the mortise and may or may not involve the syndesmosis; thus these fractures may be stable or unstable.

Type C. The fibular fracture is above the syndesmosis. They disrupt the syndesmosis and interosseous ligaments, and are thus very unstable and require ORIF.

The **Ottawa rules** state that radiographs are indicated when there is bony tenderness around (a) the medial or lateral malleolus (or 6 cm above either), (b) the navicular or (c) the 5th metatarsal, or there is (d) inability to weight-bear *both* immediately after the event and in A&E. Ankle fractures must be reduced accurately as if out of line they may cause premature osteoarthritis. Therefore, ORIF is commonly used, especially for displaced fractures.

An **ankle dislocation** is associated with extensive soft tissue damage and often a fracture, and so reduction must be performed before the patient is sent for radiographs to avoid distal ischaemia and skin damage. A **sprain** is a partial tear of a ligament, and often follows forceful inversion of the foot producing immediate pain and swelling. Treatment is conservative, although recovery may take some time since ligaments have a poor vascular supply.

Foot fractures

Avulsion fracture of the base of the 5th metatarsal is a common injury caused by inversion with plantar flexion. Since the **peroneus brevis** tendon is attached here, continued movement of the lower limb prevents healing. Consequently, a below-knee plaster cast is needed for 3–6 weeks. **Stress fractures** are overuse injuries and are common in athletes; the 2nd metatarsal is commonly affected ('march' fracture). Pain is gradual in onset and related to activity; direct palpation causes pain. Management is with rest and analgesia for 4–12 weeks followed by physiotherapy.

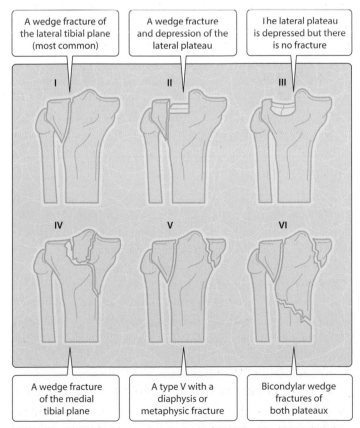

Fig. 3.49.2 Tibial plateau fractures are classified by the Schatzker system.

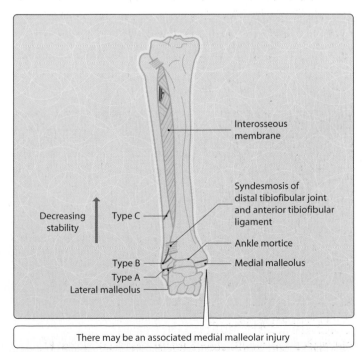

Fig. 3.49.3 Weber classification of ankle fractures (see text).

50. Neck of femur fractures

Questions
■ What are the types of neck of femur fracture?
■ Why does the type of fracture matter?
■ How may the different types be treated?

Fractures through the neck of the femur (NOF) are very common in the elderly (particularly females) and are most often caused by a fall. **Risk factors** include smoking, excess alcohol consumption, osteoporosis and positive maternal history.

Anatomy
The **hip capsule** attaches proximally to the inter-trochanteric line. The capsule is important as it carries a major part of the blood supply to the femoral head (Fig. 3.50.1).

Classification of hip fractures
Fractures of the NOF are classified as intra- or extracapsular (Fig. 3.50.2A). **Intracapsular fractures** *(subcapital and transcervical)* may interrupt the blood supply to the femoral head if they are displaced. **Extracapsular fractures** *(intertrochanteric and subtrochanteric)* lie outside the capsule and involve the trochanters; consequently, the blood supply is much less likely to be interrupted and there is a low risk of non-union.

Clinical features
The typical appearance of a NOF fracture is a shortened and externally rotated limb (the iliopsoas contracts and rotates the femoral shaft externally without the opposition of the hip joint). Elderly patients are very commonly dehydrated following this injury and they may have been injured and alone for some time, so the potential for hypothermia must be considered.

Investigations
Two plain radiographs are required (A-P and lateral views; Figs 3.50.3 and 3.50.4). An undisplaced NOF fracture may be difficult to identify. MRI and bone scan are used if radiographs are negative and hip fracture is still strongly suspected.

Management
Initial management is as for any trauma (Ch. 44); for elderly patients confusion, dehydration and comorbidities may be additional problems. Prophylaxis for DVT and infections is required.

Intracapsular fractures *are fixed with cannulated screw fixation if undisplaced and hemiarthroplasty if displaced.* Immediate hemiarthroplasty replaces the femoral head and leaves the acetabulum in place. This avoids the complications of avascular necrosis that could present if the displaced femoral head is left in place. Hemiarthoplasty also has the advantage of allowing immediate weight-bearing. If the fracture is non-displaced, the blood supply will be intact and cannulated screws can be used, although a hemiarthoplasty may be required at a later date if this fails.

Extracapsular fractures *are reduced and fixed with a dynamic hip screw.* The blood supply to the femoral head is uninterrupted and so the fracture can be internally fixed, most commonly with a dynamic hip screw (Fig. 3.50.5). This approach allows the patient to regain maximum mobility rapidly, weight-bearing in 2–3 days.

In some patients who are unfit for surgery (e.g. the very elderly and frail with severe medical comorbidities), **conservative management** with prolonged immobilization can be used, but this has many associated complications.

Prognosis
Outcome depends on the patient's age and general health; only 60% survive to 1 year. Of these, only 30% regain premorbid function; 50% do not regain their premorbid state and 20% never walk again.

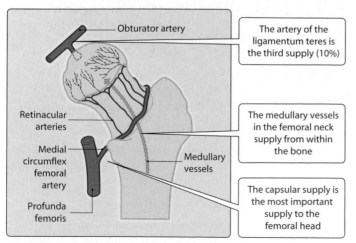

Fig. 3.50.1 Blood supply to the femoral head.

Obturator artery

The artery of the ligamentum teres is the third supply (10%)

Retinacular arteries

The medullary vessels in the femoral neck supply from within the bone

Medial circumflex femoral artery

Medullary vessels

The capsular supply is the most important supply to the femoral head

Profunda femoris

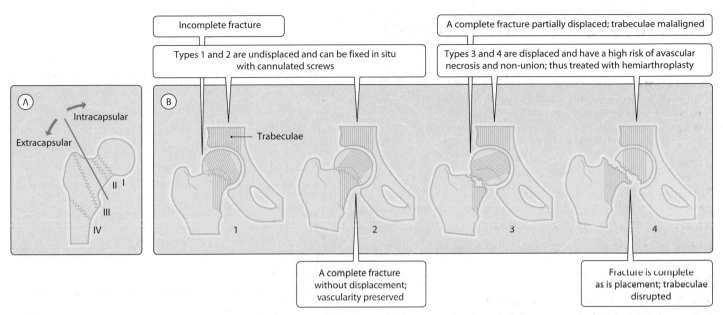

Incomplete fracture

Types 1 and 2 are undisplaced and can be fixed in situ with cannulated screws

A complete fracture partially displaced; trabeculae malaligned

Types 3 and 4 are displaced and have a high risk of avascular necrosis and non-union; thus treated with hemiarthroplasty

Trabeculae

A complete fracture without displacement; vascularity preserved

Fracture is complete as is placement; trabeculae disrupted

Fig. 3.50.2 Capsular fractures (A) Differentiation of intra- and extracapsular fractures. I, subcapital; II, transcervical; III, intertrochanteric; IV, subtrochanteric. (B) Garden's classification of intracapsular fractures.

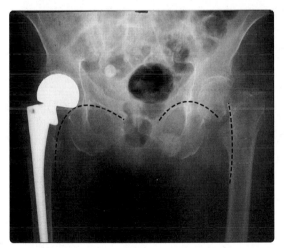

Fig. 3.50.3 A displaced, intracapsular left neck of femur fracture. Disruption of Shenton's line helps to identify less obvious fractures. A previous hemiarthroplasty is seen on the right.

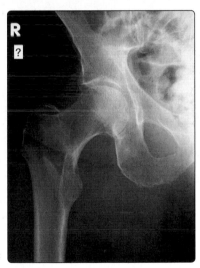

Fig. 3.50.4 Radiograph of an extracapsular neck of femur fracture.

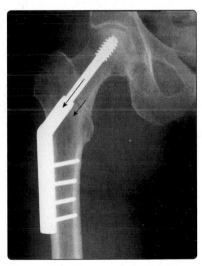

Fig. 3.50.5 The dynamic hip screw used following an undisplaced extracapsular fracture. As the fracture naturally heals and compresses (arrow in bone), the screw retracts down the barrel (arrow in the unit).

51. Axial skeleton trauma

Questions
- How would you manage a suspected spinal injury?
- How do you interpret a cervical spine radiograph?
- What is the initial management of a pelvic fracture?

All patients who have suffered trauma must be first assessed by the ABC principles including immobilization of the cervical spine and resuscitation for shock. Life-threatening injuries are treated first.

The axial skeleton comprises the skull (see Ch. 72) and spine, and it is also useful to consider the pelvis here. Trauma victims are always initially assessed by ABC principles including immobilization of the cervical spine and treatment of shock.

■ SPINAL TRAUMA AND VERTEBRAL FRACTURES

Most spinal injuries occur in accidents, primarily RTAs (50%), accidents in the home and workplace, or sports injuries. Cord injury is only seen in 5%. All unconscious patients should be assumed to have a spinal injury; *a fractured vertebra is unstable until proved otherwise*. A urinary catheter can be passed since the patient may lose filling reflexes with lower spinal injuries and go into painless urinary retention. **Clearing the cervical spine** is done with a combination of clinical, neurological and radiographical examinations. Radiographs include a lateral radiograph to show the first cervical to first thoracic vertebrae (C1 to C7/T1 junction; if it does not do this it is deemed *inadequate*) (Fig.3.51.1) and A-P views of the cervical spine and through the open mouth to show the odontoid peg (peg view). The radiographs are assessed using the ABCS system:

- **adequacy**: from C1–C7/T1 junction must be visible
- **alignment** of vertical contours formed from the vertebral bodies, spinal canal and spinous processes: a step of > 25% suggests a unifacet joint dislocation, and > 50% suggests a bifacet dislocation
- **bone margin and density**: outline of vertebral bodies and spinous processes for avulsion and wedge fractures
- **cartilage and joints**: odontoid peg fracture or dislocation
- **soft tissues**: disc spaces (prolapse may cause spinal cord compression) and soft tissue swelling.

Management of a vertebral fracture
Stable fractures generally require immobilization. Unstable fractures are reduced with traction and then external fixation or surgical stabilization.

Cervical fractures:
- atlas (C1): disruption of the bony ring may become unstable; treatment is with halo-ring or surgical fusion
- odontoid peg (C2): a loose peg may damage the spinal cord; treatment is with prolonged immobilization or fusion
- pedicles of C2 resulting in instability of the C2/C3 junction Changman's fracture; treatment is with a halo-ring or ORIF.

Cervical dislocations:
- C1–C2 subluxation: initial traction in extension with a halo ring, followed by posterior fusion
- facet joint dislocations: always unstable so treatment is with ORIF and posterior fusion.

Most thoracic spine fractures are stable because of the influence of the rib cage; conservative nursing care or surgical fusion (to prevent long bed is used stays).

Thoracolumbar fractures (T12 to L1) commonly displace, causing paraplegia. The key to diagnosis is recognizing rupture of the interspinous ligament (a boggy haematoma can be felt with a characteristic gap between the relevant spinous processes). Management is either conservative or surgical.

Compression fractures are most common in the **lumbar spine**, often following a fall from a height onto the heels (check for an associated ankle or hip injury). **Cauda equina syndrome** may occur if a bony fragment breaks off.

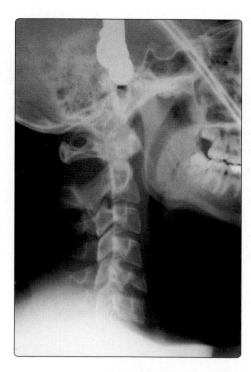

Fig. 3.51.1 A lateral cervical spine radiograph from a patient involved in a RTA. There is a fracture of the C5 vertebral body, caused by a hyperextension injury. This is an *inadequate* film as C7 and T1 are not visible and there could be fracture or dislocation that is missed. (The film must be repeated to include the C7–T1 junction or a CT scan obtained.)

Cord damage. Implications depend on the level:

L5 and below: impaired anal and urinary sphincters and sexual dysfunction, foot and ankle function

L5–L2: progressively less likely to walk

L1/2–T1: cannot walk

T1–C5: the lower the injury, the better the arm function; T1 sparing means the fine hand muscles still work

C4 and above: cannot breath as the phrenic nerve innervates the diaphragm ('*C3,4,5 keeps you alive*').

Other types of spinal injury

Osteoporotic fractures. A high index of suspicion is required in women aged over 50 presenting with sudden or low-grade pain, as only one-third of fractures are clinically apparent.

Pathological fractures. Metastatic deposits are common in the vertebrae, and the presentation may be insidious, with a low-grade pain. This should be suspected in the elderly and those with a history of or active cancer (especially prostate, breast or thyroid).

Spinal shock. Immediately after an injury, a patient may appear to have a complete cord transaction: total or partial power loss, sensory and reflex loss, urinary retention and paralytic ileus. Recovery should begin within 24 h of the initial injury; any longer than 48 h is a poor prognostic sign.

Whiplash injuries. These often result when a car strikes from behind or in a sporting injury, where the trauma causes a hyperextension injury to ligaments and muscle in the neck and shoulder. Radiographs prove normal. Rest, a collar and physiotherapy help. Some recover quickly; others have prolonged symptoms made worse by compensation.

■ TRAUMA TO THE PELVIS

The pelvis is best considered as a ring of bones; if there is one break in the circle, there is bound to be another bony or ligamentous injury. If there is a large fracture, it is important not to miss an associated smaller fracture or disruption of the sacroiliac joints. Pelvic fractures may lead to significant blood loss, which is 'hidden' in the pelvis (up to 2 litres). There is also a high risk of urological/visceral organ and neurovascular injury during high-energy impacts.

Clinical features

If there is a positive mechanism of injury and a shocked patient, there may be pelvic/perianal pain and bruising, anuria (possible ureteric or urethral damage) and vaginal or rectal bleeding.

Investigations

- rectal examination for pain, blood and bones (pelvic fracture with a tear in the rectum is considered as open)
- 'springing pelvis': pressing laterally on both sides of the pelvis produces pain if a fracture is present; this should only be done in hospital and should only be done once, as there is risk of dislodging a clot that has formed
- A-P and lateral radiographs
- intravenous urogram (following urological opinion)
- CT of pelvis.

Management

Urethral catheterization should not be attempted if there is a risk of urethral injury and no urine is being passed. This is a urological emergency requiring an experienced urologist. If needed, a suprapubic catheter is inserted and the urethral injury is repaired. Soft tissue injuries are common and important in this area. Blood loss may be significant; air surrounding the femoral head indicates that the joint has been breached; air elsewhere suggests a visceral injury.

Principles of definitive management include stabilizing the pelvis, with either internal or, usually, external fixation; a subspecialist orthopaedic surgeon may be required. Some options include:

- **fractured pubic rami:** a low-energy fall may cause one or two of the rami to break in the elderly; the patient rests and mobilization is gradual
- **'floating segment':** all four rami are broken, usually the result of a direct blow; once shock has been treated, ORIF may be indicated
- **'open book' fractures:** anterior and posterior forces disrupt the pelvis, leaving it hinged open; an internal or external fixator 'folds' the pelvis back together and controls bleeding
- **acetabular fractures:** these complex fractures are associated with compression forces or dislocations of the hip, and so bleeding may be significant; accurate ORIF is needed to realign the joint line accurately and prevent post-traumatic osteoarthritis.

52. Paediatric fractures

Questions
- How do paediatric fractures differ from those in adults?
- What is a greenstick fracture?
- What is the main complication of a supracondylar fracture?

Paediatric fractures are common, especially in the forearm. They differ in terms of structure and repair from fractures in adults. Paediatric fractures are often greenstick fractures, heal faster and remodel to a greater degree; overgrowth occurs and growth plate injuries are important.

Fracture patterns

Growth plate injuries. Injuries through a growth plate may result in complete or partial growth arrest, and thus limb length discrepancy, which may cause premature osteoarthritis. Such injuries are classified by the Salter–Harris classification (Fig. 3.52.1), where severity increases with grade.

Greenstick fractures. One side of the cortex breaks but the other stays intact (Fig. 3.52.2) as the child's bones are soft.

Buckling fractures. One side of the cortex buckles; if the force continues, the bone breaks to form a greenstick fracture.

Overgrowth. Paediatric fractures have a tendency to overgrow so some shortening is desirable when reducing the fracture.

Non-accidental injuries. The key orthopaedic features are metaphyseal fractures, posterior rib fractures, fractures at different stages of healing, complex skull fractures and spiral long bone fractures. A parent who cannot produce a corroborative history for a fracture is suspicious. **Osteogenesis imperfecta** (blue sclera and brittle bones) and **calcium deficiencies** (rickets, hyperparathyroidism) are medical conditions that should be excluded.

Common fractures
The following are the most common fractures in children.

Distal radius
The distal radius is the most commonly fractured site in children, and is often a greenstick fracture. Even though a dinner-fork deformity forms, a Colles' fracture does not occur in

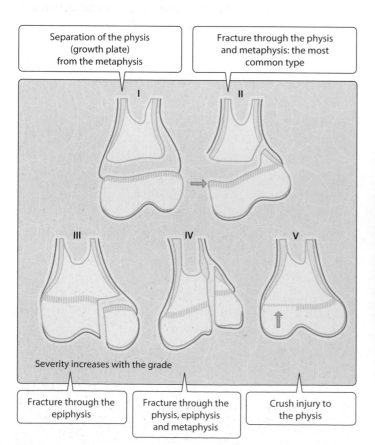

Separation of the physis (growth plate) from the metaphysis

Fracture through the physis and metaphysis: the most common type

I   II

III   IV   V

Severity increases with the grade

Fracture through the epiphysis

Fracture through the physis, epiphysis and metaphysis

Crush injury to the physis

Fig. 3.52.1 Salter–Harris classification of growth plate injuries.

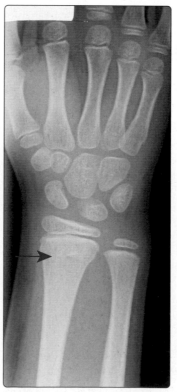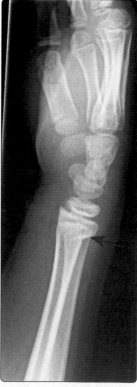

Fig. 3.52.2 A greenstick fracture of the radius. There is buckling of the posterior surface and a fracture of the anterior surface (arrows). Note that the epiphyseal plates are still visible; these will later fuse when the child reaches skeletal maturity.

children; either the radial epiphysis has separated or a greenstick fracture of the distal radius has occurred. The fracture is treated conservatively with reduction and plaster immobilization. A certain amount of displacement is allowed, since a child's growing bones remodel, and subsequently the degree of angulation decreases with age (Table 3.52.1).

Supracondylar fracture

This fracture most commonly occurs as a result of a FOOSH and has a peak age of occurrence at 7 years. It must be recognized quickly as there are numerous serious associated complications.

Neurovascular damage. The displaced fractured bones may damage the **brachial artery** and **median nerve**, and so the neurovascular status of the limb must be checked at presentation and constantly reassessed.

Compartment syndrome. There is a high risk of a compartment syndrome (Ch. 53), as the brachial artery and median nerve can both be compressed by swelling in the anterior compartment.

Volkmann's ischaemic contracture. This can follow disruption to the blood supply or a delay in treatment of a compartment syndrome. The distal limb becomes fibrosed and the joints contract (especially the fingers), leading to flexion deformity and wasting, thus severe limitation of function.

Mal-union and myositis ossificans. Myositis ossificans is an aberrant reparative process where deposition of bone occurs in an area of muscle or soft tissue, here leading to elbow stiffness.

An undisplaced supracondylar fracture is treated by holding the limb in a plaster backslab. If the fracture is displaced, closed reduction is attempted under anaesthesia and the child admitted for observation (in case of compartment syndrome). If closed reduction cannot be achieved, ORIF with K-wires is required. Any lost median nerve function almost always recovers.

Femoral fracture

Closed femoral fractures in young children are treated non-operatively. In children under 3 years, both limbs are held up in traction using a **Gallow's splint**. Older children may require external fixation, intramedullary nails or a plate.

Pulled elbow

Pulled elbow typically occurs in a child under school age who has been tugged on the arm. The head of the radius slips out of the annular ligament but then returns to its normal position (but out of the ligament). Consequently, there is no clinical deformity but the elbow is generally tender and movement is restricted. Radiographs are not required. It is relocated by pulling on the arm while flexing the elbow and supinating the hand, where the radial head clicks back into the annular ligament.

Osteogenesis imperfecta

Osteogenesis imperfecta is a genetic condition affecting collagen production; it is characterized by blue sclera, deformities from fragile bones and a high susceptibility to fractures (Table 3.52.2). It is more common in Afro-Carribeans. Radiograph shows multiple fractures at different stages of healing (so it can be confused with a non-accidental injury). Treatment is to maximize safety (teach parental handling skills, inform school), and the fractures are treated individually. Osteotomies correct deformity and intramedullary stems fix long bones.

Table 3.52.1 DEGREE OF ANGULATION ALLOWED IN A FRACTURE OF THE DISTAL RADIUS

Age (years)	Degree of angulation
4–9	20
9–11	15
11–13	10
13+	5

Table 3.52.2 TYPES OF OSTEOGENSIS IMPERFECTA

Type	Diagnosis	Characteristics	Inheritance
I	Dominant, blue sclera	Type IA has brittle bones, blue sclera, normal teeth; type IB also has dentinogenesis imperfecta (discoloured and damaged teeth) and deafness	Autosomal dominant
II	Lethal perinatal	Deformed skeleton and multiple fractures (a lethal condition in utero)	Autosomal dominant
III	Progressive deforming	Multiple fractures at birth, progressive deformities and dentinogenesis imperfecta, normal sclera	Autosomal recessive
IV	Dominant, white sclera	Similar to type I, but with white sclera; difficult to diagnose	Autosomal dominant

53. Complications of fractures

Questions
- What are potential complications of a fracture?
- What simple tests can be used for suspected compartment syndrome?
- What are the symptoms of fat embolus and when does it occur?

The complications of fractures are best considered by the time at which they occur: early general (hypovolaemic shock, acute respiratory distress syndrome (ARDS), fat embolism, DVT and pulmonary embolism, chest infection), early local (compartment syndrome, neurovascular damage, bone and joint infection (Ch. 66), blisters and plaster sores, avascular necrosis), late instability (stiffness; osteoarthritis; chronic osteomyelitis; mal-, non-, delayed union; Volkmann's ischaemic contractures).

Compartment syndrome

Compartment syndrome is a surgical emergency. The circulation and function of tissues within a fascial compartment become compromised by increased swelling within that compartment. It can occur within any muscular compartment following an open or closed fracture, crush injury or reperfusion injury. The most common site is the calf (Fig. 3.53.1) and the most common cause is an overtight backslab/plaster cast.

Pathology
Increasing swelling leads to an increase in the intracompartmental pressure; this eventually becomes higher than the venous pressure, thus preventing blood leaving the compartment. Further rise in pressure prevents the entry of arterial blood, causing rapid ischaemia with muscle and nerve necrosis. Subsequent rhabdomyolysis may cause acute renal failure and death.

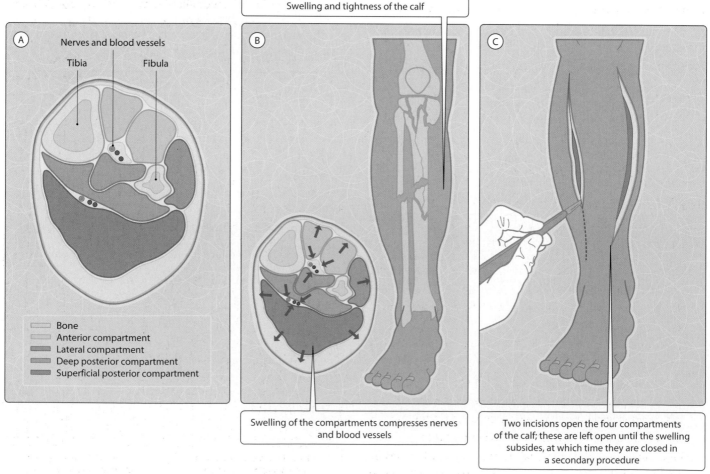

Fig. 3.53.1 Compartment syndrome. (A) Compartments of the leg; (B) fracture causes damage and swelling, increasing pressure and compression of nerves and blood vessels; (C) a fasciotomy: incisions are made in the leg and left open, which relieves pressure.

Clinical features

Pain (most important) is out of proportion to the injury or worsens after a plaster cast has been applied. Paraesthesia, loss of function (foot drop) and lack of pulses are late signs; intervention at this point is likely to be too late. There are two simple tests to form a clinical diagnosis:

- passive flexion: pushing the toes upwards will worsen a calf compression syndrome (same for flexing the fingers)
- opiate analgesia: does not control pain.

Investigation

Intracompartmental pressure measured with a compartment pressure monitor; high pressures indicate urgent surgery (normal pressure is zero). This technique is not always available and not always necessary if there is a firm clinical diagnosis.

Management

The immediate action is to split a backslab/plaster cast around the limb down to the skin. If this is not the cause (e.g. if no plaster has been applied) or does not relieve the pressure, the treatment is **fasciotomy** (Fig. 3.53.1C), which should be done immediately once the clinical diagnosis is made. All the fascias of the affected compartment are cut and split. Two incisions are made to open the four compartments of the calf. These incisions are left open until swelling subsides and risk to the limb has passed; the incisions can be closed by primary intention or with skin grafts.

Complications

If compartment syndrome is inadequately treated or missed, fibrosis and contracture (Volkmann's ischaemic contracture) can occur with neuropathy (motor and sensory). Late presentation can be with claw foot or altered sensation.

Problems with union

Mal-, non- or delayed union can occur if a fracture is inadequately treated or missed (Fig. 3.53.2).

Delayed union. If healing time has extended beyond normal, management is to try to identify and correct the cause (e.g. further monitoring, treat infection, stabilize the fracture, ensure adequate nutrition).

Mal-union. Healing in a non-anatomical position (angulation, translation or rotation) can lead to a disappointed patient and/or the potential for post-traumatic arthritis. In some cases, this is unavoidable (e.g. displaced clavicle fracture treated conservatively). Surgical correction of the abnormality can be undertaken.

Non-union. Some fractures fail to unite even when healing has ceased. Factors include interposition of soft tissues, missed fractures, incorrectly treated fractures, malnutrition

and systemic disease. Fractures through growth plates may cause non-union and so have serious growth consequences in children. Non-union results in a pseudoarthritis. Treatment is by bone grafts and internal fixation.

Other complications

Joint stiffness. Underuse of the affected joint or the affected joint on the fracture side (e.g. elbow stiffness from a Colles' fracture) can often lead to joint stiffness and early, regular physiotherapy is required. For hand and wrist fractures that require the fingers to be splinted, the fingers should be splinted at 90° to the palm to prevent permanent stiffness.

Avascular necrosis. This may present as a non-union, bone collapse or premature osteoarthritis. It occurs with fractures to the femoral neck, scaphoid, talus and proximal humerus, and with other causes (Ch. 65).

Fat embolism. Fat embolism syndrome typically follows long bone fractures (e.g. femoral shaft) and is most common in young women. It arises either from direct release from marrow fat or from peripheral fat mobilization in response to stress (catecholamine release). The clinical features are caused by a lipid embolus that blocks multiple blood vessels temporarily and incompletely; they develop 24–48 h after injury and cause hypoxia, pulmonary oedema, confusion and seizures, and petechiae. **Management** is preventative (reduce long bone fractures early) and symptomatic: supportive treatment (fluid management and ventilation) in an ITU setting.

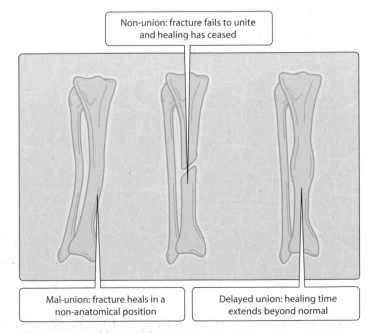

Non-union: fracture fails to unite and healing has ceased

Mal-union: fracture heals in a non-anatomical position

Delayed union: healing time extends beyond normal

Fig. 3.53.2 Problems with union.

54. Back pain

Questions
- What is the most common cause of back pain?
- What are suspicious features of back pain?
- What are the causes of cervical and lumbar pain?

Lower back pain is extremely common: 10% of the population suffer at any one time and 90% at some time in their life. However, 90% of causes are non-specific (**mechanical back pain**) and less than 10% have an underlying pathology. Other non-spinal causes should be remembered (e.g. aneurysm or visceral disorder).

Suspicious features of back pain
Tumours and acute spinal compression must not be missed; suspicious features are:

- bladder and bowel symptoms, saddle anaesthesia (buttocks), new bilateral sciatica (red flag symptoms of spinal cord compression)
- age < 20 or > 50 years; acute onset in the elderly
- weight loss (malignancy)
- fever (infection)
- active cancer or history of cancer
- recent bacterial infection
- night/rest pain
- back pain that persists for more than 3 months.

Managing back pain
Most back pain (90%) resolves in 6 weeks with or without any treatment.

Conservative management. Lifestyle adaptation, analgesia (NSAIDs, weak opiates), anaesthetic/steroid injections, heat treatments, back supports, physiotherapy.
Activity restriction. In general, the patient should limit *strenuous* activity but *remain active*, with early mobilization.
Surgery. This is almost never appropriate and so is only used for 0.5% of affected patients However, urgent surgical decompression is required for acute spinal compression.

Lower back pain: the lumbar spine
Causes of low back pain are given in Table 3.54.1.

Mechanical pain
The patient is usually 20–55 years, with pain felt in the lower back, buttocks and thighs; there are no weight loss or systemic symptoms. There may be a history of physical activity, and

neurological examination is normal. Suspicious features should be investigated further. **Management** is as above.

Prolapsed disc
Prolapse of a lumbar intervertebral disc (Fig. 3.54.1) mostly occurs at the L4/L5 or L5/S1 junction. The nucleus pulposis prolapses out of the annulus fibrosis, and compression of a nerve root causes symptoms. Onset is usually sudden, although there may be no history of trauma. Compression of a single nerve root is common, and compression of the sciatic nerve results in **sciatica**, which is characterized by shooting pain or numbness and tingling in the buttock, down the back of the knee and into the foot. The pain is worse on coughing and sneezing and is recurrent. Sensation may be altered, and straight leg raise is diminished (stretches the sciatic nerve and causes pain; see Ch. 74). Severe prolapses may compress the whole cauda equina, leading to cauda equina syndrome (Ch. 74). MRI is the best test. **Management** is initially conservative and 80%

Table 3.54.1 CAUSES OF LOWER BACK PAIN

Structural	Mechanical, facet joint osteoarthritis (spinal stenosis), prolapsed intervertebral disc, spondylolithesis/spondylolysis
Neoplastic	Primary or secondary
Infection	Osteomyelitis, discitis
Metabolic (Ch. 65)	Osteoporosis (fractures), Paget's disease, osteomalacia, ankylosing spondylitis, hyperparathyroidism (Ch. 41)

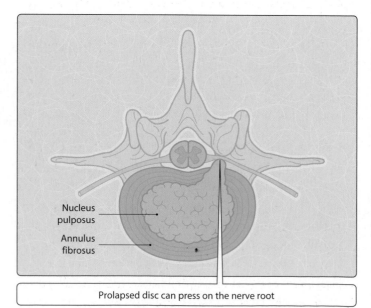

Nucleus pulposus

Annulus fibrosus

Prolapsed disc can press on the nerve root

Fig. 3.54.1 Compression of the lumbrosacral nerve root.

improve. Only if conservative measures fail is microscopic surgical excision of the disc (**microdiscectomy**) considered.

Lumbar spondylosis

Lumbar spondylosis is a common age-related, degenerative process, which also occurs in the cervical spine. Although most of those affected are asymptomatic, some may have pain and loss of movement. Characteristic radiograph changes are osteophytes and disc-space narrowing, where nerve impingement causes pain. Most settle with conservative management. Occasionally surgery is required for severe cases.

Spinal stenosis

Spinal stenosis is narrowing of the spinal canal caused by osteoarthritis and osteophyte formation. Exercise pain in the buttocks and leg is typical: **spinal claudication**. Subsequent impingement on the nerve roots produces radiculopathy and is identified on MRI. Most are managed conservatively, although surgical removal of osteophytes is required in some.

Spondylolisthesis

Spondylolisthesis is slippage of a vertebra onto the vertebra below (Fig. 3.54.2). A palpable step may be felt above the slipped vertebrae. Slippage is most common in the lumbar spine at L5/S1, where minor overuse injuries produce a stress fracture (although it may be congenital). The slip is forward, and so impingement symptoms are uncommon and the condition may be asymptomatic. However, the patient may present with chronic lower back pain or sciatica if the displacement is large. Most are treated conservatively. Large displacements may require surgical lumbrosacral fusion.

Ankylosing spondylitis

Ankylosing spondylitis should be suspected in a young man with low back pain (sacroilitis), stiffness and eye problems (uveitis). The patient must *remain active* as rest makes it worse (Ch. 65). Ankylosing spondylitis may be associated with inflammatory bowel disease but its activity is unrelated to the severity of the bowel disease.

Osteoporosis

Osteoporosis is very common, and pathological fractures can cause acute pain, chronic dull back ache or be asymptomatic.

Tumour

Most spinal tumours are metastatic (from breast, prostate and thyroid): chemotherapy and radiotherapy are the mainstay of treatment. Primary bone tumours are rare and occasionally surgical resection is possible. Spinal cord tumours are uncommon. Young patients with neurological signs are a cause for concern. MRI is the investigation.

Infection

Infection is uncommon. The signs may be mild or systemic. Infective organisms are typically pyogenic (e.g. *Staphylococcus aureus*) or tuberculous. Infection in an intraverebral disc is called **Pott's disease** (causing kyphosis). Treatment is as for acute osteomyelitis.

Neck pain: the cervical spine

Cervical spondylosis

Spondylosis is a common degenerative condition of the cervical (and lumbar) spine, where intervertebral discs degenerate and flatten and osteophytes form, producing a range of syndromes. Most are asymptomatic, and symptoms are treated conservatively.

Rheumatoid arthritis

Rheumatoid arthritis causes three main problems in the back: atlantoaxial subluxation (C1 onto C2), odontoid proximal migration and slippage of cervical vertebrae (slippage is less common at lower levels). Surgical stabilization reduces symptoms caused by nerve compression and acute spinal compression. Any patient with rheumatoid arthritis having a general anaesthetic should have a lateral radiograph of the cervical spine first, as manipulation during anaesthesia may damage the spinal cord.

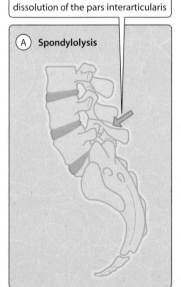
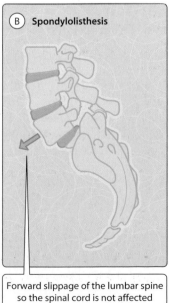

Movement results from a fracture or dissolution of the pars interarticularis

A Spondylolysis B Spondylolisthesis

Forward slippage of the lumbar spine so the spinal cord is not affected

Fig. 3.54.2 A stress fracture through the pars interarticularis is termed spondylolysis (A); if there is vertebral slippage, this is spondylolisthesis (B).

55. Shoulder pain

Questions
- What are the joints of the shoulder and the muscles of the rotator cuff?
- What are the causes of a painful arc syndrome?
- What are the other causes of shoulder pain?

Shoulder pain is the second most common cause of orthopaedic pain presentating to a general practitioner. The shoulder is composed of two bones (**humerus** and **scapula**) and three joints (**glenohumeral**, **scapulothoracic** and **acromioclavicular**). The rotator cuff is composed of four muscles, which reinforce the capsule and provide active support during movement (SITS: **s**upraspinatus, **i**nfraspinatus, **t**eres minor, **s**ubscapularis).

The glenohumeral joint is a ball and socket joint, where stability is sacrificed to allow a wide range of movement. It is a shallow joint and, although stability is improved by the glenoid labrum, joint capsule and rotator cuff muscle, it is relatively unstable compared with the hip.

Diagnosing shoulder disorders
For most disorders, diagnosis is based on the clinical features, with imaging playing a role in some. Plain radiograph (showing calcification, abnormal anatomy, joint spaces), ultrasound (cheap, can detect soft tissue damage, can guide needle-based treatments) and MRI (non-invasive, extremely sensitive and specific) are available. Shoulder arthroscopy has become increasingly used and is both diagnostic and therapeutic.

Common causes of shoulder pain
Painful arc syndrome
Pain occurs upon mid-range of active abduction (60–120°; Fig. 3.55.1) when a tendon structure (nodule) becomes painfully impinged within the subacromial space. Passive abduction is complete and painless. There are five causes.

Supraspinatus tendonitis. Acute inflammation of the supraspinatus muscle causes an acute area of swelling, which becomes painfully squashed underneath the acromion during abduction. The muscle eventually clears the nodule and pain disappears. Treatment is with rest, NSAIDs, and injection of steroid with local anaesthetic.

Calcifying tendonitis. Patients are aged 20–40 years and present as for supraspinatus tendonitis; calcification is seen within the supraspinatus tendon in a plain radiograph. 'Needling' these areas of calcification (breaking them up) while injecting steroid leads to improvement.

Rotator cuff tear. The supraspinatus tendon is the most commonly damaged, leading to sudden but brief pain and weakness of abduction. The incidence increases with age and is caused by degeneration and arthritis. There is pain on movement and at night, and movement is limited. It also often occurs in young competitive overhead throwers. Partial tears are treated with a local anaesthetic and physiotherapy. Complete tears are usually permanent and cause complete loss of abduction; repair of the cuff can be attempted in the young.

Subacromial bursitis. A subacromial bursa can become impinged. It may develop as a result of inflammatory arthropathy, local impingement (e.g. osteophyte) or trauma. Treatment is with steroid and local anaesthetic injection into the bursa.

Fracture of the greater tuberosity. Although fractures of the greater tuberosity are not uncommonly associated with anterior shoulder dislocation, isolated fracture of the greater tuberosity remains an easily overlooked injury. Confirming the presence of tenderness on the lateral wall of the greater tuberosity is a clinically effective method for preventing missed diagnosis.

Frozen shoulder (adhesive capsulitis)
Frozen shoulder is a common idiopathic condition and is characterized by painful restriction of external rotation. Reactive inflammation within the capsule is followed by adhesions, forming between the capsule and humeral head. Pain

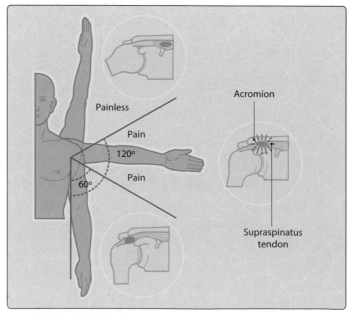

Fig. 3.55.1 Painful arc syndrome pain.

is typically at the end of the range of movement in all directions, and diagnosis is based on clinical findings. It is a self-limiting condition and is characterized by a 6-month period of recovery (Fig. 3.55.2).

Management is conservative, with analgesia and NSAID injections during the painful freezing phase and physiotherapy during recovery. Manipulation under anaesthesia (MUA) may break some of the adhesions.

Arthritis

Osteoarthritis of the shoulder most commonly occurs at the acromioclavicular joint, causing painful restriction of movements, although it is less common than in the hip or knee. Treatment is initially conservative with analgesia, physiotherapy and steroid injections. Joint replacement may be needed eventually.

Rheumatoid arthritis also occurs at the shoulder and is initially treated conservatively, although arthroplasty is effective.

Rupture of the tendon to long head of biceps

When the tendon to the long head of biceps is ruptured, there is sudden pain in the upper arm and anterior shoulder, and the patient notices a lump in the upper arm. Diagnosis is made when elbow flexion is resisted, causing a bulging of biceps fibres: the 'Popeye' sign (Fig. 3.55.3). NSAIDs and steroid injection relieve pain.

Fibromyalgia

Fibromyalgia is widespread musculoskeletal pain of unknown cause, typically in the shoulder and hip girdles. Diagnosis is formed by finding a number of separate tender points, and treatment is supportive. It is similar to **polymyalgia rheumatica**, where pain occurs in the neck, shoulder girdle and pelvis girdle.

Other causes of shoulder pain

Other causes are:

- recurrent shoulder dislocation (Ch. 47)
- cervical spondylosis: may cause neck and shoulder pain (Ch. 54)
- brachial neuritis: a rare condition of unknown aetiology causing severe unilateral shoulder pain, followed by flaccid paralysis; treatment is largely conservative, although it may take up to 2 years to resolve
- pancoast tumour: an apical lung tumour, causing brachial plexus compression and Horner's syndrome (unilateral ptosis, pupilary constriction, anhydria and enopthalmos)
- bone tumour: primary or secondary of the proximal humerus (rare)
- referred pain: can occur from an myocardial infarction or diaphragmatic irritation (e.g. visceral perforation, gallstone disease).

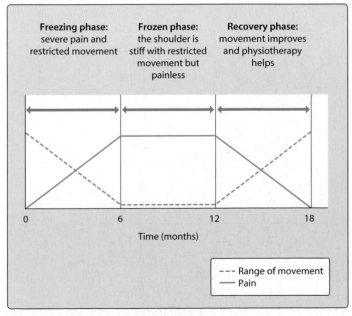

Fig. 3.55.2 Pattern of frozen shoulder

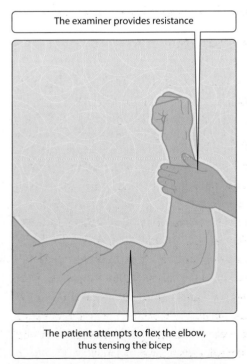

Fig. 3.55.3 Popeye's sign for a ruptured tendon of the head of biceps.

The examiner provides resistance

The patient attempts to flex the elbow, thus tensing the bicep

56. Elbow, wrist and hand disorders

Questions
- What is the difference between tennis and golfer's elbow?
- How does arthritis affect the hand and wrist?
- What is Dupytren's contracture?

The elbow

Tennis and golfer's elbow

Pain around the elbow characterizes tennis and golfer's elbow (Fig. 3.56.1). Patients are often middle aged and present with a recent history of elbow-related activity (e.g. carrying, lifting, sweeping or dusting; not only tennis or golf):

- tennis elbow: lateral epicondylitis (extensor mechanism)
- golfer's elbow: medial epicondylitis (flexor mechanism); pain is medial and is reproduced on resisted wrist flexion.

The diagnosis is clinical. Treatment is initially conservative with rest, NSAIDs and local anaesthetic creams. Local physiotherapy and steroid injections may help if the problem is persistent. If disability is severe, operative release is indicated.

Arthritis

Osteoarthritis typically follows a previous fracture, although it is rare. Treatment is initially conservative with NSAIDs. Debridement (to remove loose bodies) and arthroplasty can be used for severe cases. Rheumatoid arthritis is much more common, and management is conservative until there is secondary degenerative arthritis. The surgical options are radial head excision and synovectomy, or joint replacement.

Olecranon bursutis

Olecranon bursutis occurs in manual workers (e.g. carpet layers, 'student's elbow') and is associated with rheumatoid arthritis, gout and trauma. A fluctuant swelling around the elbow becomes painful if infected. Treatment is conservative with aspiration and culture; surgical excision is indicated for chronic cases.

The wrist and hand

Rheumatoid arthritis

Rheumatoid arthritis of the wrist and hand is common and may cause severe deformities (Fig. 3.56.2) that can severely restrict activities of daily life. Rheumatoid disease commonly presents in the hands, with morning stiffness, swelling and warmth. Note that the distal interphalangeal joint is *not* affected with rheumatoid arthritis.

Carpal tunnel syndrome may develop in rheumatoid arthritis. Conservative and medical options are considered in Ch. 57.

Surgery aims to improve functional capacity of the hands, where options include synovectomy, metacarpophalangeal arthroplasty, wrist and finger arthrodesis (fusion), carpal tunnel decompression.

Osteoarthritis

Osteoarthritis of the hand most commonly affects the carpometacarpal joint of the thumb, causing a 'square thumb'. Heberden's nodules occur at the distal interphalangeal joints and are characteristic of osteoarthritis but are rarely

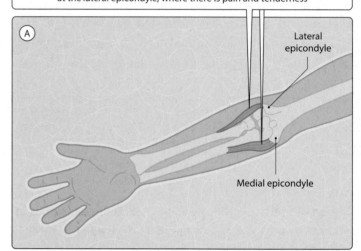

Golfer's elbow: inflammation is at the common flexor origin at the *medial* epicondyle, where there is pain and tenderness

Tennis elbow: inflammation is at the common extensor muscle origin at the *lateral* epicondyle, where there is pain and tenderness

A

Lateral epicondyle

Medial epicondyle

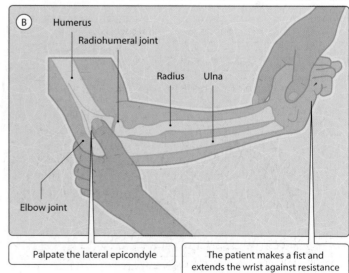

B

Humerus

Radiohumeral joint

Radius   Ulna

Elbow joint

Palpate the lateral epicondyle

The patient makes a fist and extends the wrist against resistance

Fig. 3.56.1 Elbow pain. (A) Location of pain in tennis elbow and golfer's elbow. (B) Mills' test for lateral epicondylitis; palpate the lateral epicondyle while the patient makes a fist and extends against resistance.

problematic. (Bouchard's nodes affect the proximal interphalangeal joints and are rarer.) Initial treatment is conservative with splints, NSAIDs and injections. Excision, arthrodesis and joint replacement are all possible.

De Quervain's tenosynovitis

De Quervain's tenosynovitis is inflammation of the extensor pollicis brevis and abductor pollicis longus caused by repetitive movements; it is common in women aged 30–50 years. Pain and swelling occur in the anatomical 'snuffbox'; pain is reproduced by bending the thumb into the palm (Finkelstein's test). Treatment is initially with rest and NSAIDs, occasionally with a local steroid injection or surgical decompression.

Gamekeeper's thumb

Tearing the medial collateral ligament from the metacarpophalangeal joint of the thumb by violent abduction is known as gamekeeper's thumb. Diagnosis is made on history and clinical examination. The thumb is unstable and immobilization in a cast or surgical repair of the tendon is required.

Mallet finger

Mallet finger usually results from a direct blow to an extended finger. The mallet deformity of the tip of the finger is caused by rupture or avulsion of the extensor tendon of the distal phalanx (Fig. 3.56.3). Treatment is with a mallet splint holding the phalanx in full extension for 6 weeks at all times (even when washing), where the tendon usually reunites.

Trigger finger

In trigger finger, there is thickening of the flexor tendon or tendon sheath (or both), commonly at the base of the little or index finger. A tendon nodule develops where the flexor digitorum profundus tendon enters the tendon sheath and is subject to friction. The swelling prevents the tendon passing through the sheath, where it eventually becomes trapped in flexion and must be prised open by passive extension, which may be painful. Treatment is initially rest and steroid injections; surgical division of the sheath is an immediate and permanent cure.

Dupytren's contracture

Dupytren's contracture is painless contracture of the palmar fascia. It normally starts at the base of the ring and little finger producing gradual flexion of these fingers. The hand cannot be laid flat upon a table, and the thickening of the skin of the palm and palmar fascia is palpable. Many are idiopathic, and risk factors are family history, chronic liver disease, diabetes, anti-epileptic drugs and alcoholism; there may be associated Peyronie's disease (penile fibrosis). It is more common in men aged 40–60 years and may be bilateral. Treatment is conservative until it interferes with function. The procedure of choice is a **subtotal fasciectomy** to excise the affected fascia and Z-plasty of the skin if this is badly involved. Amputation of the affected fingers is occasionally necessary.

Kienböck's disease

Avascular necrosis of the carpal lunate can present in young adults with pain and stiffness of the wrist. Treatment is with a firm splint.

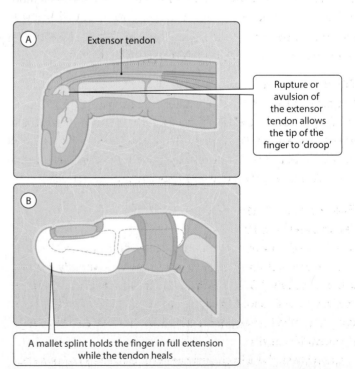

Fig. 3.56.3 Mallet finger. (A) Tendon damage; (B) a mallet splint.

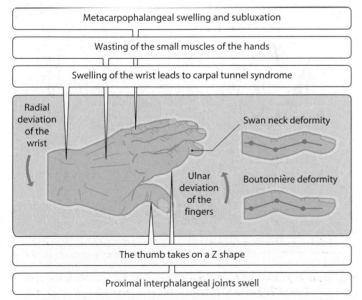

Fig. 3.56.2 Characteristic findings of rheumatoid arthritis of the hand and wrist.

57. Upper limb nerve palsies

Questions
■ What are the causes of carpal tunnel syndrome?
■ What is the sensory distribution of the hand?
■ How would you test for an ulnar nerve palsy?

Nerve palsies are particularly common around the elbow and wrist. They often present with a functional deficit, and so knowledge of the underlying anatomy is important (Fig. 3.57.1). They occur as OSCE stations so it is important to know how to examine them.

Carpal tunnel syndrome

There are 10 structures within the carpal tunnel: the median nerve and nine flexor tendons (four flexor digitorum profundus tendons, four flexor digitorum superficialis tendons and one flexor pollicis longus tendon; Fig. 3.57.2). Any process that narrows the width of the tunnel, either bony compression or fluid retention (below), will compress the median nerve as it passes through the tunnel. Causes of carpal tunnel syndrome include pregnancy (fluid retention is a common cause), repetitive strain injuries, Colles' fracture, rheumatoid arthritis, myxoedema (hypothyroidism), diabetes mellitus, idiopathic and acromegaly (rare). The median nerve innervates four muscles in the hand (LOAF): lateral umbricals (two of these),

opponens pollicis, abductor pollicis brevis, flexor pollicis brevis. The last three form the thenar eminence.

Clinical features

The patient presents with numbness, tingling ('pins and needles'), burning or pain, which is typically worse at night, in the median distribution (lateral 3.5 digits). The thenar eminence becomes wasted, and thumb abduction is weak. A nerve conduction test can be performed if there is doubt. The aims of an examination are to identify the symptoms of carpal tunnel syndrome, and to identify obvious causes.

Look. Wasting of the thenar eminence should be evident. The palmar side of the wrist might show scars from previous operations. The hands may have signs of rheumatoid arthritis, and there may be signs of systemic disease.

Feel. Ask about pain. Sensation may be reduced or altered in the radial 3.5 digits (but the condition may be bilateral). The radial pulse should be checked.

Move. These special tests identify weakness and movements:
— resisted thumb abduction is weak (thumb pointing up to the ceiling with a flat palm)

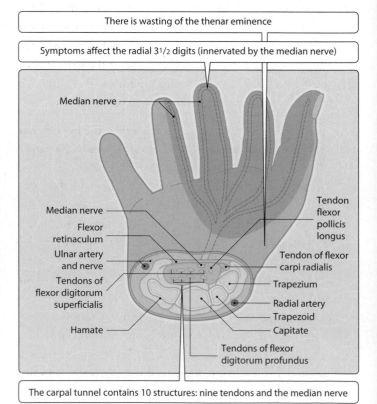

There is wasting of the thenar eminence

Symptoms affect the radial 3½ digits (innervated by the median nerve)

Median nerve

Median nerve

Flexor retinaculum

Ulnar artery and nerve

Tendons of flexor digitorum superficialis

Hamate

Tendons of flexor digitorum profundus

Tendon flexor pollicis longus

Tendon of flexor carpi radialis

Trapezium

Radial artery

Trapezoid

Capitate

The carpal tunnel contains 10 structures: nine tendons and the median nerve

Fig. 3.57.2 Carpal tunnel syndrome.

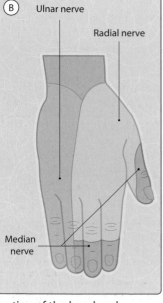

Ⓐ

Radial nerve
(C₆–C₈)

Ulnar nerve
(C₈, T₁)

Median nerve
(C₆–C₈)

Ⓑ

Ulnar nerve

Radial nerve

Median nerve

Fig. 3.57.1 Cutaneous nerve innervation of the hand and dermatomes.

— Tinel's test: the symptoms appear if the palmar aspect of the wrist (over the carpal tunnel) is tapped
— Phalen's test: the 'inverse prayer' sign (the wrist is held in flexion for 30 to 60 seconds) causes pressure in the carpal tunnel generating symptoms and weakness
— functional tests: power grasp (make a fist) and precision pinch (hold this pen, undo a button).

Management

Conservative treatment is with rest, splints, diuretics and steroid injections. Rest and diuretics are the treatment in pregnancy until delivery. Surgical decompression is used if there is no improvement, the flexor retinaculum is divided longitudinally; this is quick and reliable and recurrence is uncommon.

Ulnar nerve palsy

The ulnar nerve supplies all the small muscles of the hand (except those innervated by the median nerve (LOAF; see above)), and it also supplies flexor carpi ulnaris and half of flexor digitorum profundis in the forearm. It can be damaged where it is superficial: at the elbow as it wraps around the posterior aspect of the medical epicondyle or at the wrist. If the lesion to the ulnar nerve is at the wrist, innervation to the small muscles of the hand is lost but innervation to flexor digitorum profundis in the forearm is maintained, which can now act unopposed (since the medial two lumbricals (supplied by the ulnar nerve) can no longer extend the interphalangeal joints), leading to **claw hand** (specifically affecting the 4th and 5th fingers). If the lesion is at the elbow, all of the ulnar muscles lose innervation and so clawing is absent or mild. Consequently, clawing is worse in distal lesions (i.e. worse at the wrist than at the elbow) and this is known as **ulnar paradox** (the paradox is that typically nerve lesions are worse when proximal).

Look. There is a claw hand, with wasting of the **hypothenar eminence** and **dorsal interossi** (small muscles of the hand).
Feel. Ask about pain and assess sensation, which is altered (and may be absent) in the medial 1.5 digits; check the radial pulse.
Move. There is weakness and limited, clumsy movement. The patient loses the ability to make a fist and opening the little finger against resistance is weak. Tapping the ulnar nerve over the medial epicondyle may reproduce symptoms.
Froment's paper sign (Fig. 3.57.3). There is weak finger abduction (loss of innervation to dorsal interossi muscles) and thumb adduction (adductor pollicis) on the affected side, and so the distal phalanx of the thumb must now flex against the index finger to hold onto the paper.

Management

In acute injury the area of damage is explored and the nerve repaired. If needed, the nerve can be released surgically and possibly transposed to a new, protected position.

Radial nerve palsy

The radial nerve is most vulnerable to damage where it winds around the spiral groove in the posterior aspect of the humerus. It can be damaged through compression (e.g. falling asleep with the arm over a chair back ('Saturday night palsy')) or through humeral shaft fractures. The primary complaint is **wrist drop** (as the radial nerve supplies the wrist extensors), and the patient cannot extend the wrist. Most settle conservatively, but surgical exploration of the nerve is indicated if there is no improvement in the uncommon cases of nerve entrapment.

Erb's palsy

Erb's palsy is a traumatic damage to the upper part of the brachial plexus (C_5, C_6) from a fall onto the shoulder (or from excessive traction on a baby's arm at birth). It leads to a characteristic 'waiter's tip' sign.

Klumpke's palsy

Damaged to the lower branches of the brachial plexus (C_7–T_1) may occur during a difficult birth from excessive arm traction to the baby. There is weakness of finger flexion and intrinsic muscles of the hand. T_1 root damage may result in sympathetic involvement and a Horner's syndrome.

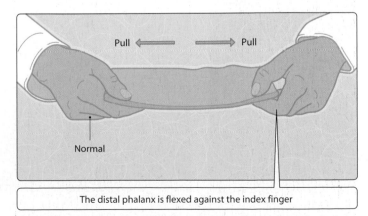

The distal phalanx is flexed against the index finger

Fig. 3.57.3 Froment's paper sign: a piece of paper is pulled.

58. Osteoarthritis

Questions
- Which joints are commonly affected by osteoarthritis?
- What are the typical features on plain radiograph?
- What are the complications of total joint replacement?

Osteoarthritis is the most common chronic joint disease and is a major cause of morbidity and disability. It commonly affects the hips, knees, hands and spine. (Rheumatoid arthritis is an autoimmune disease directed against synovial joints (see the orthopaedic chapters 54–66).)

Aetiology

Osteoarthritis is a wear and tear disease of the articular cartilage in weight-bearing joints. Where there is no clear cause, this is **primary arthritis**; the risk factors for this include:

- age: prevalence increases with age; 10% of men and 20% of women over 60 are affected
- genetic inheritance: family history, Heberden's nodes, specific gene identification
- obesity: causal relationship
- physical factors: occupations e.g. athletes.

Previous damage can cause altered joint dynamics, symptoms starting years later (**secondary osteoarthritis**). Underlying causes include:

- previous trauma or infection
- congenital: genu valgum of the knee, slipped upper femoral epiphysis, developmental dysplasia of the hip (DDH), hypermobility disorders

- bone disease: avascular necrosis, Paget's disease, neuropathic joints (Charcot's).

Pathology

The joint cartilage becomes soft, splits and fragments (**fibrillation**). The joint erodes and joint space is lost. Hypertrophy of the bone causes subchondral sclerosis and osteophyte formation. Synovial hypertrophy and capsular fibrosis leads to joint stiffness.

Clinical features

Osteoarthritis is characterized by pain of gradual onset, which ranges from mild discomfort to pain whilst weight-bearing (mechanical pain); it may prevent sleeping or require oral analgesia. Stiffness is worse after a period of rest.

Arthritis of the **hip** causes groin pain on walking (it may radiate to the knee), stiff and limited movements (initially on internal rotation), a fixed flexion deformity and a true leg length discrepancy (resulting in a Trendelenburg gait). That of the **knee** is painful and stiff. Crepitus and knee effusion are commonplace and the quadriceps muscle may become wasted. Both the tibiofemoral and patellofemoral joints are affected. Arthritis of the **hands** is described in Ch. 56.

Investigations

There are four radiograph characteristics of an osteoarthritic joint (remember with LOSS): loss of joint space, osteophytes (bony outgrowths at the joint margin), subchondral sclerosis and subchondral bone cysts (Fig. 3.58.1). Note that some patients with these changes may still be asymptomatic.

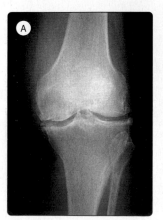
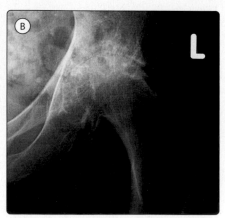

Fig. 3.58.1 Radiographs of osteoarthritis of the knee (A) and the hip (B) In end-stage hip osteoarthritis, the joint space has been totally lost, there are osteophytes of the lateral margin, the joint line is sclerosed and bone cysts are visible around the joint.

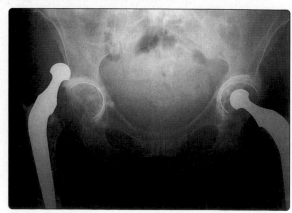

Fig. 3.58.2 Bilateral total hip replacements for end-stage osteoarthritis affecting both joints (the left side is dislocated).

Management

Early management is conservative and medical; surgery is for advanced/late disease.

Conservative management comprises exercise, activity modification, weight loss, occupational therapy (walking sticks (opposite hand for hip; same hand for knee), shoe wedges, home tools) and physiotherapy.

Medical management comprises analgesia (paracetamol or NSAIDs; ibuprofen can be used in acute episodes), intra-articular injections of steroid and/or local anaesthetic (rarely for the hip) and glucosamine (a proven alternative therapy to slow mild-to-moderate disease).

Surgical management

Surgery is indicated when disability and pain are severe. The choice of operation depends on the joint and patient.

Arthroscopic joint debridement. This is minimally invasive and does not interfere with future surgery. It is commonly used for knee osteoarthritis, where a washout is used to remove meniscal tears and loose foreign bodies, reducing pain.

Arthroplasty (total joint replacement). This is the gold standard treatment for patients with end-stage osteoarthritis (see below).

Hip resurfacing. This is used for early osteoarthritis; the damaged surface of the femoral head is replaced with a cemented metal rim and the acetabulum with a plastic cup. This reduces pain by removing the painful communicating joint surfaces. It is suitable for younger patients, as it delays a total hip replacement (the femur is left largely intact).

Osteotomy. This is suitable for younger patients (< 60 years) who have limited arthritis in the knee. The joint line is realigned to produce new weight-bearing surfaces. The patient can remain active and it defers total knee replacement until the patient is older (see Fig. 3.60.2).

Arthrodesis. This is now reserved for small joints (ankle and toes) and failed knee replacements. The joint is fused together with a bone graft to provide relief of pain, but results in severe limitation of movement.

Total hip replacement. A metal ball replaces the femoral head and is secured with an intramedullary stem (Fig. 3.58.2). A plastic cup replaces the damaged acetabulum as an articulation surface for the metal ball. Most (95%) prostheses are cemented, which allows rapid mobilization of the patient (suitable for the elderly). Uncemented stems are porous and allow bone growth into their surface; consequently, they last longer but take more time to stabilize (suitable for younger patients).

Complications of joint replacement

Early complications are wound infection (2%), dislocation (≤5%), haematoma (≤5%) and DVT (<80%, but may be asymptomatic). Late complications are aseptic loosening, deep infection and prosthesis fracture.

The best prostheses have a **revision rate** of 10% or less at 10 years. Revision can be done in one or two stages. When caused by *aseptic* loosening, the previous prosthesis is removed and a new prosthesis is placed immediately (**one-stage revision**).

Deep infection (usually *Staphylococcus epidermidis*) complicates 0.5% of hip and knee replacements and gives rise to few symptoms; low-grade fever, joint pain, swelling and a discharging sinus. Plain radiograph shows early loosening of the prosthesis and lucency around the prosthesis. Treatment is most successful with a **two-stage revision**, where the infected prosthesis is removed in the first stage and a spacer made of antibiotic-impregnated bone cement is inserted, and systemic antibiotics are started. Once signs of infection have resolved, a new prosthesis is implanted (typically 8-10 weeks later).

59. Hip examination

Questions
- What are the causes of hip pain?
- What is Thomas's test?
- What are the different types of leg length?

Hip OSCE stations most often involve a painful hip caused by arthritis or a limping child (Ch. 64). Hip pain is typically in the groin but may be referred to lower back or knee; buttock pain is associated with lower back problems.

Look

The patient is examined lying flat for muscle wasting (quadriceps), arthroplasty scars (look at the back of the hip and buttock for posterior scars), sinuses (indicating deep infection), fixed flexion deformities and obvious leg length discrepancy. The patient is examined walking to assess posture, pelvic tilt and walking aids. Gait disorders include the **Trendelenberg gait**, which is a waddle caused by swinging the affected leg out, and the **atalgic gait**, where less time is spent weight-bearing on the affected side. The Trendelenberg test (Fig. 3.59.1) assesses hip stability. Causes of a positive test include osteoarthritis and rheumatoid arthritis (hip pain), non-union of a neck of femur fracture (shortened femoral neck), weak or paralysed abductors (nerve damage, polio) or lack of a fulcrum owing to hip subluxation or dislocation.

Feel

While the patient is still standing, palpation at the back of the knee will detect a Baker's cyst and inspection will indicate scoliosis, kyphosis or lumbar lordosis. Feeling the area will indicate temperature (rarely warm, even with active inflammation in the hip since it is a deep joint) and joint tenderness (feel for greater trochanters on each side; pain indicates **trochanteric bursitis**). The anterior superior iliac spines (ASIS) should be approximately at the same level.

Move

Thomas' test (Fig. 3.59.2) examines for a fixed flexion deformity; both hips should be tested. The common causes of a fixed flexion deformity are osteoarthritis and a previous fracture of the neck of the femur.

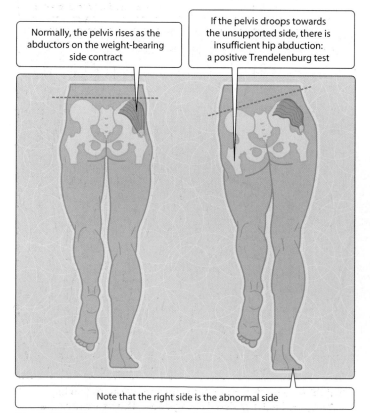

Normally, the pelvis rises as the abductors on the weight-bearing side contract

If the pelvis droops towards the unsupported side, there is insufficient hip abduction: a positive Trendelenburg test

Note that the right side is the abnormal side

Fig. 3.59.1 The Trendelenberg test. The patient is supported while standing on one leg.

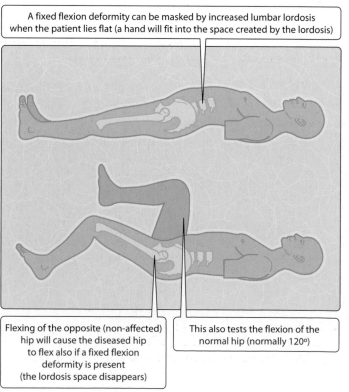

A fixed flexion deformity can be masked by increased lumbar lordosis when the patient lies flat (a hand will fit into the space created by the lordosis)

Flexing of the opposite (non-affected) hip will cause the diseased hip to flex also if a fixed flexion deformity is present (the lordosis space disappears)

This also tests the flexion of the normal hip (normally 120°)

Fig. 3.59.2 Thomas' test.

Hip movement is assessed by stabilizing the patient's pelvis with one hand while moving the leg with the other, looking for any pain during movement and for ranges of movements (normal ranges of movement are given, but there is some normal variation between individuals):

■ flexion ('Thomas' test; normal range 120°)
■ extension is performed while the patient is lying on their front or side, and so is left to the end (normal range 10°)
■ rotation (Fig. 3.59.3)
■ abduction and adduction (Fig. 3.59.4)
■ leg length (Fig.3.59.4B):
 — true leg length: measure from the ASIS to the medial malleolus on the same side
 — apparent leg length: measure from the xiphisternum to the medial malleolus on both sides; reduction occurs in pelvic tilt or fixed adduction of the hip, although the legs are still the same length.

Table 3.59.1 RADIOLOGICAL DIFFERENCES BETWEEN OSTEOARTHRITIS AND RHEUMATOID ARTHRITIS

Osteoarthritis	Rheumatoid arthritis
Loss of joint space	Loss of joint space
Osteophytes	No osteophytes
Joint line sclerosis	Erosions; subchondral erosions of the bone
Bone cysts	Porous

Concluding an examination

An OSCE station would be concluded by asking to assess the distal neurovascular status (touching the toes and checking the dorsalis pedis pulse). The most common investigation is radiography (Table 3.59.1).

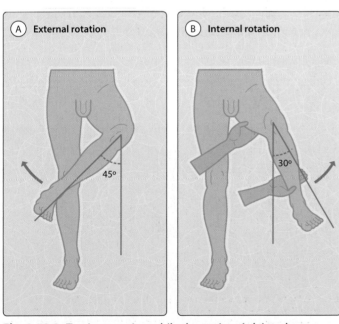

Fig. 3.59.3 Testing rotation while the patient is lying down.

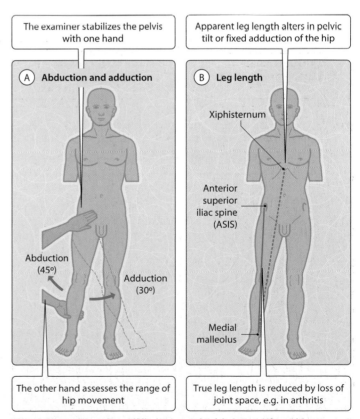

Fig. 3.59.4 Assessing abduction and adduction (A) and leg length (B), while the patient is lying down. The pelvis must be stabilized or palpated to ensure that it is the hip and not the pelvis that moves.

60. Knee pain

Questions
- What is the management of a ligamentous injury?
- What are menisci and how are they damaged?
- What are the causes of knee pain in children?

Knee pain may present suddenly after injury or as a chronic pain, and it occurs in both adults and children.

Knee pain in adults

Ligament damage
Sporting injuries are a common cause of ligament damage. Strains or isolated tears may settle with rest, analgesia and plaster or bracing; acute tears and complex or chronic injuries often benefit from surgical reconstruction.

Anterior cruciate ligaments. A tear in an anterior cruciate ligament is a common sporting injury (Fig. 3.60.1) following a twisting motion or hyperextension. The patient reports feeling something break or give way and the joint swells rapidly. There is a positive anterior draw test and Lachman's test, and an effusion may be present. Initial management is conservative with aspiration of a haemarthrosis, analgesia and physiotherapy. One-third improve with this regimen; one-third manage with the decreased level of function, but one-third need arthroscopic repair, either to achieve a higher level of function (high-level contact sports) or for severe instability.

Posterior cruciate ligament. Injury occurs with the knee flexed, when the tibia is forced backwards; another ligamental injury is common (e.g. collateral ligament). The posterior draw sign is positive. Treatment is similar to anterior cruciate ligaments although repair is more difficult.

Medial collateral ligaments. Medical collateral damage usually occurs with an associated anterior cruciate ligament and medial meniscal injury (the 'unhappy triad'). Treatment is with either immobilization in a cast for 6 weeks or surgical reconstruction to restore stability.

Lateral collateral ligament. Damage here is rarely isolated, and instability is less common than with medial collateral ligament injury. Treatment is conservative.

Meniscal injuries
Meniscal tears are common and the majority will involve the medial meniscus. They are either traumatic or degenerative. Traumatic tears are common in those whose occupation involves crouching, kneeling, turning or trauma. The majority of degenerative tears are asymptomatic and are present in 65% of those over 60 years of age. There are different types of tear, classified by their appearance (Fig. 3.60.2).

Clinical features. Patients are usually fit, young and males; there is pain, joint line tenderness and positive McMurray's test. Symptoms may settle, but episodes may be repeated.

Investigations. MRI and arthroscopy confirm the nature and location of injury.

Management. Arthroscopy and partial meniscetomy are the mainstay of treatments, and meniscal repair can be attempted. Total meniscetomy is avoided as the risk of premature osteoarthritis is high.

Chronic knee pain
Osteoarthritis. The knee is a common site for osteoarthritis,

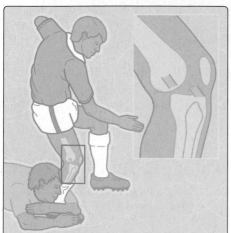

Fig. 3.60.1 Anterior cruciate ligament tear.

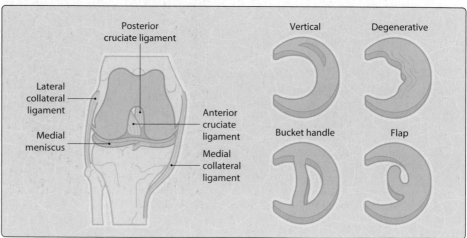

Fig. 3.60.2 Examples of meniscal tears.

which may be caused by previous injury or excessive use of the knee or an old meniscal tear. It results in pain, swelling, deformity and stiffness. General management options for osteoarthritis are discussed in Ch. 58. Knee osteoarthritis in young patients is managed conservatively for as long as possible. Steroid injections are avoided, and **osteotomies** (alteration of the joint line to allow a new-weight-bearing surface to be brought into use; Fig. 3.60.3) delay the need for knee replacement. Specific treatments for the knee include:

- **arthroscopic washout** to remove loose particles of cartilage that are causing pain
- **arthroplasty**: unicompartmental replacement is suitable for early disease, and total knee replacement (Fig. 3.60.4) for advanced 'tricompartmental' disease.

Rheumatoid arthritis.   Rheumatoid arthritis causes effusions and a valgus deformity; surgical treatment includes arthroscopic washouts, synevectomies and total joint replacements.

Localized pain and swellings.   There are several causes:

- jumper's knee: occurs at the insertion of the patellar ligament onto the patella and is similar to tennis elbow
- bursae: **prepatella bursitis** (housemaid's knee; leaning forward on the knees) and **infrapatella bursitis** (clergyman's knee; prolonged periods of kneeling); treatment is with activity modification, aspiration or excision
- popliteal cysts (Baker's cysts) usually accompany rheumatoid arthritis and may burst spontaneously; they are mostly treated conservatively.

Knee pain in children

Osteochondritis dissecans

Osteochondritis dissecans is an idiopathic disease typically affecting boys aged 8–12 years; it is characterized by partial or complete detachment of a fragment of bone (Fig. 3.60.5). It most commonly affects the lateral surface of medial femoral condyle (the talus, femoral head and first metatarsal head may also be affected). Repeated minor trauma, ischaemic changes or genetic predisposition are all implicated. Many partially separated fragments reunite conservatively with rest, although loose bodies in the joint space require surgical removal.

Anterior knee pain

Anterior knee pain is most commonly seen in adolescent girls. It is caused by softening of the cartilage on the posterior aspect of the patella, caused by stresses around the knee known as **chondromalacia patella**. Treatment is conservative as the pain usually settles with skeletal maturity.

Osgood–Schlatter's disease

Osgood–Schlatter's disease is most common in boys aged 11–15 years. The tibial tuberosity is lifted off the tibia when young athletes exert too great a traction in their underdeveloped apophysis (**traction apophysitis**). There is pain on activity; swelling and a painful lump may be found. Radiographs may show fragmentation of the tubercle. Spontaneous recovery is usual but takes time (up to 2 years), and periods of rest may have to be reinforced with a plaster cast. Loose fragments in the joint require surgical removal.

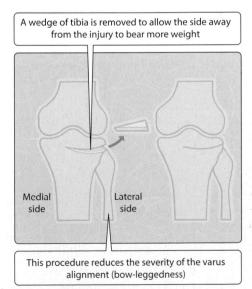

A wedge of tibia is removed to allow the side away from the injury to bear more weight

Medial side   Lateral side

This procedure reduces the severity of the varus alignment (bow-leggedness)

Fig. 3.60.3 Tibial osteotomy shown on an anterolateral view of the knee.

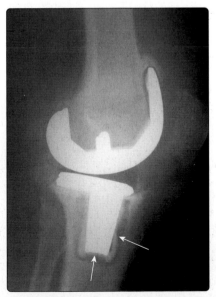

Fig. 3.60.4 Total knee replacement in lateral view. Infection has caused septic loosening around the prosthesis (arrows).

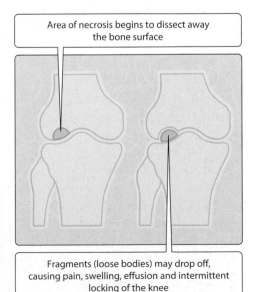

Area of necrosis begins to dissect away the bone surface

Fragments (loose bodies) may drop off, causing pain, swelling, effusion and intermittent locking of the knee

Fig. 3.60.5 The disease process in osteochondritis dissecans.

61. Knee examination

Questions
- What are the signs of active inflammation in the knee?
- What tests indicate anterior ligamentous stability?
- What tests indicate a meniscal tear?

Knee problems can give rise to altered gait, active inflammation and swelling.

Active inflammation is indicated by heat, rubor (redness or erythema), swelling caused by effusions and pain. Knee swelling can be caused by general effusions: rheumatoid arthritis, osteoarthritis, septic arthritis (hot and swollen; uncommon). Posterior swelling could be a Baker's cyst, bursitis or popliteal aneurysm. Anterior swelling can be bursitis (common) or Osgood–Schlatter's disease.

Introduction
Knee pain may be referred to the hip or lower back (or referred from the hip). An OSCE station might cover knee pain (commonly osteoarthritis or rheumatoid arthritis), knee swellings, ligamental instability or meniscal tear.

Look
With the patient standing assess gait (a step comprises heel strike, stance, toe-off and swing), look for posterior scars and palpate in the popliteal fossa for a Baker's cyst.

With the patient lying down look for:

- scars: longitudinal midline scar indicates total knee replacement; arthroscopy portals
- effusions and redness: normal joint contours may be lost
- wasting: of the quadriceps can be quantified by measuring the circumference of both thighs with a tape measure, 10 cm from the top of the patella
- genu valgum (knock-kneed) and genu varum (bow legged)
- deformity of the foot (e.g. club foot).

Feel
Assessment will be for temperature, effusions and joint line tenderness. The knee will feel warm if active inflammation is present (e.g. rheumatoid arthritis, septic arthritis).

Small effusions can be assessed with the **bulge test** (Fig. 3.61.1). Large effusions can be assessed by a **patellar tap**, although this is less sensitive. The effusion is again drawn towards the knee and without removing your hands, press down on the patella; an effusion has a 'boggy' feeling under the knee, and the patella gently 'bounces'.

Joint line tenderness is assessed when the patient is on the bed with the knee placed at 90% and the ankle on the bed. Feel in the soft area between the patella and tibial tuberosites, moving backwards towards the thigh. This presses against the joint line and if painful indicates a meniscal tear.

Move
Internally rotating the hip will cause hip pain when there is coexisting hip pathology. Movement is assessed as both active and passive movement with the patient lying down:

- active
  - flexion: the patient bends the knee as far up to their chest as possible (135° in a normal knee)
  - extension: lift both limbs up by the ankles (with the knees locked); most knee joints do not extend backwards but some normal knees still bend by 10°
  - while the knee is bending, a hand over the patella can feel joint **crepitus** (cracking of the knee joint, indicating damage to the articular surfaces
- passive movement
  - when active flexion is at its maximum, the clinician carefully attempts to flex the knee further; it should be possible to elicit another 10° of flexion.

Special tests
Ligamentous stress tests

Anterior draw sign for the anterior cruciate ligament. The knee is flexed to 90° with the legs stabilized by the clinician sitting at the patient's toes (Fig. 3.61.2). A ruptured anterior cruciate ligament will allow the tibia to move forward to a greater degree than normal, usually defined as > 1 cm.

Lachman's test for anterior cruciate ligament instability. The knee is held in 20° flexion off the bed, and the calf pulled forward while the thigh is held firm. This means that the tibia is moving forward against the femur, stressing the anterior cruciate ligament).

Posterior draw sign for the posterior cruciate ligament. From the position of the anterior draw test, the knee is pushed firmly back. Again, there may be some natural give, but with a ruptured posterior crutiate ligament, the tibia will move backwards > 1 cm.

Stability test for the medial and lateral collateral ligaments. The knee is flexed to 20–30°, with the thigh held in one hand and the calf in the other (Fig. 3.61.3). Pushing the calf medially (inwards) and thigh laterally (outwards) stresses the lateral collateral ligaments. In the opposite direction, it stresses the medial collateral ligaments.

Testing for meniscal tears. **McMurray's test** is a difficult and unreliable test to detect meniscal tears. It is performed only if joint line tenderness is present. The knee is flexed fully and the foot externally rotated with the lower leg abducted. If the joint is extended smoothly, there will be a click with pain over medial joint line if there is a meniscal tear.

Concluding an examination

Further examination would be for the neurovascular status of the limb (sensation and distal pulses) and the joint above and below the knee (hip and ankle).

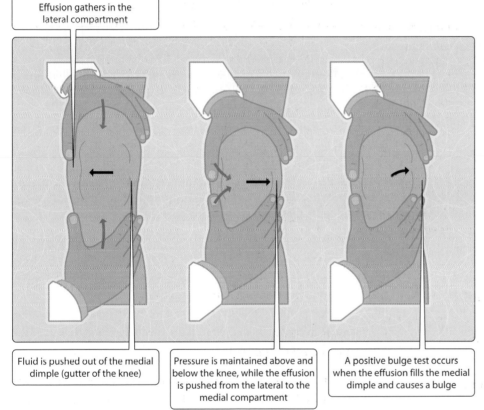

Effusion gathers in the lateral compartment

Fluid is pushed out of the medial dimple (gutter of the knee)

Pressure is maintained above and below the knee, while the effusion is pushed from the lateral to the medial compartment

A positive bulge test occurs when the effusion fills the medial dimple and causes a bulge

Fig. 3.61.1 The bulge test.

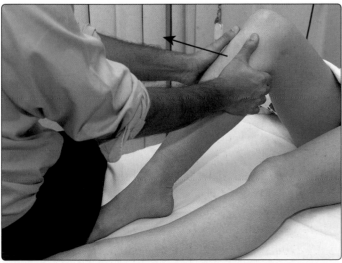

Fig. 3.61.2 The anterior draw test. With the hands on the tibial tuberosities, the knee is pulled firmly forward to test the anterior cruciate ligament; pushing backwards tests the posterior cruciate ligament.

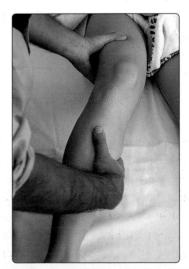

Fig. 3.61.3 Testing for stability of the medial collateral ligament; swapping over the hands and pushing in the opposite direction tests the lateral collateral ligaments.

62. Ankle and foot disorders

Questions
- What are the treatment options for hallux valgus?
- What might be the underlying abnormality in pes cavus?
- How can you test for an Achilles tendon rupture?

Hallux valgus

Hallux valgus is the most common deformity of the foot (Fig. 3.62.1); it is a valgus deformity of the big toe and is often bilateral. It typically affects two groups: adolescent/young and elderly women. Associations include a positive family history, wearing tight-fitting pointed shoes and rheumatoid arthritis. Problems are related to pain when wearing footwear, which is typically the pointed footwear and high heels more commonly worn by young women.

A weight-bearing radiograph is the key investigation and diagnosis is formed by finding a hallux valgus angle of > 15° and an intermetatarsal angle > 9°.

Surgery is indicated for continuing pain and significant deformity; it is not indicated for cosmesis alone. Conservative treatments with orthoses and well-fitting shoes are more acceptable in older patients, although surgery is typically more acceptable to the younger patient; there are many procedures available (numerous osteotomies; Keller's procedure is an arthrodesis that may be suitable for severe deformities).

A **bunion** is a bursa that develops over a prominent first metatarsal head. The bunion may become infected, which can become complicated in conditions such as diabetes mellitus, resulting in infection of the underlying joint and gangrene. Conservative treatment with comfortable shoes solves most, although **bunionectomy** can be performed; treatment of an underlying hallux valgus is needed.

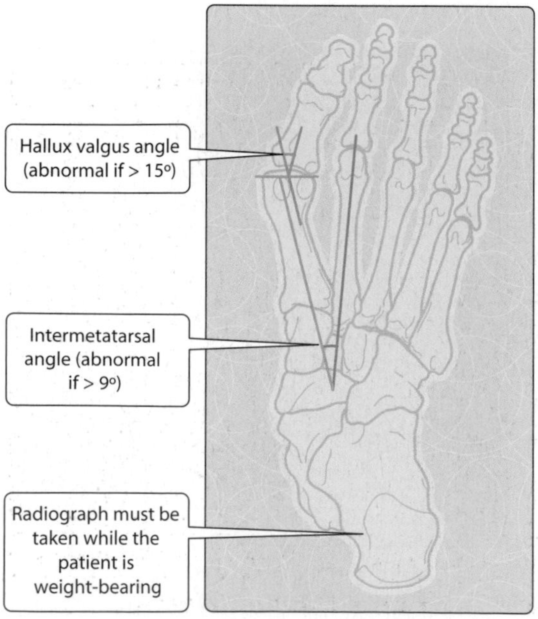

Hallux rigidus

Hallux rigidus is the common name for osteoarthritis of the first metatarsal. Osteophytes form on the head of the first metatarsal, which causes a 'stiff big toe': movement (especially dorsiflexion) and normal walking are restricted. Radiographs show the severity of changes and helps to guide management.

Conservative management is with shoes containing a pressure-relieving metatarsal bar; steroid injections may help. Early surgery to trim the osteophytes also helps (**cheilectomy**), and arthrodesis or replacement may be required for advanced disease.

Rheumatoid arthritis

Rheumatoid arthritis of the foot and ankle is common. The changes are similar to those found in the hand. The metatarsal heads come to lie underneath the toes as the fat pad is drawn forward, and this brings them close to the skin on the sole of the foot. Walking is difficult and bone is easily eroded; infection can occur. Hallux valgus develops, and tendon ruptures may cause deformity of the ankle and flat foot.

Treatment is initially conservative with moulded footwear and skin care. If these measures are ineffective, arthrodesis of the affected joints can be attempted; forefoot arthroplasty removes the metatarsal heads, reliably relieving pressure.

Fig. 3.62.1 Angles of deformity in hallux valgus assessed in a weight-bearing radiograph.

Hallux valgus angle (abnormal if > 15°)

Intermetatarsal angle (abnormal if > 9°)

Radiograph must be taken while the patient is weight-bearing

Lesser toe deformities

The deformities of the lesser toes (Fig. 3.62.2) are very common. Treatment is either conservative, modifying footwear to fit the toe, or surgical to straighten the toes, usually by removing the affected joint and fusing it.

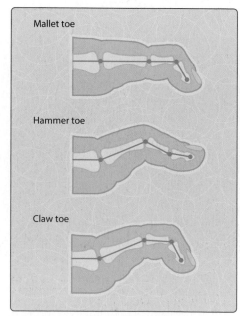

Mallet toe

Hammer toe

Claw toe

Fig. 3.62.2 Lesser toe deformities.

Pes cavus

In pes cavus there is a high-arched foot, and a claw toe may be present. The majority of cases are caused by a neuromuscular condition, although there is occasionally a congenital bony abnormality. Examples of spastic neurological conditions are cerebral palsy, muscular dystrophy, Charcot–Marie–Tooth disease, Friedreich's ataxia and spina bifida.

A full neurological examination should be performed, to include the lumbar spine to search for dimpling or hairy patches of spina bifida. MRI of the spine should be performed. If there is pain from the foot, a corrective osteotomy or soft tissue release is needed.

Achilles tendon rupture

Rupture of the Achilles tendon is a relatively common sporting injury, where the patient feels the tendon 'give' or 'snap', with sudden-onset pain. There is a palpable gap in the tendon, and when the calf is squeezed, the foot does not move (Simmond's test; Fig. 3.62.3). **Management** is controversial. Conservative treatment is with a plaster case, and surgery involves rejoining the ends of the tendon (although this can prove difficult); both have associated problems.

Flat foot

In adults, flat foot may be associated with osteoarthritis, where it is painful, or with general ligamentous laxity. Treatment is with comfortable shoes; rarely surgical correction is needed. In children, flat foot is flexible or rigid:

- flexible flat foot occurs when the child stands on tip-toes and the foot returns to normal; this is caused by ligamentous laxity and generally requires no treatment (general ligamentous laxity may be present)
- rigid flat foot occurs when the foot remains flat when the child stands on tip-toe and is caused by joint abnormalities and muscle spasticity; treatment depends on the pathology but occasionally corrective subtalar fusion is required.

Plantar fascitis

Plantar fascitis is a common condition caused by a strain of the attachment of the plantar fascia to the calcaneum. Pain occurs when the heal strikes the ground when walking; examination reveals a tender point on the heel. A firm pad in the shoe relieves symptoms, and a steroid injection may be advised.

Gout

Gout most often presents initially with a hot, red and swollen first metatarsophalangeal joint. Circulating uric acid is high and urate crystals are deposited in the joint. It may be precipitated by red meat, alcohol and thiazide diuretics. Septic arthritis is an important differential to exclude, especially if the larger joints are affected. Colchicine or NSAIDs are used in the acute phase, with allopurinol for long-term prevention.

Congenital talipes equinovarus (club foot)

Congenital talipes equinovarus is a congenital deformity (Fig. 3.62.4). It is apparent at birth; ultrasound will confirm the diagnosis. It is bilateral in 50%, and more common in males. The spine and other limbs should be examined for other abnormalities. In the first 6 weeks of life, the deformity is gradually corrected with gentle, regular stretches or manipulations, with strapping of the foot. If this fails, surgery may be needed to lengthen ligaments, release soft tissues or fuse bones (wait until the infant is 6 months of age).

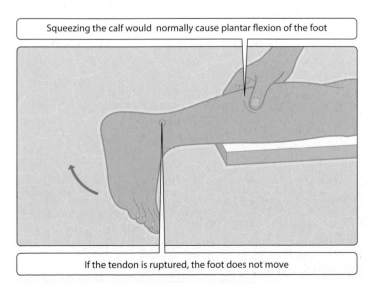

Squeezing the calf would normally cause plantar flexion of the foot

If the tendon is ruptured, the foot does not move

Fig. 3.62.3 The squeeze test (Simmond's test).

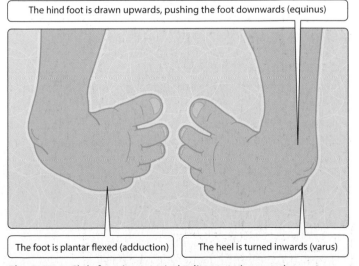

The hind foot is drawn upwards, pushing the foot downwards (equinus)

The foot is plantar flexed (adduction)

The heel is turned inwards (varus)

Fig. 3.62.4 Club foot (congenital talipes equinovarus).

63. Miscellaneous orthopaedic examinations

There are specific things to assess for each joint and it is vital *always* to examine the neurovascular status and the joints above and below.

Shoulder

Look: the shoulder should be viewed for deformity (e.g. fractured clavicle), shoulder and neck positioning, spine alignment, deltoid wasting (axillary nerve damage) and winging of the scapula (serratus anterior wasting).

Feel: the shoulder should be palpated for **winging** of the scapulae and for the rotator cuff defects and pain.

Move: the range of movement of the shoulder is assessed with the occurrence of pain (Fig. 3.63.1 and Ch. 55). The scapula should not move until the arm has abducted 90°.

Special tests: for specific defects.

Apprehension test for unstable shoulder. Both shoulder and elbow are put to 90° and externally rotated; at the end of the range of movement, the patient will become apprehensive as their shoulder will soon dislocate (stop pushing at this point), compare with the other side.

Sulcus sign for recurrent shoulder dislocations. Pulling the patient's arm gently downwards while they are sitting will reveal a sulcus.

Popeye's sign for ruptured tendon of long head of biceps. Flexing the arm against resistance will elicit an abnormal prominence of the belly of biceps; this may cause pain around the shoulder near the scapular origin of the biceps.

Elbow examination

Look: rheumatoid nodules, carrying angle: 10–15° in males, and > 15° in females.

Feel: assess pain at the lateral humeral epicondyle (tennis elbow), and the medial humeral epicondyle (golfer's elbow).

Move:

- extension and flexion: 0–150°; when the elbow is fully extended, check for hyperextension
- suppination and pronation: should be 90°

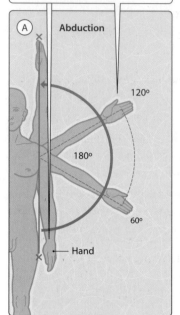

Failure of active abduction while passive abduction is normal indicates rotational cuff tear

Painful arc syndrome indicated by pain at 60–120°

A Abduction
120°
180°
60°
Hand

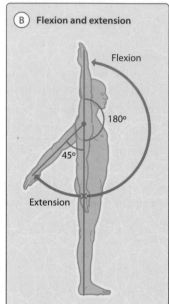

B Flexion and extension
Flexion
180°
45°
Extension

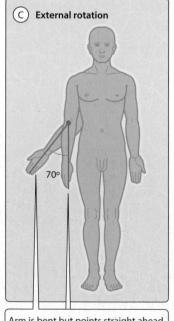

C External rotation
70°

Arm is bent but points straight ahead

Normal movement (70°) may be lost in frozen shoulder

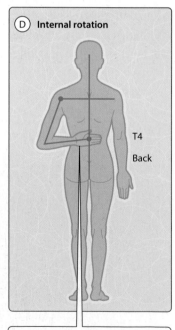

D Internal rotation
T4
Back

The hand is moved to the small of the back and then up the back as far as possible (normal is to T4)

Fig. 3.63.1 Shoulder movements.

- tennis elbow: pain on resisted *pronation* of the wrist (Mills' test)
- golfer's elbow: pain on resisted *suppination* of the wrist.

Special tests: Tinel's test over the ulnar nerve: tap over the medial epicondyle to elicit pins and needles or numbness in the ulnar fingers (medial 1.5 digits); if positive, examine for ulnar nerve irritation (Ch. 57).

Ankle and foot examination

Look: with the patient standing, and then either sitting or lying; the patient should remove trousers and socks:

- obvious deformity: hallux valgus, club foot, hammer toe, claw toe
- flat feet in children: the arch returns if the patient stands on tip-toes in a flexible (muscular) flat foot but remains flat if it is a rigid flat foot
- pes cavus: is a high arched foot.
- gait: for abnormalities
- shoes: for signs of uneven wear

Feel: for warmth, pulses and sensation and to see if pain is elicited in joints, bones of the feet, ligamentous insertions.
Move: active movements: assess the ankle, hindfoot and toes. Passive movements: grasping the heel to move

- ankle: dorsiflexion and plantar flexion
- subtalar joint: inversion and eversion
- mid-foot: adduction, abduction
- metatarsophalangeal joints: flex and extend each toe.

Special tests: Simmond's test assesses an Achilles tendon rupture (Fig. 3.62.3).

Back examination

The patient is examined in their underwear and standing up. In lower back pathology, pain refers to the buttock and posterior thigh; in hip pathology pain refers to the groin.

Look: assess gait, posture (kyphosis, scoliosis or lumbar lordosis), knee and hip (problems in these joints may cause back pain) and lower limbs (compare for muscle wasting).
Feel: palpate down each vertebra; pain may indicate ligamental injury or acute disc prolapse and steps may indicate cervical spondylolithesis.
Move: (Fig. 3.63.2).
Special tests:

Straight leg raise to identify sciatica: see Fig. 3.74.1.

Schober's test to measure flexion. A vertical line is drawn on the patient's back at the level of the posterior iliac spine (i.e. approximately at L5) extending 10 cm above L5 to 5 cm below it. When the patient bends forward (with their knees straight), the lumbar spine should extend and lengthen and the line should extend by at least 5 cm. If not, there is a limitation of flexion of the lumbar spine.

Concluding a back examination: neurological status (tone, power, sensation) and pulses of the upper and lower limbs should be examined.

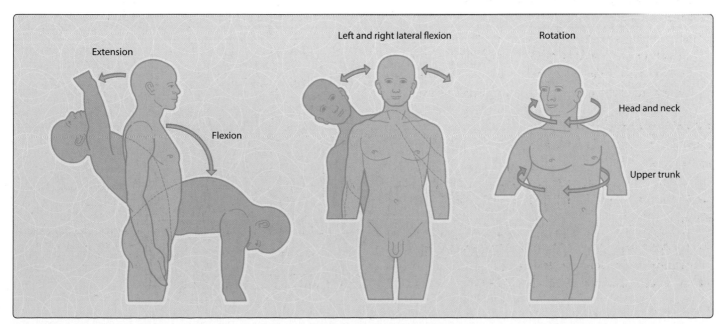

Fig. 3.63.2 Movements of the spine (repeat for the cervical spine).

64. Paediatric hip conditions

Questions
- What is the most likely diagnosis of acute onset hip pain in a 7-year-old boy, without a history of trauma?
- What are the risk factors for developmental dysplasia of the hip?
- What is slipped upper femoral epiphysis?

The 'limping child' is a common problem presenting to general practice and A&E, and the age of a child is key to forming a differential diagnosis. In the absence of trauma, transient synovitis is the next most common cause of a limp. Table 3.64.1 compares the specific features of the different paediatric hip conditions. *Transient synovitis* (the irritable hip) may be triggered by a recent viral infection and septic arthritis and any underlying pathology should be excluded.

Developmental dysplasia of the hip

DDH is a spectrum of disease where the femoral head is dislocated, subluxed (partially dislocated) or located normally but with mild acetabular changes (dysplasia) (Fig. 3.64.1). The underlying pathology is a shallow acetabulum. Risk factors for DDH are first born, female, positive family history (30 times increased risk), breech birth, other congenital abnormalities (particularly foot) and left hip involvement.

Clinical features

Neonates are screened soon after birth, when an asymetrical groin creases may be visible.

- Barlow's test: flex, adduct and depress the hip to detect a dislocatable hip
- Orlanti's test: flex and abduct the hip reduces a dislocated hip with a 'clunk'.

A toddler may present with delayed walking, painful or painless limp or unilateral toe walking. Occasionally a young adult will present with an extremely painful limp (caused by premature osteoarthritis) or painless Trendelenburg gait.

Management

In the neonate, a **Pavlik harness** or **von Rosen splint** holds the hip in place where it fixes in reduction, and there are no long-

Table 3.64.1 DIFFERENTIATING SPECIFIC HIP CONDITIONS

	Developmental dysplasia of the hip	Septic arthritis	Transient synovitis	Perthes' disease	Slipped upper femoral epiphysis
Typical age at presentation (years)	Neonates (screening); toddlers/adults if missed	< 2	3–10	4–8 (> 8 has a poor prognosis)	Boys 14–16; girls 11–13
Sex	Female	Equal	Male	Male (typically social class 4 or 5)	Male (obese)
Bilateral (%)	20	Uncommon	5	< 10	25
Presentation	Screening at birth; delayed walking/limp if missed	Painful hip; infants with decreased movement or systemic signs (fever, rigors, tachycardia)	Acute painful limp, effusion, limited hip movement	Limp (painful or painless); hip or knee pain	Acute with painful limp; chronic with gradual onset limp
Summary of pathology	Shallow acetabulum	Infection	No underlying abnormality	Osteochondritis of the femoral head	Slipping of the epiphyseal plate between the femoral head and neck
Key investigation	Ultrasound in neonate (radiograph in children/adults)	Aspiration	Radiograph	Frog leg lateral radiograph	Frog leg lateral radiograph
Investigation shows	Abnormal hip anatomy, femoral head dislocation	Culture and sensitivity	No abnormal pathology	Early presentation shows widened joint space; late shows flattened femoral head or collapse	Widened femoral growth plates
Treatment	Control hip	Aspiration, washout and antibiotics	Observe, NSAIDs	Observe, NSAIDs	Surgery

term consequences. If diagnosis is late, the older the child, the more likely the need for surgical open reduction. A missed DDH by this stage is a disaster:

- 6 months: a Pavlik harness can be tried; closed reduction and a plaster cast may be needed; occasionally open reduction is necessary
- over walking age: open reduction, soft tissue releases and osteotomies increase cover of the femoral head (maintaining reduction) and reduce pain
- adult: a pseudo-acetabulum has formed where the femoral head has impacted higher up in the pelvis; relocating the femoral head may be possible.

Perthes' disease

Legg–Calvé–Perthes disease is an osteochondritis of the femoral head (Fig. 3.64.2); it typically presents in boys between 4 and 8 years of age. The exact cause is unknown, but it is an **osteochondritis** where recurrent infarctions interrupt the femoral head blood supply. It is self-limiting and will stop after 3–4 years, although severe deformity of the femoral head often results in premature osteoarthritis.

Management aims to contain the femoral head, although many patients do not require surgical intervention and bed-rest with NSAIDs at times of pain is adequate. In severe cases, an osteotomy relocates and secures the femoral head, allowing a longer pain-free period.

Slipped upper femoral epiphysis

SUFE occurs when the epiphysis between the femoral head and neck slips as the bone grows (Fig. 3.64.3). It typically presents between 12 and 14 years in hypogonadal obese boys (although it does occur in the tall and thin). It is more common in Afro-Caribbeans, and there may be associated renal osteodystrophy, hypogonadism and hypothryroidism. SUFE must be considered in any child presenting with knee pain.

Pathology

The epiphyseal growth plate between the femoral head and neck fails to grow properly (**dehiscence**), and the epiphysis slips away as the bones grow. The head remains in the acetabulum, but the neck of the femur rotates and displaces, eventually avascular necrosis with early-onset arthritis may develop (unusual).

Clinical features

Presentation may be acute or chronic. Pain may be present in the groin, hip or knee. The child holds the affected limb in external rotation, which is also shortened. Internal rotation is restricted, and when flexing the hip it moves into gross external rotation.

Management

Urgent surgical stabilization is needed to fix the growth plate in place and prevent further slips. If the slips are minor, the growth plate is fixed in situ with screws. In chronic severe presentations, a femoral osteotomy may be needed.

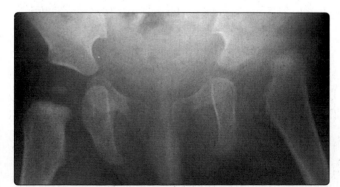

Fig. 3.64.1 The ossification centre of the femoral head does not appear until 5 months. On the left side, the ossification centre is not present and would not lie within the acetabulum, the acetabular angle is large and Shenton's line is broken.

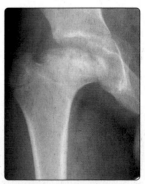

Fig. 3.64.2 Perthes' disease. The femoral head is flattened, enlarged, subluxed and uneven in density.

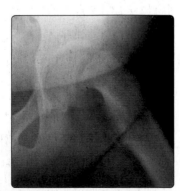

Fig. 3.64.3 The epiphysis between the femoral head and shaft has 'slipped' out of place in slipped upper femoral epiphysis.

65. Metabolic bone disorders

Questions
- What is the definition of osteoporosis?
- What is the abnormality in Paget's disease?
- What must you consider in a 20-year-old man who presents with lower back pain?

The metabolic bone disorders alter bone metabolism itself (Table 3.65.1).

Osteoporosis

Osteoporosis is a systemic skeletal disease with an increased risk of low-intensity fractures:

- osteoporosis: bone mineral density more than 2.5 standard deviations below the mean
- osteopenia: bone mineral density 1–2.5 standard deviations below the mean.

Osteoporosis is more common in women: 80% of those affected are women and 25% of women over 50 years have osteoporosis.

Aetiology

Primary osteoporosis is most common and occurs in postmenopausal women or the elderly. Risk factors include females, age, family history, sedentary lifestyle, smoking and excess alcohol intake. Secondary osteoporosis can occur (e.g. in malnutrition, cancer, hyperparathyroidism, rheumatoid arthritis, steroid use).

Clinical features

The most common first presentation is with fractures following low-energy impact. Vertebral fractures present with back pain (which may be mild), although only one-third of vertebral fractures actually present. Some patients are identified incidentally while investigating other problems.

Investigations

Bone density scan is the diagnostic test (dual radiograph absorptiometry (DEXA)). Spinal radiographs are performed for all suspected cases.

Management

Conservative treatment is with exercise, high-calcium diet and risk factor modification. Medical approaches include hormone replacement therapy for perimenopausal women (controversial), calcium and vitamin D supplements, calcitonin and bisphosphonates.

Osteomalacia (rickets)

Osteomalacia is a failure of bone mineralization; it is called rickets when it occurs in children. The most common causes are renal disease and dietary insufficiency of vitamin D, although they themselves may be caused by genetic disease or malabsorption syndromes (e.g. partial gastrectomy, caeliac disease).

Clinical features

In **adults** there is bone pain and tenderness plus the characteristic pseudofractures through Loosers' zone (areas of sclerosis on the concave surfaces of bones, typically the pelvis and femur).

In **children**, presentation is with failure to thrive, developmental delay and characteristic skeletal changes:

- skull: flat occiput, frontal bossing, dental caries
- thorax: rachitic rosary (prominence of the costal cartillages), pectus carinatum, Harrison's sulcus (the diaphragm detaches from the soft ribs)
- limbs: bowing, fractures, joint deformity.

Investigations

Plain radiographs identify 'fraying, splaying and cupping' of the metaphysis of the wrist or knee. Other skeletal changes and Loosers' zone are identifiable.

Table 3.65.1 METABOLIC BONE DISORDERS

	Disease principle	Calcium	Phosphate	Alkaline phosphatase	Parathyroid hormone
Osteoporosis	Low bone density (mineralization normal)	Normal	Normal	Normal	Normal
Osteomalacia	Lack of mineralization (normal density)	Low or normal	Low	High	High
Paget's disease	Two-stage: bone resorption and remodelling	Normal	Normal	Very high (a marker of activity)	Normal

Management

Treatment is with vitamin D and calcium supplements, and treatment of malabsorption syndromes. Surgery may be needed for fractures, slipped upper femoral epiphysis and deformities.

Paget's disease

In Paget's disease coordination between osteoclasts (resorption) and osteoblasts (remodelling) is lost, and osteoblasts lay down weak and disorganized woven bone. Paget's disease typically affects the axial skeleton—skull, spine, pelvis, femur and tibia—although any bone may be affected.

Clinical features

Presentation is either incidental (radiograph for another reason) in asymptomatic patients or with bone pain. Bowing of the tibia is characteristic. There may be nerve compression/entrapments (cranial nerves causing hearing loss, dizziness; spinal roots causing paraplegia; back pain; peripheral nerve entrapments), pathological fractures and premature osteoarthritis.

Investigations

Plain radiograph shows thickened cortex, osteosclerotic bone, pseudofractures and bowing of the long bones (femur and tibia). ALP is very high and is the most widely used marker. A bone isotope scan shows increased uptake at sites of involvement; a useful screening test.

Management

Medical treatment is with calcitonin and bisphosphonates to reduce bone resorption.

Surgical treatment includes arthroplasty for premature osteoarthritis, osteotomy for deformity, fixation of fractures, nerve entrapment release and treatment of malignancy (< 0.5% develop osteosarcoma).

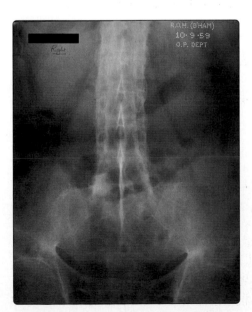

Fig. 3.65.1 Characteristic 'bamboo spine' showing fusion of the vertebrae in ankylosing spondylitis.

Ankylosing spondylitis

Ankylosing spondylitis is an uncommon inflammatory condition primarily affecting young males between the ages of 15 and 30 years.

Clinical features

Lower back stiffness, deformity and pain in a young man are the key presenting features. The spinal column may become fused, causing kyphosis (bending over) and spondylosis (curved spine). Chest fusion leads to limited chest expansion and recurrent chest infections and may lead to respiratory failure. There may be coexisting sacroiliitis and the patient may have associated inflammatory bowel disease, usually ulcerative colitis, and uveitis (97% carry HLA-B27).

Investigations

Plain radiographs show a bamboo spine and the above bone defects (Fig. 3.65.1). The ESR is raised.

Management

Exercise makes it better but may not be tolerated because of the pain (rest makes it worse). NSAIDs are taken for pain.

The long-term aim is to fuse the patient in a functional position: fusing the spine in an upright position (preventing a severe kyphosis). Osteotomy of the spine may be used to correct severe defects, and arthroplasty for premature hip osteoarthritis. Early death is often caused by chest infection as a result of the thoracic deformity.

■ AVASCULAR NECROSIS

Avascular necrosis is the death of bone following a reduction in oxygen delivery. It may affect the femoral head, proximal humerus, scaphoid, talus and lunate. It typically presents with progressively severe pain from non-union, bone collapse or premature osteoarthritis. Common causes include trauma (neck of femur fractures, scaphoid fractures), idiopathic, alcohol, steroids and sickle cell disease. Rare causes are caisson disease (*the bends*, from deep sea diving) and radiation therapy.

MRI is the most sensitive and specific test for the hip, allowing bilateral involvement to be identified (in 50%). Early treatment is with core decompression or osteotomy. Late collapse and degeneration in the hip may require total hip replacement.

66. Bone and joint infections

Questions
- What is the differential diagnosis of a hot swollen joint?
- What are the treatment principles of septic arthritis?
- What are the treatment principles of osteomyelitis?

Joint infections (**septic arthritis**) and bone infections (**osteomyelitis**) have devastating consequences if missed or inadequately treated. Both are more common with extremes of age (<3 years and the elderly), diabetes mellitus, arthritis, immunosuppression, alcoholism, in those with prosthetic replacements and following open fractures. Gangrene (p. 8) can occur in surrounding tissues.

Pathogens reach the joints and bones by varied routes (Fig. 3.66.1). *Staphylococcus aureus* accounts for up to 90%; other causative organisms are more likely in certain age groups:

- *Haemophilus influenzae*: incidence has rapidly declined through vaccination in children
- *Neisseria gonorrhoeae*: the most common cause of septic arthritis in adults under 30 years; this is a sexually transmitted organism
- *Pseudomonas aeruginosa*: implicated with intravenous drug abusers
- *Salmonella* spp.: a common cause of osteomyelitis in patients with sickle cell anaemia
- *Staphylococcus epidermidis*: the most common organism in infected total joint replacement (Ch. 58).

Clinical features
Presentation is with:

- a hot, swollen painful joint: septic arthritis is the presumed diagnosis until proved otherwise
- loss of function: limp or decreased movement of the limb (infants)
- systemic upset: malaise, pyrexia, weight loss, failure to thrive, tachycardia with or without locomotor symptoms (systemic features occur especially in children)
- pyrexia of unknown origin: especially in patients with a prosthetic joint
- localized bone pain: the local joint may have a mild effusion (pain may be chronic): likely osteomyelitis.

Septic arthritis
The hip and knee joints are most commonly affected (Fig. 3.66.2; the hip in infants).

Investigations. The following investigations are needed:
- ESR, CRP and white cell count
- blood culture: *before* antibiotics
- aspiration of the joint until dry: for both diagnostic and therapeutic purposes
- plain radiograph: often is normal in early infection
- ultrasound for detection of a suspected hip effusion in a child, which guides aspiration.

Management. Urgent aspiration is required until the joint space is dry; this is repeated daily until the joint remains dry. If symptoms persist, arthroscopic lavage is indicated. Intravenous antibiotics are initiated; initially 'best guess' is for *S. aureus* with flucloxacillin (with fusidic acid) for 4–6 weeks. Culture results may require a change in antibiotic. Splints immobilize the joint early on and thereafter physiotherapy maintains joint function. Infection of a joint replacement is best treated with a two-stage revision (Ch. 58).

Complications. If the diagnosis is not prompt or treatment is inadequate, septic arthritis can lead to osteomyelitis, joint stiffness, loss of function, contactures, growth abnormalities in children and premature (secondary) osteoarthritis.

Osteomyelitis
Osteomyelitis (Fig. 3.66.2) is either acute or chronic. **Acute osteoarthritis** presents with acute bone pain, adjacent joint effusion, systemic symptoms, as a complication of an open fracture. **Chronic osteoarthritis** presents as a chronic sepsis after penetrating trauma, open fracture, internal fixation or elective orthopaedic surgery; as non-resolution of acute osteoarthritis; or as chronic sepsis with sinus formation.

Investigations. Acute osteoarthritis is investigated by:
- ESR, CRP and white cell count
- blood culture, *before* antibiotics (positive in 50–75%)
- aspiration is only required if an abscess or effusion is present.

Plain radiograph is not useful in acute or early disease as it is often initially normal. In late osteomyelitis, a **sequestrum** (dead bone surrounded by granulation tissue) and an **involucrum** (new bone formed around old bone or sequestrium) may become visible. Bone scans and MRI are required if tumour is a differential diagnosis.

Management of acute osteomyelitis:
- antibiotics: 2 weeks of intravenous antibiotics (initially flucloxacillin against *S. aureus*), followed by oral antibiotics for a minimum of 6 weeks

■ surgery: required to drain abscesses, debride the infected site (removing any sequestrum) or if antibiotics fail.

Management of chronic osteomyelitis. When infection of the bone is long standing, there may be periods of normality (sometimes years) followed by repeated exacerbations. Treatment is difficult:

■ antibiotics are continued for at least 12 weeks (intravenous followed by oral) but will not be enough alone

■ surgical debridement: a significant cavity may be left (may be treated with Ilizarov bone-lengthening techniques); amputation is occasionally necessary.

Subacute osteomyelitis. A low-grade infection disappears and recurs, possibly without swelling. A **Brodie's abscess** may be visible on plain radiograph (a sharply delineated radiolucent area that contains pus within a well-established lesion). Treatment is with intravenous antibiotics and surgical debridement of the pus and dead bone.

Tuberculosis of bone

The incidence of tuberculosis of the bone is increasing in the UK as a result of HIV infection and international travel. It primarily affects the vertebrae (**Pott's syndrome**), and only one-third have evidence of pulmonary tuberculosis (chest radiograph is mandatory). Tuberculous arthritis may affect other joints particularly where tuberculosis is endemic. Treatment is with standard antimycobacterial drugs usually in a multidrug regimen to counteract resistance.

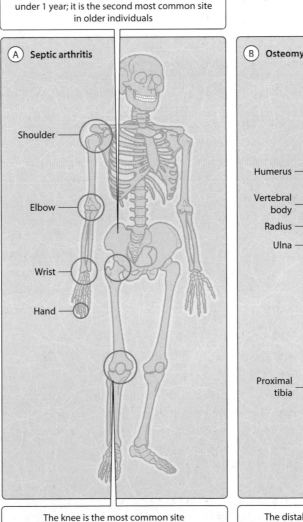

The hip is the most common site in infants under 1 year; it is the second most common site in older individuals

(A) Septic arthritis

Shoulder
Elbow
Wrist
Hand

The knee is the most common site

(B) Osteomyelitis

Humerus
Vertebral body
Radius
Ulna

Proximal tibia

The distal femur is the most common site

Fig. 3.66.2 Common sites of infection (given in descending frequency of occurrence). (A) Septic arthritis: knee, hip, shoulder, elbow, wrist, hand. (B) Osteomyelits: distal femur, proximal tibia, humerus, radius, ulna, vertebral bodies. The most common site is at the metaphysis of long bones, with infections of the lower limbs being more common than of the upper limbs.

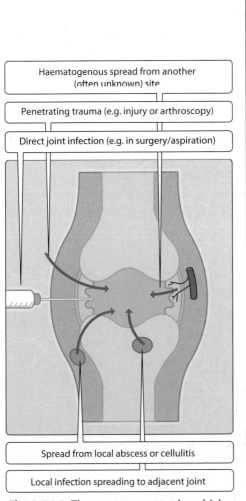

Haematogenous spread from another (often unknown) site

Penetrating trauma (e.g. injury or arthroscopy)

Direct joint infection (e.g. in surgery/aspiration)

Spread from local abscess or cellulitis

Local infection spreading to adjacent joint

Fig. 3.66.1 The common routes by which pathogens reach the joints and bones.

67. Bone tumours

Questions
- How do bone tumours present?
- What is the most common type of bone tumour?
- What are the common tumours which metastasize to bone?

Primary bone tumours are either benign or malignant, primary or secondary. Primary tumours are extremely rare; the most common type is **osteosarcoma**. Secondary **metastatic bone tumours** are much more common. Both primary and secondary bone tumours may present with:

- pain: the most common presentation; it is typically *non-mechanical* and not related to activity (as opposed to arthritis, which is *mechanical*)
- swelling
- loss of function
- pathological fracture: a fracture through a weakened or diseased area of bone.

The **differential diagnosis** of a bone lesion identified by radiography is:

- metastatic bone tumour
- primary bone tumour: osteosarcoma, chondrosarcoma, Ewing's sarcoma
- myeloma
- lymphoma
- infection
- developmental abnormality, e.g. fibrous dysplasia.

▪ MALIGNANT PRIMARY TUMOURS

Osteosarcoma
Osteosarcoma mainly affects adolescents, with a peak at the age of 16 years, and presents as above. The most common site of osteosarcoma is the distal femur (Fig. 3.67.1); other sites include the proximal and distal tibia, proximal humerus and pelvis (very rare). It is typically found in the metaphysis. Tumours of the pelvis are rare and have poor prognosis. Osteosarcoma is associated with:

- retinoblastoma: pRB mutation
- Li Fraumeni syndrome: p53 mutation, causing breast cancers, osteosarcomas, neurofibromatomas and leukaemias (which affect multiple members of the same family)
- radiotherapy
- Paget's disease (< 1%).

Investigations:
- myeloma screen: for paraproteins
- alkaline phosphatase (a marker of bone activity): the higher the value, the worse the prognosis
- plain radiograph
- chest radiograph: to identify lung metastases; typical spread is haematogenous
- bone isotope scan: shows increased uptake at the site of the tumour, further lesions or bone metastases
- biopsy: confirms the diagnosis; normal tissue should not be contaminated (refer to a specialist centre before biopsy).

Management

Chemotherapy. Neo-adjuvant (before surgery) chemotherapy aims to eliminate micrometastases and to shrink the tumour size before resection. it can also be given adjuvantly (after surgery) to prevent local recurrence.

Surgery. The tumour is removed with wide margins and a custom-built massive **endoprosthesis** is fitted with soft tissue reconstructions so as to preserve cosmetic and functional status of the limb; this is limb salvage. However, if a wide margin of excision is not achievable, amputation is indicated.

Prognosis

With chemotherapy and new biomechanical devices, 5-year survival for osteosacoma may be as high as 65%.

Other malignant primary tumours

Chondrosarcoma, This is the second most common type of primary tumour; it arises from cartilage cells and is treated in a similar way to osteosarcoma.

Ewing's sarcoma. This tumours arises within the diaphysis of long bones (arm, thigh, pelvis and ribs) and usually affects children. The exact cells of origin are unknown. The tumour is radiosensitive and 5-year survival is 60%.

Multiple myeloma. This malignant proliferation of plasma B cells in the bone marrow leads to Bence-Jones proteinuria, abnormal electrophoretic pattern of blood proteins, and multifocal radiographic changes. Pathological fractures are common. Treatment is with chemotherapy and radio-therapy plus fixation of any fractures.

Non-Hodgkin's lymphoma. This can present as a solitary area of bone involvement; it responds well to chemotherapy and radiotherapy.

Giant cell tumours. These benign tumours are treated as a malignancy because of their rapid rate of growth.

■ METASTATIC BONE DISEASE

Metastatic bones tumours are much more common than primary tumours and tend to affect older patients (Fig. 3.67.2). They present with similar features to primary bone tumours, although hypercalcaemia is more of a problem. The common sites of bony metastases (in decreasing order of frequency) are spine, proximal long bones, pelvis, ribs.

Tumours of breast, prostate, lung, kidney and thyroid commonly metastasize; spread to bone is haematogenous. The other common sites for metastatic deposits are brain, breast, liver and lung.

Investigations

Investigations are as for primary tumours but would also include:

- identification of the primary tumour
- serum calcium: rapidly growing metastatic lesions may displace large amounts of calcium from the bone, resulting in hypercalcaemia; this may require emergency treatment with high levels of intravenous fluids and bisphosphonates
- biopsy: to confirm diagnosis if in doubt
- assessment of other metastatic spread, and to find other asymptomatic skeletal metastases: chest radiograph, lung CT and bone isotope scan (Fig. 3.67.3).

Management

The aims of surgery are palliative, to relieve pain and restore function:

- stabilization or reconstruction of pathological fractures: initially use analgesia and splintage, while the cause is identified; metastatic deposits are best managed with internal fixation, using intramedullary nails, plates or pins (followed by radiotherapy)
- radiotherapy: a single palliative fraction may be effective in reducing pain
- bisphosphonates: to treat hypercalcemia and prevent pathological fractures
- prophylactic fixation: of an impending fracture site
- spinal cord compression (Ch. 74).

Prognosis

Some patients survive 3 or more years. Prognosis is related to the natural history and response to treatment for the primary tumour, and whether there are liver or lung metastases.

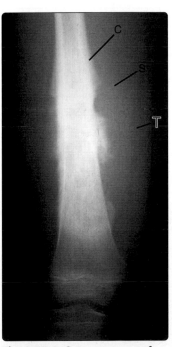

Fig. 3.67.1 Osteosarcoma of the distal femur. There is new bone formation, sunray spickles (S), periosteal elevation, Codman's triangle (C) and soft tissue swelling (T).

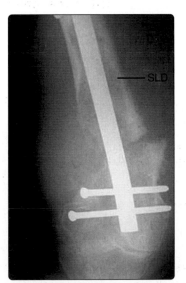

Fig. 3.67.2 A pathological fracture of the distal femur in an elderly patient caused by metastatic bone disease (secondary lytic deposit, SLD).

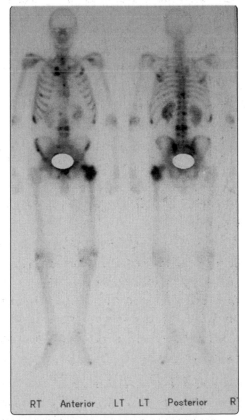

Fig. 3.67.3 Bone isotope scan in an 80-year-old man presenting with lower back pain only. Deposits could be seen in the left hip and throughout the spine, ribs, pelvis and the left scapula.

68. Burns and skin loss

Questions
- How are burns classified?
- What is the initial management of a burn?
- How can you replace major losses of skin and tissue?

Burns are defined as a coagulative destruction of the skin. They are caused by four main mechanisms:

- thermal: flame or friction (dry) or scalds (wet)
- chemical: alkalis burn for hours; acids are short lived
- electrical: causing a deep burn that heals slowly; a small skin defect may mask a large underlying trauma
- radiation: ionizing radiation (uncommon).

Estimation of body surface area
The 'rule of nines' (Fig. 3.68.1) allows an estimation of the body surface area that is affected and decides management. Mortality increases with increasing percentage body surface area affected: a major burn is > 15% body surface area in an adult (> 10% in children); the patient should be admitted to hospital. Minor burns of < 2% can be dealt with in casualty.

Classification of burns
Burns are classified by their depth (Fig. 3.68.2).

Superficial partial thickness. The burns are very painful, red and blistered and they blanch easily to light touch. Burns may progress to become full thickness and should be reexamined at 48 h. The basal layer where growth of skin takes place is intact and so regrowth occurs.

Deep partial thickness. The dermis is lost, but hair follicles and sweat glands remain and regrowth still occurs. Burns are painful to pinprick but blanch less easily. There is a high risk of hypoperfusion and infection.

Full thickness. All skin layers are totally destroyed, and underlying structures may be damaged. The lesions are painless since all free nerve endings are destroyed, and the area is discoloured (white/grey) but not blistered. There is a very high risk of infection. Regrowth will not occur.

Management

Initial resuscitation
It is vital to maintain the airway. Burns to the face and mouth, stridor and hoarseness indicate smoke inhalation. Inflammation follows the burn and laryngeal oedema may occlude the airway quickly; consequently, early intubation is preferred to emergency tracheotomy. This type of inhalation injury can be difficult to diagnose but can be rapidly fatal. Humidified high-

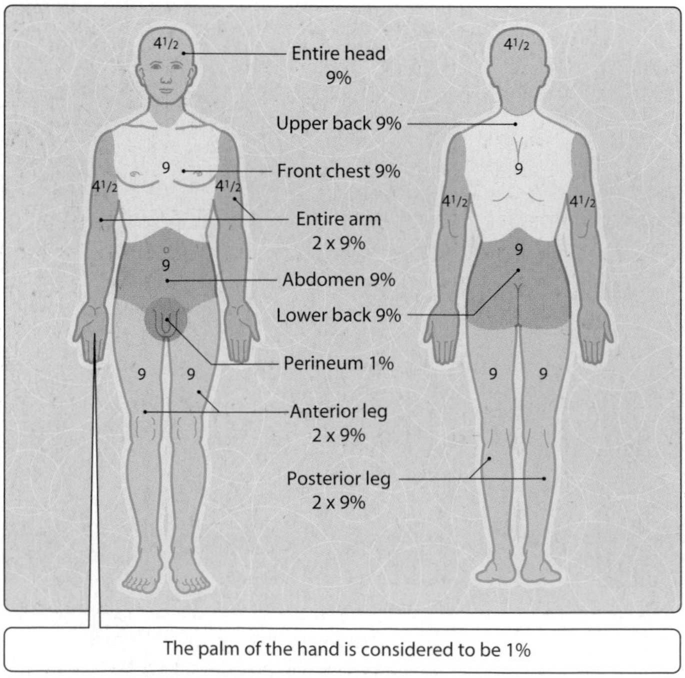

Entire head 9%

Upper back 9%

Front chest 9%

Entire arm 2 x 9%

Abdomen 9%

Lower back 9%

Perineum 1%

Anterior leg 2 x 9%

Posterior leg 2 x 9%

The palm of the hand is considered to be 1%

Fig. 3.68.1 The 'rule of nines' to assess body surface area.

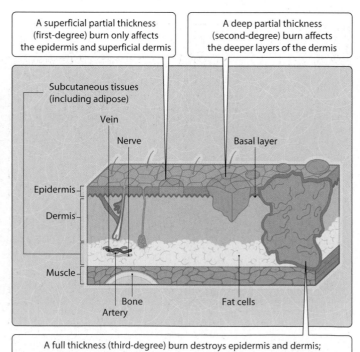

A superficial partial thickness (first-degree) burn only affects the epidermis and superficial dermis

A deep partial thickness (second-degree) burn affects the deeper layers of the dermis

Subcutaneous tissues (including adipose)

Vein

Nerve

Basal layer

Epidermis

Dermis

Muscle

Bone

Artery

Fat cells

A full thickness (third-degree) burn destroys epidermis and dermis; it is painless and underlying structures and organs may be damaged

Fig. 3.68.2 The depth of burns.

flow oxygen should be given, and arterial blood gases and chest radiograph are indicated.

It is vital to secure early intravenous access rapidly and maintain circulation. Circulatory collapse is expected with burns affecting ≥ 30% body surface area, and fluid management is a high priority.

Initial burn management

Prevention of infection. Routine antibiotics are not given unless there are signs of sepsis or for those at high risk (e.g. prosthetic heart valves). Clingfilm is used to cover serious burns to prevent infection and allow for future inspection.

Fluid replacement. Fluid resuscitation is indicated when burns are > 15% body surface area in adults (10% in children). The **Parkland formula** is used to calculate the *additional* fluid replacement beyond normal requirements from the time of injury (not admission), usually with Hartmann's solution. The volume of fluid/h for the first 8 h after the burn is given by:

$$0.25 \text{ ml} \times \% \text{ body surface area affected} \times \text{weight (kg)}.$$

Subsequent burn management

Superficial partial thickness burns. These heal in 7 to 10 days without scarring. Infection is prevented with a non-adherent sterile dressing. Analgesia is needed. Blisters should not be *deroofed* (burst).

Deep partial thickness burns. These take 14 to 21 days to heal and will scar. Skin regenerates from adjacent tissues and the basal layers of intact sweat glands and hair follicles.

Full thickness burns. Skin grafting is almost always required to prevent scarring and contraction deformities.

Escharotomy. This is an incision made through a burn that is threatening to occlude the circulation to a distal limb (e.g. a circumferential burn) or the expansion of the chest. The procedure is best undertaken *prophylactically* before complications occur.

Complications of burns

Early complications are:

- hypovolaemic shock
- inhalation injury/carbon monoxide poisoning
- infection/septicaemia
- distal ischaemia, especially with circumferential burns
- ileus/electrolyte imbalance.

Late complications are gastrointestinal stress ulceration (**Curling's ulcer**; prevented with proton pump inhibitors), DVT and hypertrophic scars, contractures (especially across joint flexures) and Marjolin's ulcer (Ch. 69).

Skin loss

Skin losses need to be covered or replaced to reduce pain, infection, scars and contracture formation. Therapy is guided by a reconstructive ladder (Fig. 3.68.3). Open wound management is needed if there is underlying swelling, infection, necrosis or tissue loss. Significant skin loss requires cover with a skin graft when the wound is not infected and is clean. Large tissue loss needs to be covered with a skin flap or a myocutaneous flap.

A **skin graft** derives its blood supply and nutrients from its recipient bed. Grafts are taken from an unburnt or healthy donor site (usually the buttocks or thigh), without its own vascular supply, and so require a well-vascularized bed at the recipient site. If a good bed is available, a full-thickness skin graft may be used. If the bed is poor, a thin split-skin graft is used.

A **skin or myocutaneous flap** is a piece of tissue taken with its own blood supply and is often formed from skin or muscle or both. They are independent of the recipient bed and can be used to cover areas of more significant skin and tissue loss.

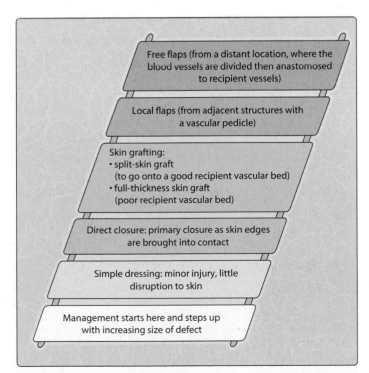

Fig. 3.68.3 Reconstructive ladder.

Free flaps (from a distant location, where the blood vessels are divided then anastomosed to recipient vessels)

Local flaps (from adjacent structures with a vascular pedicle)

Skin grafting:
- split-skin graft (to go onto a good recipient vascular bed)
- full-thickness skin graft (poor recipient vascular bed)

Direct closure: primary closure as skin edges are brought into contact

Simple dressing: minor injury, little disruption to skin

Management starts here and steps up with increasing size of defect

69. Skin cancer

Questions
■ What are the different types of skin cancer?
■ How is the prognosis of melanoma determined?
■ Who is at risk of skin cancer?

The incidence of skin cancer is increasing in the developing world and it is the third most common cancer worldwide. The most important types are melanoma and the non-melanoma skin cancers: basal cell carcinoma (BCC) and squamous cell carcinoma (SCC), also rare skin cancers such as skin lymphoma and Merkel cell carcinoma.

Basal cell carcinoma

BCC is the commonest form of skin cancer and is most common in those over 55 years. It occurs on white sun-exposed skin and is common on the face, head and neck (Figs 3.69.1 and 3.69.2). BCC grows slowly over years and rarely metastasizes.

Clinical features

The patient typically notices a crusting or bleeding papule which does not heal.

The lesions characteristically have a telangiectatic, translucent edge with a depressed, ulcerated centre and are usually nodular. They may present as persistent, destructive, ulcerated lesions without any more specific features.

Management

Treatment options include surgery (with a minimum of 4 mm margins), cryotherapy (not for head and neck) and radiotherapy (over 60 years and head and neck lesions). With appropriate selection, cure rates are over 95%.

Squamous cell carcinoma

SCC is a malignant tumour that occurs on white sun-damaged skin, particularly the head and neck but also on the arms and legs. It mostly occurs in those over 55 years and is particularly common in immunosuppressed patients. SCC arises from keratinocytes within the epidermis and it occasionally metastasizes, especially in the immunosuppressed. In situ SCC (**Bowen's disease**) may develop into invasive SCC.

Clinical features

The lesion is typically a rapidly growing (few weeks to a few months) pink/red nodule and it may be ulcerated with a central keratin plug or scab. Without prompt treatment, it may become deeply invasive with extensive tissue distruction and may metastasize.

Management

Surgery or radiotherapy provides cure rates of 95%. A surgical margin of excision of at least 6 mm is required. SCC metastasizes in 5–10% of patients.

Melanoma

Melanoma is an uncommon skin cancer; although its incidence is increasing, it only accounts for 1–2% of all cancer deaths. Approximately 50% occurs in those under 50 years of age. The **risk factors** are mole count (risk is directly proportionate to number), skin type (pale skin is at higher risk; especially those who burn easily/tan poorly: type I skin), family history (in up to

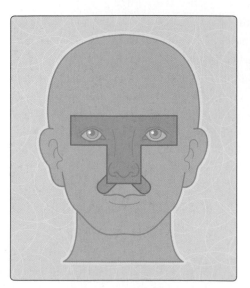

Fig. 3.69.1 Distribution of basal cell carcinomas. These typically occur on sun-exposed areas.

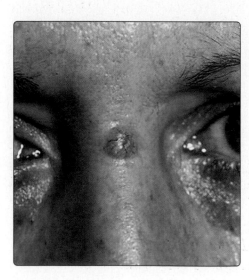

Fig. 3.69.2 A nodulo-cystic basal cell carcinoma.

5%) and sunlight exposure (unlike non-melanoma skin cancers, there is no dose–response relationship between ultraviolet exposure and incidence).

Clinical features

The history provides important clues to the diagnosis: for example a new, small mole that has rapidly appeared over a few months in someone aged, say, > 50 years, itching, bleeding and a scaly edge suggest melanoma. Changes in an existing mole or development of a new mole especially over the age of 30 may suggest a melanoma (Fig. 3.69.3).

Pathology

Melanoma arises from melanocytes; 50% arise de novo and 50% in a preexisting mole. Tumour thickness is the most important prognostic factor (Table 3.69.1) and it determines treatment.

- *Superficial spreading melanoma* (50%). This is the most common type and may grow over several months or years. It is most common on the lower limb in women and the trunk in men. It typically affects those aged 20–60 years.
- *Nodular melanoma* (25%). This presents as a raised papule/nodule, often rapidly growing.
- *Lentigo malignant melanoma* (15%). This is common on sun-damaged skin of the face of the elderly.
- *Acral lentiginous melanoma* (10%). A form that occurs on the extremities.

Metastasis occurs in 20–49%; this is usually first loco-regional (around primary site and lymph nodes) and then distant. Distant metastases may appear early in liver, lungs, brain, bowel—indeed alomost anywhere.

Management

Excisional biopsy with 2 mm margins and a cuff of subdermal fat is essential to allow histological sampling at the time of investigation. Surgery is the only cure for melanoma. Excision down to muscle fascia must include a wide lateral skin margin (Table 3.69.1) to minimize the risk of loco-regional recurrence.

Table 3.69.1 BRESLOW THICKNESS TO GUIDE MARGINS OF EXCISION AND SURVIVAL FOR MELANOMA

Thickness (mm)	Margin of excision (cm)	5-year survival (%)
< 1	1	> 90
1–2	2	70–90
> 2	3	< 70

Other types of skin tumour

Bowen's disease. This is an intraepithelial/in situ SCC and is most common on the lower limb in elderly women. The lesions are often multiple and infrequently transform into invasive SCC. An incisional biopsy confirms the diagnosis, and the lesion is treated locally with cryotherapy, 5-fluorouracil or excision.

Solar/actinic keratosis. A patch of pink, scaly rough skin on sun-exposed sites that occasionally develops into SCC; treatment is with cryotherapy or topical 5-fluorouracil.

Keratoacanthoma. This characteristically begins over a few weeks as a pink nodule with a central keratin plug (so very much like SCC). However, it regresses completely within 6–8 weeks to leave a depressed scar. It is not invasive, hence bleeding or ulceration indicates an SCC.

Marjolin's ulcer. An SCC may develop in a chronic scar (e.g. an old burn) or a chronic venous ulcer. These tumours usually present late and have a poor prognosis.

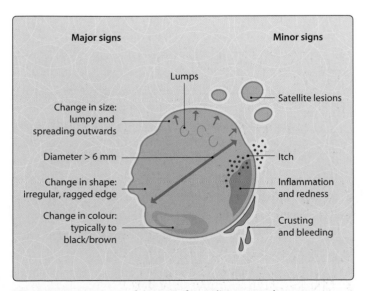

Fig. 3.69.3 Suspicious features of a malignant melanoma.

70. Lumps and bumps

Questions
- What are sebaceous cysts and lipomas?
- What is a ganglion and how can it be treated?
- What are dermoid cysts and where do they occur?

There is a wide range of 'lumps and bumps' that patients can present with and these frequently form part of an OSCE station. An examination will follow the standard steps of introduction, obtaining consent and then exposing the relevant area. The patient should be asked about any pain and is examined using the look, feel, move scheme. Lumps and bumps can be found anywhere on the body (Fig. 3.70.1). Lumps in the abdomen, groin, scrotum, breast and neck are covered in Chs 6, 33, 39 and 42, respectively.

Sebaceous cyst

A sebaceous cyst is derived from the outer sheath of the hair follicles. It is *not* a cyst of sebaceous glands and it does *not* contain sebum. It mainly contains keratin and its breakdown products, and its wall is formed from squamous epithelium. Sebaceous cysts are situated in the dermis and attached to the skin by the sebaceous duct. They are commonly found on the face, neck (especially around the posterior hairline), shoulders and chest, and also the scrotum and vulva; 50% have a punctum,

which is pathognomonic. A sebaceous cyst is firm (although often fluctuant) but not transilluminable.

Definitive treatment is with surgical excision. If it is infected, early treatment is with antibiotics, but if the infection is established, incision and drainage is indicated.

Lipoma

Lipoma is a common benign tumour of adipose cells. It occurs anywhere on the body where fat is present, but mostly on the head, neck, abdominal wall and thighs. It is mobile underneath the skin (but not attached to it), and if large may be fluctuant and transilluminable. It is extremely slow growing and very rarely undergoes malignant change. Most are well circumscribed but a few are diffuse and difficult to excise completely. If multiple and painful lipomas occur this is **Dercrum's disease**. Treatment is either conservative or surgical to excise the lump locally, for either cosmetic reasons or for lumps greater than 5 cm.

Lymph nodes

Enlarged lymph nodes (**lymphadenopathy**) are extremely common (see Ch. 41) An enlarged lymph node in the supraclavicular fossa may be a Virchow's node, indicating a gastric tumour (**Troisier's sign**).

Ganglion

A ganglion is an abnormal lump of unknown origin, commonly found within the tendon sheaths or attached to synovium on the dorsum of the wrist but are also found on the hand and ankle. They are occasionally painful and some may burst spontaneously or upon trauma (they were traditionally hit with a Bible). Otherwise treatment is dependent on patient's preference; if it is left alone, it will regress with time, or simple surgical excision can be undertaken (although recurrence is common).

Furuncle (boil)

A furuncle is an acute infection of a hair follicle, usually caused by *Staphylococcus aureus*. It most commonly occurs on the back and on the neck but may occur anywhere. It may discharge pus from its centre, and it is acutely painful. Patients are often diabetic or immunosuppressed (if presenting for the first time, the patient's urine should be tested glucose).

A **carbuncle** is deep infection with necrosis, and after a few days discharge occurs through multiple sinuses. Treatment is with prompt antibiotics (flucloxacillin), and surgery to debride and drain abscesses.

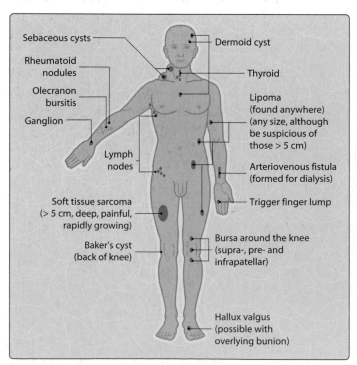

Fig. 3.70.1 Occurrence of lumps on the body.

Dermoid cysts

Dermoid cysts are lined by squamous epithelium and occur in the midline because of faults in embryonic fusion. They are found in the midline of the trunk and are also common on the head and neck (e.g. behind the ears; outer end of the eyebrow). The **sacrococcygeal dermoid** is fluctuant and occurs over the tip of the coccyx in the midline; it may be attached to the central canal, contain cerebrospinal fluid and be surrounded by a part of the lumbosacral nerve roots. Excision should never be undertaken in this region wihtout an MRI to define the anatomy.

Basal cell papilloma (aka seborrhoeic wart)

Basal cell papilloma is an extremely common benign tumour that develops as the patient ages, becoming multiple in the elderly. It is often pigmented and occurs anywhere, but mostly on the trunk and arms. It may be treated conservatively (although malignant transformation can occur) or removed with simple surgery.

Dermatofibroma

A dermatofibroma is a slow-growing benign tumour of fibroblasts in the dermis, typically occurring in young and middle-aged adults. Treatment is conservative.

Neurofibroma

Neurofibroma is a benign tumour of the nerve sheath forming a dumbell shape in the spine, with nerve root signs and occasionally spinal cord involvement. It is firm, subcutaneous and sometimes painful. Neurofibroma is mobile but still attached to the nerve sheath, and paraesthesia may occur if it is squeezed. Neurofibroma is difficult to remove without removing the nerve. Malignant change may rarely occur (**neurofibrosarcoma**), often in the pelvis.

Neurofibromatosis type I (**von Recklinghausen's disease**) is characterized by six or more **café au lait patches** (flat coffee-coloured patches) and two or more neurofibromas (which are, in fact, often multiple). These lesions are progressive, causing pain and localized paresis from nerve involvement.

Haemangioma

Haemangioma is a benign vascular tumour that can occur in several forms:

- strawberry naevi: congenital bright red lesions

- port-wine stains: a congenital flat deep-red pigmentation of the skin, often on the face; in **Sturge–Weber syndrome**, the port-wine stain occurs in the trigeminal distribution and is associated with developmental delay and epilepsy
- Campbell de Morgan spots: small bright red spots in those over 50 years.

Fibroma

Fibroma is a benign tumour of fibrous connective tissue. It can be hard or soft and may be found anywhere in the subcutaneous tissues.

Soft tissue sarcomas

Soft tissue sarcomas are malignant lumps (Ch. 71). Deep, large, rapidly growing lumps are suspicious.

Arteriovenous fistula

An arteriovenous fistula is a communication between a vein and an artery. It can be either congenital or surgically fashioned to allow for dialysis, most commonly in the forearm. It feels firm, expansive, has a pulsation and thrill; a bruit (machinery murmur) is audible upon auscultation.

Around joints

Baker's cyst.   This is a synovial pouch in the popliteal fossa that communicates with the knee joint. It is associated with knee rheumatoid arthritis, where an effusion forms into the cyst as the knee swells. These cysts often burst spontaneously, which causes self-limiting acute pain and calf swelling. No treatment is required, although anticoagulation is contraindicated in these patients. This painful rupture can be confused with a DVT, where an arthrogram is diagnostic of the ruptured cyst.

Rheumatoid nodules.   They are localized subcutaneous pockets of synovium, often found at the elbows, tendons, in the sclera of the eye and in various viscera, particularly the lung. They are rubbery in consistency.

Trigger finger.   A localized swelling of the tendon or tendon sheath at the base of the little finger causes a lump and trigger finger (Ch. 56).

Bursitis.   A large fluctuant swelling can arise around a joint as a result of repeated low-grade trauma. These swellings are painful if infected.

71. Soft tissue sarcomas and lump examination

Questions
- What are the features of a suspicious lump?
- What is a wide local excision?
- How do you examine a lump?

Patients worried about a lump usually present to their GP (Fig. 3.71.1). While less than 1% of lumps are malignant, all clinicians need to be aware of the features of a suspicious lump.

Suspicious features are:

- size > 5 cm
- rapidly increasing in size: if a lump has been present for many years, has never changed and is not painful, it is unlikely to be malignant
- pain: raises the risk of malignancy
- deep seated (in deep muscle)
- recurrence of a previously excised lump.

A lump that has grown rapidly over 6 months and is painful has a higher chance of being malignant. If it is clear that the lump is benign, a patient can be offered no treatment or in some cases surgical excision for confirmation of diagnosis and reassurance.

If a malignancy is suspected, it should be referred to a specialist before biopsy.

■ EXAMINATION FOR A LUMP

The position of the lump and the same position on the opposite side of the body should be examined. The following scheme

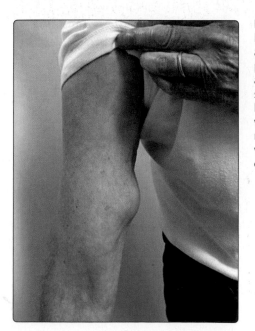

Fig. 3.71.1 This lump grew rapidly and was tender to palpation. Biopsy and MRI scan showed it to be a liposarcoma. It was successfully removed with a wide local excision.

would be suitable in an OSCE station for any general lump on the body (commonly for arm, leg, trunk head and back of the neck). Other lumps have their own examination schemes (breast (Ch. 39), neck (Ch. 42), scrotal sac and groin (Ch. 33)). Likely cases in an OSCE station are sebaceous cyst, lipoma, multiple lipomas and dermoid cyst.

Inspection
A full description of the lump (uses the 6S's):

- size
- shape
- site, including position in relation to other structures
- surface: change in skin texture or colour; any discharge or sinus
- smoothness: apparent nodularity
- surrounding tissues: change in skin, bones, joints, arteries, veins.

Palpation
Palpation will determine:

- surface: smooth, nodular or irregular
- consistency: solid, fluid or gas, pulsatile or a thrill, compressible, fluctuant or reducible
- depth: deep or superficial to surrounding muscles
- tethering: gently pinch the overlying skin
- temperature: feel with the back of the hand
- cough impulse.

Transilluminability should also be assessed.

Percussion
A lump over the abdomen should be percussed to see whether it contain loops of bowel (for a hernia, the scheme in Ch. 33 is followed).

Auscultation
Auscultation examines for a bruit, indicating narrowing of a vessel (an **arteriovenous fistula** formed surgically to aid renal dialysis, commonly in the forearm), as a machinery murmur.

Concluding an examination
A history must be taken (see the suspicious features above) either before or after examining the lump. In an OSCE station, a student may be expected to offer other relevant systems that should be examined, for example the regional lymph glands: checking the axillary lymph nodes is sensible for an arm lump (query malignant). Conversely, if an enlarged lymph node is

found in the axilla, the breast should be examined and then the neck and groin for general lymphadenopathy.

SOFT TISSUE SARCOMAS

Soft tissue sarcomas (STS) are tumours of the connective (soft) tissues, including bone, muscle, fat, nerves, blood vessels and fibrous tissue; they can be benign or malignant. Benign STS are much more common than malignant STS (Table 3.71.1) and include lipomas, fibromas, haemangiomas and neurofibromas (Ch. 70). Early referral of a malignant lump to a specialist sarcoma centre (to a specialist orthopaedic oncology surgeon, rather than a general surgeon) improves the prognosis.

Investigations

A patient with a suspicious lump should be referred to a specialist centre before biopsy. Clinical examination assesses size, site, fixity, involvement of adjacent tissues and evidence of metastases.

MRI assesses the size and neurovascular involvement. A **Trucut biopsy** is taken, where a small tissue core is removed through a large-bore needle surrounded by a sheath (thus not 'seeding' malignant cells elsewhere) and sent for histology. The biopsy track is later removed with the lump at surgical excision.

More extensive imaging is warranted if the patient has pulmonary metastases on radiography or bone pain.

Pathology

STS is most common in middle age, although it can occur at any age. It can also occur anywhere but is most frequent in large muscle masses such as the thigh, and usually presents at about 10 cm. A liposarcoma is the most common type. Some tumours are poorly differentiated spindle cell tumours, which may involve the retroperitoneum or pelvis.

Management

The main principle of treatment is to obtain wide margins where possible at surgical excision to ensure removal of all tumour cells including those surrounding the main tumour that are not visible (thus preventing them causing local recurrence) (Fig. 3.71.2). Chemotherapy and radiotherapy are used in conjunction with surgery and may achieve resolution of resectable locally advanced disease.

Table 3.71.1 THE MORE COMMON TYPES OF MALIGNANT SOFT TISSUE SARCOMA

Type	Tissue of origin	Characteristicss
Liposarcoma	Adipose tissue	Found in fat tissue anywhere in the body; this is the most common type
Synovial sarcoma	Unknown	Not related to the synovium in joints; usually found in arms or legs
Leiomyosarcoma	Smooth muscle	Involuntary muscle as found in uterus and gastrointestinal tract; less commonly in arms and legs
Rhabdomyosarcoma	Skeletal muscle	More common in children than adults; usually arms and legs, also head and neck
Malignant fibrous hystiocytoma	Connective tissue	Tendons and ligaments of arms, legs and trunk

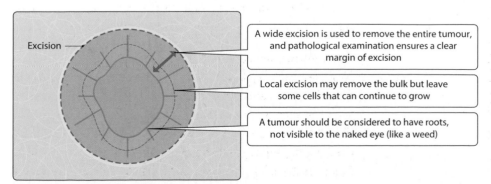

Fig. 3.71.2 Principles of wide local excision.

Excision

A wide excision is used to remove the entire tumour, and pathological examination ensures a clear margin of excision

Local excision may remove the bulk but leave some cells that can continue to grow

A tumour should be considered to have roots, not visible to the naked eye (like a weed)

72. Head injury

Questions
- What are the types of brain injury?
- What are the treatment priorities?
- Which patients with head injuries should be admitted to hospital?

Head injury is a frequent presentation to the A&E department and is commonly caused by an RTA, fall or assault. All unconscious patients are admitted into hospital from A&E, but difficulty arises in deciding which conscious patients require further investigation and admission. Prognosis after a severe head injury is:

- one-third recover
- one-third are left with residual disability (motor, neuropsychiatric or epilepsy)
- one-third die.

Brain injury is classified as:

- **primary damage**: occurs at the time of injury (impact injury) and cannot be reversed
- **secondary damage**: occurs after the injury and is preventable; treatable conditions include intracranial haematomas, hypoxia (airway obstruction, shock), infections and epilepsy.

Figure 3.72.1 shows the types of skull fracture that can occur.

Management of head injuries

Initially the emphasis is always upon resuscitation: ABC principles with cervical spine immobilization. **Associated injuries** are then assessed. The cervical spine will need careful assessment in any case of multiple injury, particularly if there is a history of head trauma; the chest, abdomen, pelvis and limbs must also be assessed. A rapid assessment of head injury is made with:

- history: mechanism of injury (including timings of events), loss of consciousness, epilepsy
- Glasgow Coma Scale (GCS; Table 3.72.1): assesses conscious level by eye, motor and verbal responses
- focal neurological signs: pupil size and reactions
- a falling pulse and increasing blood pressure: indicative of raised intracranial pressure (**Cushing response**).

Investigations

During the initial resuscitation and stabilization, the following will also be done:

- FBC, U&E, cross-match, arterial blood gases
- cervical spine radiograph: mandatory for all head injuries and must include C7/T1
- urgent head CT scan: may be indicated within 1 h.

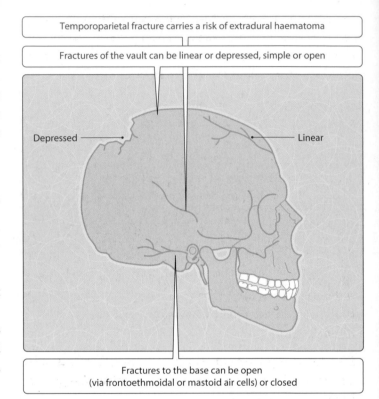

Temporoparietal fracture carries a risk of extradural haematoma

Fractures of the vault can be linear or depressed, simple or open

Depressed

Linear

Fractures to the base can be open (via frontoethmoidal or mastoid air cells) or closed

Fig. 3.72.1 Types of skull fracture.

Table 3.72.1 THE GLASGOW COMA SCALE

Assessment	Score
Eye opening	
Spontaneous opening	4
To speech	3
To pain	2
None	1
Best verbal response	
Orientated	5
Confused	4
Inappropriate words	3
Incomprehensible sounds	2
None	1
Best motor response	
Obeys commands	6
Localizes pain	5
Withdraws to pain	4
Abnormal flexion to pain	3
Extension response to pain	2
None	1

Maximum score is 15 and minimum score is 3.

Fully conscious patients may require a skull radiograph:

- if the injury is high velocity or with a weapon
- if there is a history of loss of consciousness at any time
- if there is marked scalp bruising or wounds.

Only 5% of patients have a skull fracture, but when present there is a greatly increased risk of secondary complications developing.

Base of skull fractures are associated with high-energy impacts, primary brain damage and an increased risk of complications. As these may not be clear on skull radiograph, the clinical signs are vital for identification:

- racoon sign: periorbital haemtomas
- battle sign: bruising around the mastoid process
- leakage of cerebrospinal fluid: rhinorrhoea (from the nose) or otorrhoea (from the ear)
- haemotypanum: blood behind the eardrum.

Further management

There is no specific treatment for skull fractures in their own right, unless the fracture is open or depressed, where surgery may be required. Patients can be considered in three groups:

- those fit for discharge home
- conscious but requiring admission
- unconscious.

All unconscious patients are admitted, but a decision has to be made as to who to admit within the conscious group. The criteria for admission are:

- confusion
- decreased level of consciousness
- skull fracture
- penetrating brain injury
- cerebrospinal fluid leak from nose or ear

- seizures
- neurological signs
- severe headache or vomiting
- difficulty in assessment (alcohol, drugs, very young/elderly)
- medical disorders (clotting disorders, diabetes).

Patients may need to be transferred to a neurosurgical centre and if this is a possibility, their advice needs to be sought promptly.

Patients fit for discharge home

Bleeding from a scalp wound is controlled with external pressure; it is cleaned with irrigation and closed with steri-strips or sutures. A general head injury note is given to a responsible accompanying adult.

Conscious patients requiring admission

Neurosurgical observations are the mainstay of management: conscious level, pupil size, limb movement, blood pressure, heart rate and respiratory rate.

Unconscious patients

Adequate oxygenation is ensured and hypercapnia is prevented (causes brain swelling). Ventilation may be needed to protect the airway and prevent hypoxia. Arterial blood gases, saturation levels and blood pressure are monitored. Transfer to the neurosurgical centre must be controlled; the patient must be resuscitated and stabilized before transfer and escorted and monitored on the way. The airway must be protected, haemorrhage controlled and spinal injuries identified. **Mannitol** is a diuretic that is used in emergencies only to buy time pending transfer to a neurosurgical unit.

A head CT scan identifies intracranial haematomas (Ch. 73) and areas of cerebral contusion. At a neurosurgical unit, neurosurgery is used to evacuate haematomas and sometimes areas of cerebral contusion.

73. Intracranial haemorrhage

Questions
- What are the clinical features of an extradural haematoma?
- What are the clinical features of a subarachnoid haemorrhage?
- How is a diagnosis of subarachnoid haemorrhage confirmed?

Intracranial haemorrhages may be traumatic (extradural, subdural) or spontaneous (e.g. subarachnoid, intracerebral).

Traumatic intracranial haematomas
After a head injury, extradural and subdural haematomas must be considered as possible causes of secondary brain injury (Figs 3.73.1–3.73.4).

Extradural haematoma
Extradural haematoma involves rupture of the anterior branch of the middle meningeal artery, which lies beneath the **pterion** (thinnest part of the skull vault). A skull fracture almost always coexists. Although this injury is rare, it must be identified early to prevent *secondary* damage.

Clinical features
The haematoma develops over a period of hours (rarely more than 6 h), during which period the victim will be awake and appear normal (the *lucid interval*). After this, intracranial pressure increases and the patient rapidly declines and may die without intervention. Clinical features are headache, vomiting, impaired consciousness, focal neurological signs and pupillary inequality.

Management
The key is to notice the reduction in conscious levels at an early stage. CT scan identifies a classical lens-shaped haematoma (Fig. 3.73.2). A craniotomy is made through the skull to evacuate the clot and secure the bleeding artery. In a dire emergency, without immediate access to neurosurgical facilities, a single burr hole to evacuate part of the clot may be life saving.

Subdural haemorrhage
Acute subdural haemorrhages most commonly occur in association with high-energy injuries, such as an RTA. There is usually a high level of primary damage and this generates a poorer prognosis. Bleeding occurs when bridging veins in the subdural space tear. Chronic subdural haematomas most commonly occur in the elderly following minor head injury, where presentation may be several weeks later, perhaps without a clear history of head injury.

Clinical features
Patients with more severe head injuries present in a coma. With more minor trauma, clinical features can vary, from subtle cognitive impairment through to drowsiness with focal signs.

Management
CT scan will show a diffuse haemorrhage that follows the surface of the brain (Fig. 3.73.3). Surgical evacuation is similar to that used for an extradural haematoma.

Spontaneous intracranial haemorrhages

Subarachnoid haemorrhage
Subarachnoid haemorrhage is bleeding into the subarachnoid space, where blood mixes with CSF. Patients are often in the prime of life. Mortality is 30% in the first week, there is a 30% risk of rebleed in the first month and only 30% fully recover function.

Aetiology
Subarachnoid haemorrhages are caused by berry aneurysms (70%), arteriovenous malformations (10%), tumours/trauma (5%) and unknown causes (10%), although hypertension and atherosclerosis are important risk factors. Berry aneurysms form through weakness in the tunica media of the cerebral arteries commonly at the bifurcation of large arteries in the circle of Willis. Occasionally they are associated with hereditary

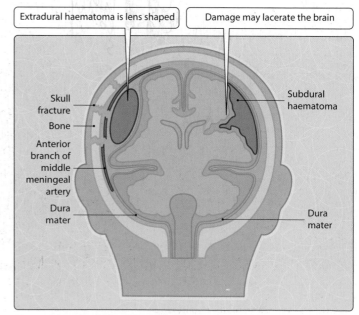

| Extradural haematoma is lens shaped | Damage may lacerate the brain |

Skull fracture

Bone

Anterior branch of middle meningeal artery

Dura mater

Subdural haematoma

Dura mater

Fig. 3.73.1 Extradural and subdural haematoma.

conditions of abnormal collagen formation, such as Marfan's disease and Elhlers–Danlos disease.

Clinical features

In some patients, subarachnoid haemorrhage causes sudden death. The signs are sudden severe headache ('felt like I was hit around the back of the head'), nausea and vomiting, altered rating on Glasgow Coma Scale (Table 3.72.1), collapse and focal signs (hemiparesis, palsy of cranial nerve III) and neck stiffness (common). If these symptoms resolve, this may be a 'warning leak' before a fatal leak. In childhood, this type of meningism is more likely to be a bacterial meningitis.

Investigations

CT scan. This identifies 98% of subarachnoid haemorrhages (Fig. 3.73.4). If CT is negative in someone with a suspected subarachnoid haemorrhage, a **lumbar puncture** is required to confirm the diagnosis.

Lumbar puncture. CSF contaminated by blood has a yellow colour 12 h after a bleed from xanthochromia (red cell breakdown products). Waiting 12 h ensures that a bleed can be distinguished from current red blood cells generated if a vessel is nicked during the puncture. A lumbar puncture is contraindicated in the presence of a mass lesion (e.g. an intracranial clot or tumours).

Cerebral angiography. This produces a detailed image of the intracranial vascular anatomy preoperatively.

Management

The primary bleed cannot be treated directly and so the patient is stabilized and measures undertaken to avoid secondary complications of chest infection, electrolyte disturbances and development of hydrocephalus. The key aim is to prevent a rebleed. Nimodipine, a vasodilator, relieves the vasospasm that occurs after bleeding (caused by local toxins), maintaining cerebral flow. Surgery to close off an aneurysm uses coils (placed endovascularly with interventional radiological techniques) or clips (placed through a craniotomy; less popular now).

Intracerebral haemorrhage

Intracerebral haemorrhages occur in older patients (> 60 years) and accounts for 10% of all strokes. The most common associated factor is hypertension, which causes spontaneous rupture of tiny microaneurysms (Charcot–Bouchard aneurysms). Presentation is with sudden headache, nausea, vomiting and focal neurological signs. Large, accessible haematomas may be evacuated surgically via craniotomy, but the value of such intervention is open to debate. Small haematomas are treated conservatively.

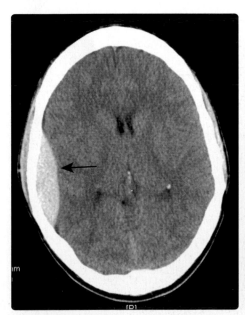

Fig. 3.73.2 A CT scan showing a characteristic lens-shaped extradural haemorrhage, following a head injury. There is an associated skull fracture.

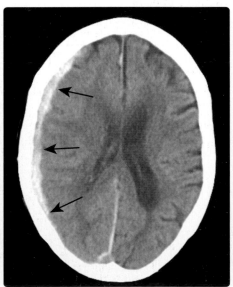

Fig. 3.73.3 A characteristic acute subdural haematoma following a fall in an elderly woman.

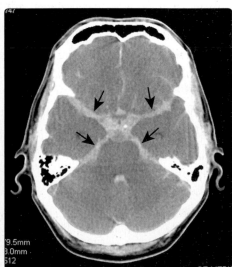

Fig. 3.73.4 A large subarachnoid haemorrhage in a CT scan. The four arrows highlight the white area, which is blood.

74. Spinal cord compression

Questions
- What are the causes of acute spinal cord compression?
- What are the signs of acute spinal cord compression?
- How is it managed?

Acute spinal cord compression is a surgical emergency, and since it often presents to the GP or casualty officer, diagnosis must not be missed at this early stage. If compression of the spinal nerves occurs below L2 (where the spinal cord ends), this is termed **cauda equina compression**.

Causes

There are a number of potential causes:

- congenital: spina bifida
- tumour: metastatic spinal cord tumours are much more common than primary cord tumours; prostate, breast and lung tumours are the most common primaries, whereas renal cell carcinomas, myeloma and lymphomas are less common
- trauma: fracture, subluxation or penetrating trauma
- prolapsed intervertebral disc: cervical and thoracic disc prolapses can compress the cord; lumbar disc prolapses can compress single nerve roots (e.g. the sciatic nerve, leading to sciatica), but occasionally central prolapse can compress the whole cauda equina (cauda equina syndrome)
- spinal stenosis: severe Paget's disease, ankylosing spondylitis or spondylolithesis may occasionally cause compression.
- infection, e.g. epidural abscess.

Clinical features

The symptoms of spinal cord compression are:

- pain: local spinal pain and/or root pain (e.g. sciatica (Fig. 3.74.1),with unilateral or bilateral leg radiation)
- neurological deficit: typically lower limb weakness and loss/change of sensation; lower motor neuron signs may occur at the level, but upper motor neuron signs below the level of cord compression predominate
- sphincter disturbance: bladder and bowel disturbance, leading to urinary retention and bowel constipation or incontinence; painless urinary retention may present to a urologist as acute urinary retention.

If spinal (central) damage is suspected, the **dermatomes** (Fig. 3.74.2), areas of skin on the limbs and trunk that are supplied by a pair of spinal nerves or spinal cord segments, are tested. Spinal cord compression is indicated by saddle (buttock) anaesthesia and alterations in the perianal dermatomes and anal sphincter tone (lax, determined by rectal examination). Motor distribution to myotomes can also be tested: lower motor neuron signs may occur at the level of the compression but upper motor neuron signs will predominate below the level of compression.

Investigations

Patients with suspected spinal cord compression must be urgently referred to hospital for a neurosurgical opinion. An urgent MRI scan is the test of choice (Fig. 3.74.3).

Management

Traumatic spinal cord compression requires spinal immobilization. The patient may need to be catheterized; a full bladder with no sensation for the need to pass urine is indicative of a neuropathic bladder and possible spinal cord compression.

Further treatment may be surgical (surgical decompression) or conservative by continued immobilization. Treatment in a specialist centre is required.

Urgent **surgical decompression** within 6 h is the definitive treatment for non-traumatic spinal cord compression. The compressing agent is removed where possible and space created in the spinal canal.

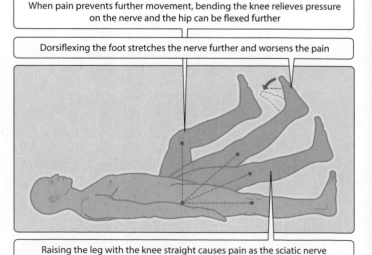

When pain prevents further movement, bending the knee relieves pressure on the nerve and the hip can be flexed further

Dorsiflexing the foot stretches the nerve further and worsens the pain

Raising the leg with the knee straight causes pain as the sciatic nerve (L₄–S₃) is stretched

Fig. 3.74.1 Straight leg raise to detect sciatica. Possible cauda equina syndrome is indicated by severe pain on the affected side when the unaffected side is flexed, and severe and bilateral symptoms.

Steroids (dexamethasone) and **radiotherapy** may be useful alternatives for treating several metastases if disease is widespread, neurology is advanced or if the patient is unfit for surgery. In these cases, the aim is to alleviate pain and to provide some degree of functional independence. Major surgery, when there is an already poor prognosis, is not warranted.

■ SPINA BIFIDA

Spina bifida is a congenital developmental disorder that involves the lower lumbar spine, sacrum, spinal nerves, spinal canal and skin. It can be detected in utero. Severity of the defect varies enormously from an open defect with paresis and bowel and bladder denervation, with a high risk of meningitis, hydrocephalus and neonatal death, to much more minor defects. In favourable cases, the defect should be repaired at birth. Long-term mangement of deformities and bowel and bladder dysfunction is needed throughout life, with life expectancy varying from mid-teens to as much as 40 years in some.

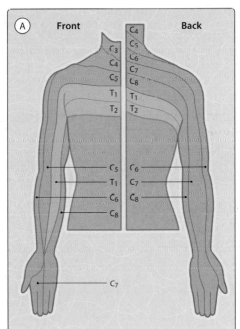
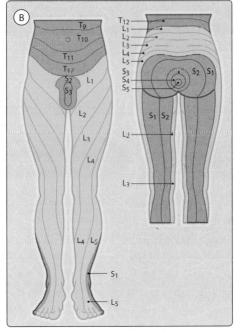

Fig. 3.74.2 Dermatomes of the upper (A) and lower (B) limb.

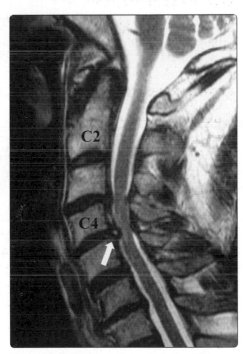

Fig. 3.74.3 Prolapsed cervical disc: This mid-sagittal MRI scan of the cervical spine reveals a prolapsed disc between the C4 and C5 vertebrae (arrow). It is visibly compressing the spinal cord, which is the grey structure outlined by the surrounding cerebrospinal fluid. On this T_2-weighted image, the cerebrospinal fluid is white and is displaced from around the cord at C4/C5 by the disc prolapse.

75. Brain tumours

Questions
- How do brain tumours present?
- What are the principles of treatment for brain tumours?
- What is hydrocephalus and how can it be treated?

Brain tumours account for 3.5% of all malignancies and 2% of cancer deaths; they form 20% of paediatric tumours. The most *common brain tumours are metastatic* (30%). The important issues are what is the lesion and where is it.

■ TUMOURS

Pathology
Brain tumours are benign or malignant, primary or secondary. Primary tumours are classified according to the types of cell from which they arise, of which there are many.

Primary brain tumours are either benign or malignant; they tend to present as space-occupying lesions and they do not metastasize.

Gliomas.   These are the most common type of primary brain tumour (50%) and are usually malignant; subtypes are:
— astrocytomas: commonest type (80%); **glioblastoma multiforme** is an uncommon aggressive subtype, with a poor prognosis (7–32 months)
— oligodendrocytomas: slow growing, better prognosis
— ependyomas.
Meningiomas.   These make up 10% of brain tumours and arise from the meninges; they are most often benign and slow growing.
Acoustic neuromas.   These are benign **schwannomas** (derived from Schwann cells) of the vestibulo-cochlear nerve (cranial nerve VIII), and so tinnitus is often the first symptom. Bilateral acoustic neuromas may be a part of neurofibromatosis II. These make up 7.5% of brain tumours.
Pituitary adenomas.   These benign tumours (5% of primary tumours) may secrete hormones and exert endocrine effects or may be non-functional (Ch. 40).

Tumours in children are usually malignant and include astrocytomas (the most common), craniopharyngioma and medulloblastomas (highly malignant and occur mostly in children under 10 years).

Clinical features
Brain tumours grow to form space-occupying lesions, which exhibit three groups of signs (Fig. 3.75.1).

1. *Raised intracranial pressure.* Symptoms of raised intracranial pressure are a common presentation of this pathology. Symptoms occur as a result of the mass effect of the tumour and/or because of **hydrocephalus** if the ventricles are obstructed. *Headache, vomiting* and *papilloedema* are the classical signs and are *progressive*. Headache is characteristically worse in the morning and on sneezing and coughing and is not relieved by lying down (opposite for migraine).
2. *Focal damage.*   Symptoms depend on the location of the tumour: personality change (frontal lobe), hemipareisis and dysphasia (parietal lobe), visual field defects (occipital lobe), ataxia and brainstem signs (cerebellum).
3. *Epileptic fits.*   New-onset epilepsy in an adult should be investigated further and may be an early symptom of intracerebral tumour.

Investigations
Investigations are central to management of these patients:

■ CT/MRI: these are the crucial tests to determine tumour growth and extent (Fig. 3.75.2)

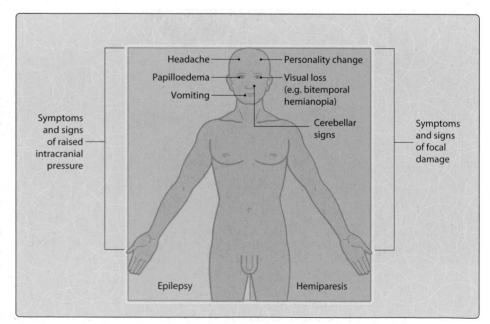

Fig. 3.75.1 Presenting features of brain tumours.

- angiography: used occasionally to delineate the blood supply to the tumour
- biopsy: either through a craniotomy or stereotactic biopsy (a frame is used to stabilize the head and CT guides a biopsy needle through a burr hole into the brain).

Management

The specific management depends on patient age, functional status and specific tumour. The general principles of treatment are as follows.

Conservative and medical management. Steroids (which decrease cerebral oedema) are often started following initial diagnosis. Anticonvulsants may be required to control seizures.

Surgery. Surgery aims to remove the entire tumour but this is not always possible as brain tumours are often highly infiltrative. 'Debulking' removes as much of the tumour as possible. Surgery can also be performed to palliate symptoms, and shunts may be inserted to treat any associated hydrocephalus. Solitary metastatic deposits may sometimes be removed surgically.

Radiotherapy. This is often used after surgery to destroy any remaining tumour cells, but frequently this is only palliative.

Radiosurgery. A focused beam of high-dose radiation can be delivered to a specific point within the brain (only in specialist centres). It is suitable for small, well-defined tumours (e.g. acoustic neuromas, secondary deposits).

Chemotherapy. When surgery and radiotherapy have failed to prevent tumour growth, and in children, chemotherapy is an option. Examples are carmustine and the 'PCV' regimen (procarbazine, lomustine and vincristine).

Prognosis

Prognosis is determined by the type of tumour, the age of the patient and the degree of presenting neurological disability. Low-grade tumours have a better prognosis, and young patients do better than elderly patients.

◼ HYDROCEPHALUS

Hydrocephalus is defined as an increase in CSF volume. It typically presents with signs of raised intracranial pressure as above. Causes include:

- non communicating hydrocephalus (*obstructive*): tumours, congenital abnormalities (e.g. spina bifida)
- communicating hydrocephalus: failure of the extracerebral CSF circulation and/or reasbsorption; this can follow meningitis, subarachnoid haemorrhage and tuberculosis
- normal pressure hydrocephalus: a specific syndrome, usually affecting elderly people; there is a classical triad of gait apraxia, dementia and incontinence
- arrested hydrocephalus: patients with large ventricles in large heads, who have reached equilibrium and have a normal intracranial pressure.

Treatment is commonly with ventricular shunts (draining to the peritoneal cavity or an atrium; Fig. 3.75.3). Endoscopic cerebrospinal fluid diversions (**third ventriculostomy**) are sometimes possible. Occasionally an underlying tumour (e.g. colloid cyst of the third ventricle) can be removed.

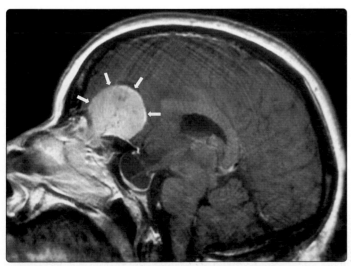

Fig. 3.75.2 Intracranial meningioma: This mid-sagittal contrast-enhanced MR image of the brain shows a large subfrontal meningioma arising from the skull base in the region of the cribriform plates. It is well encapsulated (arrows) and displaces and compresses but does not invade the surrounding brain tissue.

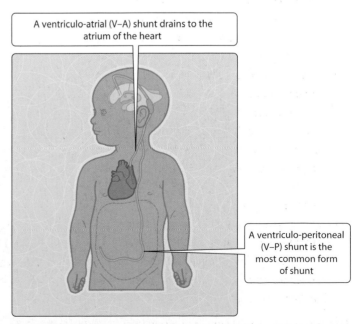

A ventriculo-atrial (V–A) shunt drains to the atrium of the heart

A ventriculo-peritoneal (V–P) shunt is the most common form of shunt

Fig. 3.75.3 Hydrocephalus and shunts: ventriculo-atrial and ventriculo-peritoneal shunts.

76. Cardiac surgery

Questions
- What is a cardiopulmonary bypass graft?
- What are the different types of replacement heart valve?
- How is congenital heart disease classified?

Cardiothoracic surgery involves surgery of the thoracic cage and its contents (see Ch. 77 for thoracic surgery). Figure 3.76.1 shows approaches to the thoracic cavity. **Cardiopulmonary bypass** (CPB) is a key factor in making cardiac surgery possible. Chest drains inserted following surgery prevent haemo- or pneumothorax.

Indications for cardiac surgery

Ischaemic heart disease

Ischaemic (or **coronary**) heart disease is the leading cause of death in Western and many Asian societies. Symptomatic disease is usually treated medically, with nitrates, beta-blockers and calcium channel antagonists. Cardiac catheterization allows assessment of severity and confirms the diagnosis. Balloon angioplasty (**percutaneous transluminal coronary angioplasty**; PTCA) with or without stent insertion may be indicated for some coronary lesions. In some cases cardiac surgery is still necessary: angina refractory to medical treatment, triple vessel disease and left main stem disease (long segment stenoses or diffusely diseased vessels may not be technically suitable for PTCA) and acute ischaemia during coronary artery stenting or PCTA.

The mainstay of surgery is the **coronary artery bypass graft** (CABG; Fig. 3.76.2). **Total arterial revascularization** with use of other arterial conduits (e.g. radial artery, bilateral mammary arteries) is an increasingly popular strategy because of the superior patency rates. Approximately 20% of CABG procedures in the UK are currently performed on a 'beating heart' without use of cardioplegia (off-pump CPB).

Valvular heart disease

The aortic and mitral valves most commonly require surgery because they are subject to higher pressures. Common causes of valvular diseases are inflammatory (rheumatic heart disease) and degenerative (dystrophic calcification), and less commonly infection (infective endocarditis). Surgery is indicated when symptoms are limiting and not controlled by medical therapy or if there is evidence of progressive cardiac chamber dilatation or hypertrophy. The most commonly used valves are **mechanical** and **xenografts** (from pigs or cows); homografts (from cadavers) are used less frequently. Mechanical valves last longer but require lifelong anticoagulation with warfarin.

Ventricular aneurysms

A saccular space may develop following healing of an myocardial infarction. Left ventricular function is impaired and long-term survival is poor. There is persistent ST elevation;

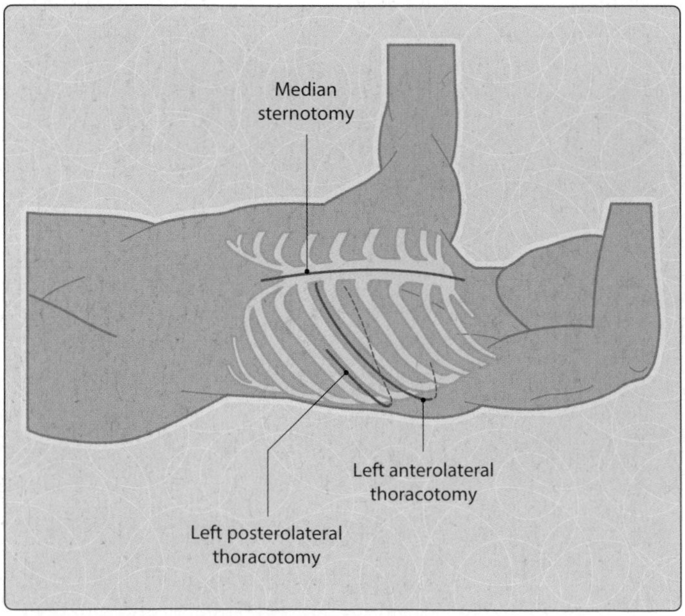

Fig. 3.76.1 Surgical approaches to the thorax.

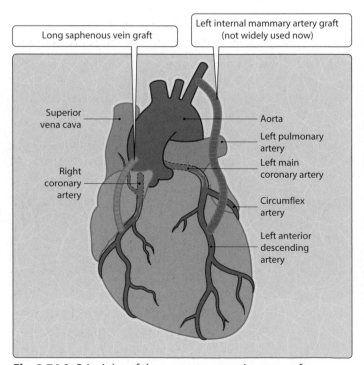

Fig. 3.76.2 Principles of the coronary artery bypass graft.

Table 3.76.1 SUMMARY OF THE MORE COMMON CONGENITAL HEART DISEASES.

Disease	Defect	Murmur	Presentation	Treatment
Ventricular septal defect (most common)	In the ventricular membranous septum Left to right shunt	Pansystolic murmur at the left sternal edge	Murmur at birth; congestive cardiac failure	Small defects may close spontaneously (25–50%); otherwise surgical closure
Atrial septal defect	Between the atria Left to right shunt	Fixed splitting of the second heart sound; pulmonary ejection systolic murmur	Asymptomatic until 20–30 years of age; development of Eisenmenger's syndrome, causing progressive heart failure	Close the defect with a patch of pericardium or Dacron
Coarctation of the aorta	Narrowing of the thoracic aorta Ventricular outflow	Systolic murmur audible over the back	Absent/ weak femoral pulses at birth, congestive cardiac failure	Open surgical correction via a left thoracotomy
Tetralogy of Fallot (Fig. 3.76.3)	DROP: defect in ventricular septum (VSD); right ventricular hypertrophy; overriding aorta; pulmonary stenosis Right to left shunt	Harsh systolic murmur at the left sternal edge	Cyanosis either at rest or during activity; breathlessness; clubbing ('boot-shaped' heart on radiograph)	Open 'total surgical correction'; a palliative shunt between the subclavian and pulmonary arteries (**Blalock–Taussig**) boosts blood delivery to the lungs so correction can wait to ~ 4 years
Patent ductus arteriosus	Failure of the ductus arteriosus to close Left to right shunt	'Machinery' murmur to the neck and precordium	Failure to thrive, breathlessness	Intravenous indometacin at birth ; otherwise surgical clipping

chest radiograph shows an enlarged heart, and echo and cardiac catheterization confirm the diagnosis. Management is either medical (angiotensin-converting enzyme inhibitors, diuretics) or surgical (excision of the aneurysm, CABG).

Cardiomyopathy and chronic ischaemic heart disease

Cardiac pump failure in the absence of serious comorbidity, particularly in cardiomyopathy, may be an indication for cardiac transplantation (Ch. 78).

Congenital heart disease

Congenital heart disease affects 8 in 1000 births, and most patients now survive until adulthood with modern surgical techniques. Congenital heart disease is either *cyanotic* or *acyanotic* and the direction of the shunt varies (Table 3.76.1). Some acyanotic conditions may eventually become cyanotic (secondary pulmonary hypertension) and 10% are attributable to a genetic or environmental cause (e.g. Down's syndrome (trisomy 21), Turner's syndrome, congenital rubella, maternal alcoholism). In **Eisenmenger's syndrome**, a left-to-right shunt through an atrial septal defect is initially acyanotic. However, the shunt enlarges over time until pulmonary hypertension develops and the shunt reverses to become a right-to-left shunt producing cyanosis with polycythaemia. There is no curative treatment by this stage.

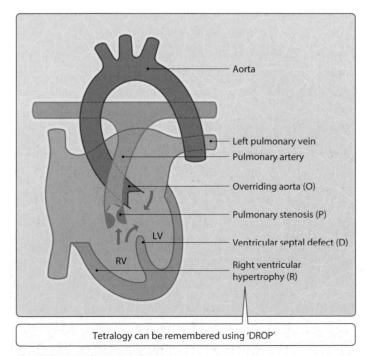

Tetralogy can be remembered using 'DROP'

Fig. 3.76.3 Fallot's tetralogy.

77. Thoracic surgery and tracheostomy

Questions
■ What proportion of lung cancers are resectable?
■ What is a 'flail chest'?

Indications for thoracic surgery

Lung cancer

Only 10% of lung tumours are surgically resected because the disease presents late as there is no suitable test for screening (Table 3.77.1). Complete surgical resection is most effective for peripheral tumours away from the hilum, most commonly for stage I or II non-small cell lung cancer. Incomplete resection may palliate symptoms or 'down-size' the tumour for better response to adjuvant chemotherapy or radiotherapy.

Resectable tumours can be identified with plain radiograph, CT, positron emission tomography (PET) with rigid or flexible bronchoscopy but overall health state of the patient (*operability*) must be considered. Lung resections usually involve removal of an entire lung (**pneumectomy**), lobe (**lobectomy**), broncho-pulmonary segment (**segmentectomy**) or a wedge resection. Surgery is performed through a thoracotomy or, less invasively, thoracoscopically when technically feasible.

Empyema

An empyema is a collection of pus in the pleural space and may be life threatening. A preceding pneumonia, a swinging fever and weight loss may be present. Empyema is a potential complication of chest drains. Established empyemas should undergo a prompt **decortication** procedure via a thoracotomy (the infection is drained and the pleural layers freed), with perioperative intravenous antibiotic therapy.

Rib fractures and flail chest

A double fracture, usually caused by a compression force, results in a floating section of the rib (**flail segment**; Fig. 3.77.1), which may damage underlying contents and cause paradoxical respiration. Treatment depends upon the severity of the injury:

■ simple rib fracture: analgesia and physiotherapy
■ flail segment: positive pressure ventilation until stable (a tracheostomy may be needed)
■ underlying pneumothorax: chest drain and observation
■ major airway damage (trachea or bronchi) or bleeding: emergency thoractomy and repair.

Pneumothorax

A pneumothorax is air in the pleural space (Fig. 3.77.2). It can occur spontaneously or be caused by trauma (penetrating injury, fractured ribs, damaged trachea or bronchi), iatrogenic (pleural taps causing lung damage), infection (rupture of a cavity), positive pressure ventilation, asthma, chronic bronchitis (with apical bulbae that rupture), cystic fibrosis or post-pulmonary surgery (air leak).

A chest radiograph shows the extent of the pneumothorax and management depends on the type. Both simple pneumothorax and haemopneumothorax require a chest drain.

Spontaneous pneumothorax often occurs in tall, thin young men and has an excellent prognosis (but may be recurrent);

Table 3.77.1 TYPES OF LUNG CANCER[a]

Type	Proportion (%)	Location	Notes
Adenocarcinoma	45	Peripheral	
Squamous cell	30	Central/hilar	Usually associated with smoking
Small cell (oat cell)	20	Central	Usually associated with smoking; chemosensitive
Large cell	5–10	Peripheral	Poor prognosis owing to early spread

[a]*Five-year survival remains at 5%. Median survival for small cell cancer is 8–12 months.*

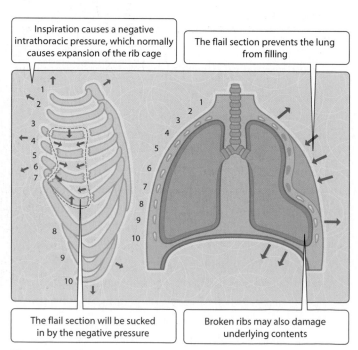

Inspiration causes a negative intrathoracic pressure, which normally causes expansion of the rib cage

The flail section prevents the lung from filling

The flail section will be sucked in by the negative pressure

Broken ribs may also damage underlying contents

Fig. 3.77.1 Flail segment: a floating section is formed.

treatment is supportive. It may also occur in the elderly with chronic obstructive pulmonary disease, where mortality is high. Surgery is indicated for patients with recurrent unilateral or bilateral pneumothorax or those in 'at-risk' occupations such as deep-sea divers or airline pilots. Surgical options include either an open or a thoracoscopic pleurectomy and/or pleural abrasion.

Tension pneumothorax is a life-threatening emergency. A 'one way valve' exists so with each breath more air is drawn into the pleural cavity, increasing the 'tension' and shifting the midline of the mediastinum causing airways obstruction. Eventually the increasing pressure impairs venous return to the heart (see Ch. 44).

Open pneumothorax is life-threatening as gas exchange is immediately diminished. It requires immediate closure with a square dressing closed on three sides to act as a valve (converting it to a 'simple' pneumothorax), with subsequent chest drain insertion.

Surgery may occasionally be needed in recurrent or bilateral pneumothorax, with **pleurodesis** (pleural fusion with chemicals) or **pleurectomy** (stripping of the pleura).

Tracheostomy

Tracheostomy (between tracheal cartilages 2 and 3) is used to relieve airway obstruction and to protect the airway. It may be a necessary part of radical surgery following pharyngolaryngectomy for malignant disease and as a means of providing respiratory support in neurological disease. **Indications** for tracheostomy are:

- emergency: acute upper airway obstruction (Ch. 44)
- potential airway obstruction: major surgery on the oropharynx, larynx or neck
- trauma: inhalation, faciomaxillary injuries, head injuries
- neurological disease: tetanus, polio, acute bulbar palsy
- prolonged artificial ventilation
- radical pharyngolaryngectomy or laryngectomy.

There are a number of potential complications: haemorrhage, injury to peritracheal structures (carotid artery, recurrent laryngeal nerve, oesophagus, great veins), trachea damage, subcutaneous emphysema, pneumomediastinum, pneumo- thorax, accidental extubation, infection and swallowing dysfunction.

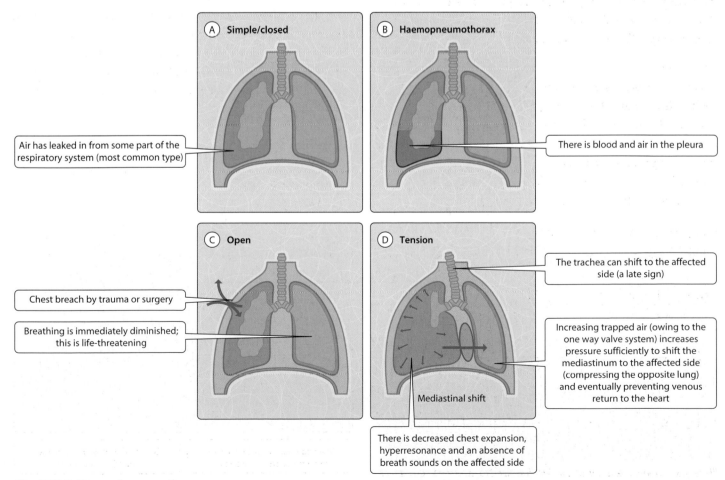

Fig. 3.77.2 Types of pneumothorax.

78. Transplantation

Questions
- What is the indication for heart–lung transplant
- What are the main complications of organ transplantation?

The major limiting factor for transplantation in the UK and worldwide is the availability of donated tissues. Cadaver organs, usually from individuals who have suffered a lethal head injury, require prior consent, matching for recipient tissue, careful harvesting, distribution to transplant centres and the shortest possible ischaemic time. Live related donor organs or segments are more complex to retrieve and transplant and there are complex ethical issues including complications and donor death. However, immunosupression may not be necessary and the availability of organs is more predictable.

Indications for common transplantations

Most transplants are **allotransplants**: from different members of the same species. Donors must be well matched for size and ABO blood grouping (vital). HLA matching decreases the chance of rejection but is not totally necessary. Current transplant options include:

- **heart**: cardiomyopathy, ischaemic heart disease, myocarditis and congenital heart disease
- **lung**: end-stage chronic lung diseases (fibrosis, chronic obstructive pulmonary disease, chronic sepsis, pulmonary hypertension)
- **kidneys** (the most common type of transplantation): chronic glomerulonephritis, chronic pyleonephritis, diabetic nephropathy
- **liver**: cirrhosis secondary to viral hepatitis, biliary cirrhosis, primary sclerosing cholangitis, some metabolic diseases, fulminant liver failure; a liver can be split into its two lobes and donated to two recipients
- **pancreas**: type 1 diabetes mellitus (usually coupled with a renal transplant for diabetic nephropathy)
- **small bowel**: under trial following major resections (e.g. ischaemic enteritis where there is insufficient bowel to sustain life or because of inadequate venous access; occasionally in extensive Crohn's disease)
- **cornea**: corneal scarring/irregularity
- **skin**: burns.

Heart and lung transplantation is a relatively new procedure, where options include:

- heart transplantation
- single/double lung transplantation
- heart–lung transplantation.

Complications for transplantation

There are two key complications: infection and rejection.

Infection

The early postoperative period is the most common time for infection, although these immunosuppressed patients are susceptible at any time. Cytomegalovirus is a very common causative pathogen, causing influenza-like symptoms and significant morbidity if not treated with ganciclovir. Donors are screened for cytomegalovirus. There is an increasing risk of opportunistic infections: multiresistant *Staphylococcus aureus* (MRSA), pseudomembranous colitis (*Clostridium difficile*) and tuberculosis (*Mycobacterium tuberculosis*).

Rejection

The characteristics of rejection and its significance depend on when it occurs after the transplantation:

hyperacute: minutes to hours postoperatively; the greatest period of risk
acute: a few weeks to months
chronic: months to years.

All patients undergoing transplantation will require lifelong immunosuppression unless their organ or part organ is from an identical twin or an immunologically tolerant sibling. The most common regimens include:

- ciclosporin: the mainstay of immunosuppression; side-effects include nephrotoxicity, hypertension, hepatotoxicty and lymphoma
- tacrolimus: for patients refractory to ciclosporin or who suffer severe side-effects
- azathioprine
- prednisolone: side-effects are numerous, although Cushing's syndrome and osteoporosis are amongst the most significant.

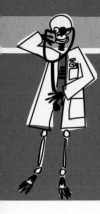

Glossary

Abbreviations

ABC	airway, breathing and circulation
A-P	anterioposterior
ARDS	adult respiratory distress syndrome
ASIS	anterior superior iliac spines
CRP	C-reactive protein
CSF	cerebrospinal fluid
CT	computed tomography
DVT	deep vein thrombosis
ERCP	endoscopic retrograde cholangiopancreatography
ESR	erythrocyte sedimentation rate
FBC	full blood count
FOOSH	fall on an outstretched hand
GCS	Glasgow Coma Scale
LFT	liver function tests
MRCP	magnetic resonance cholangiopancreatography
MRI	magnetic resonance imaging
MSOF	multiple system organ failure
NSAID	non-steroidal anti-inflammatory drug
OGD	oesophago-gastro-duodenoscopy
ORIF	open reduction with internal fixation
PSA	prostate specific antigen
PVD	peripheral vascular disease
RTA	road traffic accident
TNM	tumour, node, metastases staging system
U&E	urea and electrolytes

Terms

Adjuvant
The use of a treatment after the main treatment, usually either *chemotherapy* or *radiotherapy* after surgery; the aim is to destroy any cancer that has spread

Alkaline phosphatase
Enzyme measured in plasma as a marker of bone activity (raised after fractures, Paget's disease, metastases, hyperparathyroidism, osteomalacia) and liver disease (suggests cholestasis)

Aneurysm
Permanent, localized dilatation in an arterial wall

Arteriovenous fistula
Communication between a vein and an artery, either *con-genital* or *surgically fashioned* to allow for dialysis, most commonly in the forearm; they feel firm, have a pulsation and thrill, and a bruit is audible upon auscultation

Arteriovenous malformations
Abnormal connections between the venous and arterial systems. Almost all are congenital, and some may cause no problems. Others may cause significant complications, including cardiac failure and major bleeding. Embolization is the mainstay of treatment

Bisphosphonates
Drugs that 'stabilize' bone matrix by inhibiting osteoclast activity and number, curtailing bone formation and resorption. Used in treatment of osteoporosis, Paget's disease and metastatic bone disease

Bone density scan (DEXA)
Assessment of the density of bone (commonly for osteoporosis), determined by the proportion of photons that pass through the bone

Bone isotope scan
Intravenous technetium isotopes are detected as concentrated 'hot spots' in bones where there is pathological activity. It is used to assess spread of metastatic bone tumours, for tumour staging, assessment of primary bone tumours and microfractures

Carcinoma in situ (CIS)
Malignant cells that have not yet spread beyond the basement membrane, e.g. ductal CIS in the breast and bladder CIS

Colour duplex scan
B mode ultrasound and Doppler ultrasound produce a colour picture illustrating direction of blood flow (blue forward, red back)

Coning
Raised intracranial pressure forces the brainstem through the foramen magnum and is usually immediately fatal; this is why lumbar puncture is contraindicated when intracranial pressure is raised, to prevent inadvertent coning

Contusions
Area of skin discolouration (bruise) caused by the escape of blood from damaged blood vessels, e.g. brain and lung contusion

Critical limb ischaemia
Rest pain, ulceration or gangrene that has been occurring for 2 weeks or more and requires strong analgesia

Dislocation
Complete loss of contact between the articular surfaces of a joint, e.g. anterior dislocation of the shoulder

Disseminated intravascular coagulation (DIC)
Overstimulation of the clotting system in response to disease or injury (e.g. severe infection, asphyxia, placental abruption); coagulation factors are rapidly used up and the resulting deficiency causes spontaneous, widespread bleeding

Dyspepsia
Encompasses a range of symptoms: pain (epigastric or retrosternal), heartburn, bloating

Dysphagia
Difficulty in swallowing

Dysplasia
Abnormal development of a tissue

Endoscopy
Use of an instrument to visualize the inside of the body (typically a fibreoptic tube with a light, connected to a video camera), e.g. colonoscopy, sigmoidoscopy, oesophago-gastro-duodenoscopy

Enteral feeding
Feeding using the patient's own gastrointestinal tract, e.g. oral intake, nasogastric tube, gastrostomy

Fibrous dysplasia
Developmental abnormality of the bone, where trabecullar bone is replaced by fibrous tissue, causing aching bone pains and a susceptibility to fractures

Fistula
Abnormal communication between two epithelial surfaces

Haematuria
Blood in the urine; either macroscopic (*frank*), where blood is visible to the naked eye, or microscopic, where blood is only detectable on dipstick

Haematemesis
Vomiting of blood, from bleeding in the oesophagus, stomach or duodenum

Intermittent claudication
A cramp-like pain that occurs in a group of muscles upon exercise and is relieved by rest

Intraosseous line
Fluid resuscitation by insertion of a line into the bone, typically in paediatric trauma victims (with soft bone)

Lipoma
Common benign tumour of adipose cells that can occur anywhere on the body where fat is present, but mostly on the head, neck, abdominal wall and thighs

Melaena
Passage of dark, tar-like stool caused by upper gastrointestinal bleeding; the blood mixed into the stool appears black as it is partially digested. Melaena occurs when at least 500 ml of blood enters the gut

Metaplasia
Change in cells to a form that is not normally found in the tissue concerned

Myelopathy
Symptoms caused by compression, inflammation or irritation of the spinal cord

Necrotizing fascitis
Bacterial infection of the fascial layer beneath the skin, with type A streptococci. Tissue necrosis and toxin production cause shock and organ failure. The elderly and postsurgical patients are susceptible, and treatment is with prompt antibiotics and surgical debridement

Neo-adjuvant
Treatment given before the main treatment: usually chemotherapy or radiotherapy before surgery

Neoplasia
New or abnormal growth of a tissue, resulting in a neoplasm (a tumour)

Open reduction and internal fixation (ORIF)
Method of treating fractures where at open surgery the fracture is reduced and then fixed in place, e.g. with a plate and screws or an intramedullary nail

Osteoporosis
Bone mineral density of 2 standard deviations below the mean for the population

Paget's disease
Metabolic disease of bone that is characterized by increased uptake of bone, followed by disorganized remodelling of bone

Panproctocolectomy
Resection of the entire colon, rectum and anus and formation of a permanent end-ileostomy

Pericardiocentesis
Needle aspiration to remove excess fluid (which is compressing the heart) from within the pericardium

Pericarditis
Acute or chronic inflammation of the membranous sac that surrounds the heart (the pericardium). It has many causes, including viral infection and cancer. A friction rub may be heard

Polycystic kidney disease
Autosomal dominant disorder where both kidneys are filled with numerous cysts. Haematuria, urinary tract infection and hypertension develop at ages 20–40 years and are associated with chronic renal failure

Polyp
Outgrowth from a mucus membrane (usually benign)

Prostate-specific antigen (PSA)
Protein produced by the prostate that turns semen into liquid; men with prostate cancer tend to have higher levels of PSA in their blood

Radiculopathy
Symptoms caused by compression, inflammation or irritation of a nerve root

Reactive hyperaemia
Rapid blood flow into a hypoxic area, typically causing a marble red-appearance in the foot when performing Beurger's test. It is influenced by the build up of metabolites while the tissue is hypoxic

Saphenous cutdown
Method of gaining venous access by dissecting down to the great saphenous vein behind the medial malleolus, typically when other methods have failed in the shocked trauma patient

Sarcoma
Malignant tumour that has arisen from 'mesenchymal' tissues such as bone, muscle, connective tissue, cartilage and fat

Shock
Syndrome in which the perfusion of tissues is inadequate for metabolic requirements

Sinus
Tract connecting an epithelial surface to a blind-ending pouch

Skin graft
Used to replace skin loss (e.g. after burns), deriving its blood supply from its recipient bed; it is either a split-skin graft or a full-thickness graft, depending on the quality of the recipient bed

Sprains
Injury to a ligament caused by sudden overstretching; healing is gradual

Stoma
Surgically created opening in the body between the skin and a hollow viscus (Greek *stoma*, mouth), e.g.colostomy (large bowel), ileostomy (small bowel)

Strains
Damage to a muscle caused by excessive working or stretching, resulting in pain and swelling of the muscle

Subluxation
Partial loss of contact between the articular surfaces of a joint, e.g. of a metatarsophalangeal joint of the hand in rheumatoid arthritis

Tissue flap
Piece of tissue taken with its own blood supply to replace a site of significant tissue loss; most often formed from skin or muscle

Total parenteral nutrition (TPN)
Feeding directly into a central vein (e.g. subclavian vein) when the gastrointestinal tract must be avoided. Less commonly used than enteral feeding and it has associated risks

Ulcer
Break in the continuity of an epithelial surface

Varicose veins
Tortuous dilatation of veins, commonly affecting the lower limbs

Volvulus
Twisting (*malrotation*) of the bowel around its mesentery, commonly at the sigmoid or caecum; more common in the elderly

Wound dehiscence
Complete breakdown of a wound; it complicates 2–10% of abdominal wounds, following infection or when sutures tear through weak tissues

Laws and rules

Beck's triad
Hypotension, raised jugular venous pressure and muffled heart sounds: classically present in patients with cardiac tamponade

Buerger's test
The leg is elevated and becomes pale; when hung over the side of the bed it turns a marbled, deep-red colour (reactive hyperaemia, the sunset sign); this indicates critical limb ischaemia

Charcot's triad

Rigors, obstructive jaundice, pain: indicating ascending cholangitis

Courvoisier's law

A painless, palpable gallbladder in the presence of jaundice is unlikely to be caused by gallstones; the mass is more likely to be cancer of the head of the pancreas

Finkelstein's test

Pain of de Quervain's tenosynovitis is reproduced by bending the thumb into the palm

Froment's paper sign

The patient holds a piece of paper between the thumb and index finger, with both hands at the same time; flexing the distal phalanx of the thumb on the side of the index finger indicates an ulnar nerve palsy

Goodsall's rule

Fistulae that open onto the anterior half of the anus are likely to be direct and those that open onto the posterior half tend to be indirect

Mills' test

Pain reproduced on resisted wrist extension indicates tennis elbow

Phalen's test

The wrist is held in flexion for 30–60 s, which causes pressure in the carpal tunnel and symptoms and weakness in an affected wrist ('inverse prayer' sign)

Popeye's sign

Resisted elbow flexion causes a bulging of muscle fibres; this indicates rupture of the tendon to long head of biceps

Rigler's sign

Plain radiography of the bowel showing that it is lined by gas on its interior and posterior surface indicating perforation of the bowel

Rovsing's sign

Pressing in the left iliac fossa causes pain in the right iliac fossa: indicates acute appendicitis

Thomas' test

The clinician's hand is placed in the small of the patient's back and the patient flexes the hip; a fixed flexion deformity is indicated if the other hip flexes and the lumbar lordosis is maintained

Tinel's test

Tapping over a nerve reproduces symptoms of a compression syndrome, e.g. over the volar aspect of the wrist to reproduce carpal tunnel syndrome

Tourniquet test

Assesses for incompetent perforating veins in varicose vein assessment

Troisier's sign

The presence of an enlarged lymph node in the left supraclavicular fossa (**Virchow's node**)

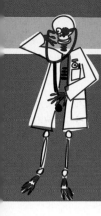

Index